Green Fertility:
Nature's Secrets For Making Babies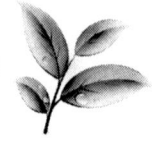

A Powerful, Proven Plan
To Help You
Get Pregnant Fast
& Have A Healthy Baby

What the experts are saying about Green Fertility

" Green Fertility is a unique and groundbreaking lifestyle guide for any couple who wants to get pregnant. The concepts featured in the book have been proven in multiple studies, and I have personally seen many couples improve their fertility profiles by following this plan. It works for both natural conception as well as to enhance assisted reproductive technologies such as IVF and ICSI, and I highly recommend it."

        Carlo Acosta, B.Sc.
        Embryologist & Reproductive Technology Specialist
        New York City, NY

" Using the power of nature Green Fertility teaches every couple how to safely and gently maximize their ability to get pregnant. It's a must-read for the health conscious mother-to-be, which should be all mothers. Green Fertility may eventually become the only way."

        Patricia Conrad, M.D., F.A.C.O.G.
        Board Certified Gynecologist & Reproductive Endocrinologist
        Fellow of the American College of Obstetrics and Gynecology
        New York City, NY

"I highly recommend Green Fertility - an all natural, holistic approach to improving a couple's fertility. The authors have thoroughly researched this subject and present information that is of ground breaking importance for any couple trying to get pregnant, and for those who wish to conceive faster and easier and have a healthier baby. The combination of vitamins, minerals, supplements, foods and the relaxation techniques have been proven in studies to bring about extraordinary results."

        Linda Chard, D.C,
        Board Certified Doctor of Chiropractic,
        Holistic Consultant for the NHS Fertility Clinics,
        President of the London based clinic WantToBeWonderful, Ltd.
        London, England

Green Fertility:
Nature's Secrets For Making Babies!

By Niels H. Lauersen, M.D., Ph.D.
& Colette Bouchez

Ivy League Press
New York, NY

ILP

Green Fertility: Nature's Secrets For Making Babies
Copyright 2010 Niels H. Lauersen & Colette Bouchez

All rights reserved. No part of this book may be reproduced or transmitted in any form or by any means, electronic or mechanical including photocopying, recording or any information storage or retrieval system without express written consent from the publisher or author. For further information contact: Info@IvyLeaguePress.com

Green Fertility: Nature's Secrets For Making Babies may be purchased for business or promotional use or special sales. For information please contact Info@IvyLeaguePress.com or visit www.IvyLeaguePress.com

This book is not intended as a substitute for medical advice from your physician. The reader should regularly consult with a physician in matters pertaining to her health & fertility, particularly in regard to
symptoms that may require medical attention.

The authors or Ivy League Press cannot be responsible for any results obtained or derived from information in this book. The information in this book is not considered medical advice and is offered only as a guide to getting optimal care.

Printed in the United States of America
10 9 8 7 6 5 4 3 2 1
First Edition Published 2010

ISBN: 978-0-615-39351-3

Library of Congress Cataloging in Publication Data:
Green Fertility: Nature's Secrets For Making Babies
/Niels Lauersen -Colette Bouchez

1. Conception - Popular Works
2. Reproductive Health - Popular Works
3. Natural Treatments - Popular Works

Interior and Cover Design by Elle Media
www.ElleMediaNetwork.com

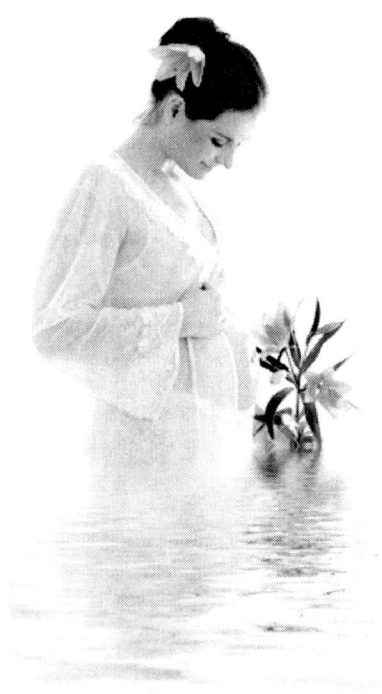

This book is dedicated to all the parents who have recognized the power of natural living as well as the power of combining ancient Chinese wisdom with modern Western medicine to change their lives and to help them bring into the world a new generation of healthier children.

And to our own parents:

"As we all go forward to shape our planet into a healthier and greener place to live we are blessed by those who have gone before us, and honored by those who follow in our path."

We dedicate this book to all of you.

Grateful Acknowledgements

First and foremost we would like to thank all the thousands of patients as well as the readers of all our previous books, who believed in our natural health ideals and throughout the years supported and encouraged our continuing mission to safely and naturally bring healthier, stronger babies into the world. To those who have helped us perfect this brand new Green Fertility program, we are grateful and thankful for your suggestions and insights, and for helping us to spread the word about the awesome power of nature to change your life.

We also want to acknowledge the many medical organizations , who as we do, believe that science and nature can work hand in hand. We applaud you and we thank you for your dedication and for sharing your knowledge and research.

We would especially like to thank those organizations who so generously shared with us their expertise including The American Society of Reproductive Medicine, The New York Society for Reproductive Medicine; The American Dietetic Association, The American Diabetes Association, The American College of Obstetricians and Gynecologists, The Endometriosis Association, The American Botanical Society, WebMd, The Journal of Complementary and Alternative Medicine, The American Association of Oriental Medicine, The National Certification Commission for Acupuncture and Oriental Medicine.

To all our colleagues in the brave new world of Green Fertility who are helping to carry our message of hope and natural help to so many patients, we are grateful for your support and encouragement. Special gratitude goes to embryologist Carlo Acosta for his expertise in assisted reproductive technologies; to Dr. Linda Chard, for her extraordinary knowledge of natural and holistic health techniques and treatments; to Patricia Conrad, MD, for her continued support and knowledge of women's health care and reproductive medicine; to Norbert Gleicher M.D., and David Barad M.D. for their research and lecture series on DHEA and research into fertility in older women; to Poula Helth and Hans Jorn Filges for their important work on the emotional side of infertility; to Professor Niels Jorgen Secher, M.D., for sharing his knowledge and contributions to women's health care; to John Zhang, M.D, Ph.D., and Lyndon Chang, M.D. for their dedication to natural fertility treatments.

Our thanks also goes out to our special friends Michelle and Robert Szakacs, Bruce & Svetlana Kowal, Cecilia Simmons, Debbie Ciraoloa, M.A., and Tyler Evans, M.D., for their continued loyal support and friendship. And to Elaine Trebek Kares for her creative inspiration and support.

Our deepest gratitude also goes to our legal team, attorney David Field, and Albert Terranova. And to the staff of Ivy League Press: Thank you for the hard work, support and dedication .

To Eleanor Rawson - The Duchess of Book Publishing: We are forever indebted to you for bringing us together, and for standing with us through all the years. We will miss you always.

And to Mary B ... for the wisdom & the love that gives us all hope for a brighter future.

And finally, to St. Jude: Thank you for bringing us through it again.

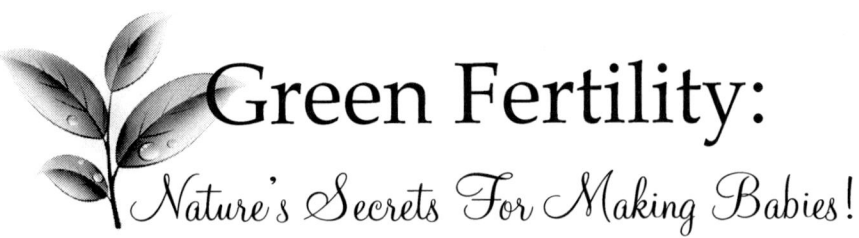

Green Fertility:
Nature's Secrets For Making Babies!

By Niels H. Lauersen, M.D., Ph.D.
& Colette Bouchez

TABLE OF CONTENTS

INTRODUCTION   *PAGE 12*
HOW MOTHER NATURE CAN HELP YOU GET PREGNANT FASTER!
Getting Pregnant Naturally: Yes You Can! - Overcoming Unexplained Infertility - How This Book Will Help You - Green Fertility Treatments: An Extra Surprise

---

CHAPTER ONE: *PAGE 20*
UNDERSTANDING YOUR FERTILITY -
HOW CONCEPTION REALLY OCCURS
Sex, Hormones & Getting Pregnant - Introducing Sperm To Egg : How Conception Really Occurs - Why Timing Is Everything - When Pregnancy Doesn't Happen: What Can Go Wrong & How To Beat It - The Green Secret To Getting Pregnant

---

CHAPTER TWO: *PAGE 32*
PROTECTING YOUR FERTILITY -
WITH THE NEW PRECONCEPTION EXAM
The New Preconception Counseling Exam : What It Must Include - Your Pre Conception Physical - The Fertility Pelvic Exam - Fertility Blood Tests - Fertility Protection Diagnostics - Why Your Fertility Intuition Matters

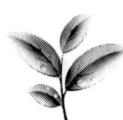

CHAPTER THREE
INCREASING YOUR FERTILITY ODDS -

PAGE 44

How Ovulation Prediction Works - 5 Proven Systems To Help You Get Pregnant Fast - How To Choose A Fertility Monitor - Having Sex & Making Babies: Some Practical Advice - Sex Do's & Don't's To Increase Fertility - Douching & Fertility - Sex & The Sex of Your Baby.

CHAPTER FOUR
ENHANCE YOUR FERTILITY -
WITH WEIGHT CONTROL STRATEGIES THAT REALLY WORK!

PAGE 78

- How Weight Affects Fertility - Inflammation: The New Link To Infertility - Belly Fat & Infertility - The New Blood Test That Measures Fertility - Using Your BMI To Help You Get Pregnant - Are You Too Thin To Conceive? - The Breakthrough Natural Fertility Hormone - 6 Simple Steps For Optimizing Your Fertility Weight

---

CHAPTER FIVE
STRENGTHEN YOUR FERTILITY -
WITH A PROVEN PRE CONCEPTION FITNESS PLAN

PAGE 96

- How Fitness Affects Fertility - Metabolism & Conception: An Important Connection - How Your Thyroid Affects Your Fertility - Exercises To Boost Your Metabolism - Exercises To Optimize Fertility - Your Fertility Fitness Prescription - Yoga & Fertility - The Anti-Fertility Workouts: What To Avoid

---

CHAPTER SIX
IMPROVE YOUR FERTILITY -
WITH STRESS REDUCTION STRATEGIES THAT REALLY WORK

PAGE 112

Stress & Infertility: Causes and Effects - Ancient Eastern Technique Reduces Stress & Increases Fertility - Stress & Miscarriage - Chronic Stress Vs. Acute Stress - The Stress Busters That Boost fertility - 10 Ways To Reduce Stress & Get Pregnant!

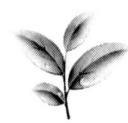

CHAPTER SEVEN *PAGE 141*
BOOST YOUR FERTILITY -
WITH FOODS THAT MAKE A REAL DIFFERENCE!

- Comfort Carbs & Getting Pregnant - The Food Allergy That Can Block Conception - Fats That Fuel Fertility - Omega-3: The Super Sonic Fertility Booster - The Fats That Harm Fertility - Inflammatory Foods: What Blocks Conception - How Ice Cream Can Boost Your Fertility - Super Protein Fertility Power - The New Fertility Protein

---

CHAPTER EIGHT *PAGE 179*
SUPPORT YOUR FERTILITY -
WITH THE AMAZING POWERS OF FRUITS, VEGGIES, NUTS & SEEDS

- The Fertility Super Fruits & Vegetables - & Why You Need Them! - Protect Your Fertility With These Natural Foods - The Nuts That Boost Fertility Odds - The Special Food Nutrients That Can Help You Get Pregnant Faster - What To Eat Today To Get Pregnant Tomorrow - Six Super Fertility Food Boosters - Food & Sex: What Turns Fertility On!

CHAPTER NINE *PAGE 207*
ENCOURAGE YOUR FERTILITY -
WITH POWER PACKED VITAMIN SUPPLEMENTS

- Is Your Fertility In Nutritional Jeopardy? - The 7 Super Nutrients Every Woman Needs To Get Pregnant - Want Twins? Take This Vitamin! - Multi Vitamins Vs Pre-Natal Vitamins - Give Your Eggs A Vitamin Bath: Here's How! - The One Vitamin That Prevents Birth Defects - Vitamin C & Common Fertility Problems - The "Beach Vitamin" That Increases Fertility

---

CHAPTER TEN *PAGE 244*
INCREASE YOUR FERTILITY -
WITH MOTHER NATURE'S MINERAL SECRETS

- The Road To Pregnancy Is Paved With Minerals! - 6 Super Fertility Minerals & Why You Need Them - Fertility & The Calcium Connection - Soda, Minerals & Getting Pregnant - The One Mineral You Should Never Skimp On - Minerals That Protect Your Baby Before You Conceive! -

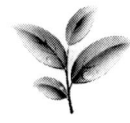

CHAPTER ELEVEN
SUPPLEMENTING YOUR FERTILITY
WITH NATURAL HERBS THAT REALLY WORK!

PAGE 266

- 6 Super Fertility Herbs & Why They Work! - The Chinese Fertility Cocktail-- Bee Pollen, Royal Bee Jelly & Your Fertility - Omega-3 Supplements: How They Help You Get Pregnant - Evening Oil of Primrose & Fertility - How DHEA Can Help You Get Pregnant Faster - The New Fertility Supplements: What You Should Know - Choosing A Fertility Supplement: What To Look For!

CHAPTER TWELVE
ENSURING YOUR FERTILITY
THE SMALL LIFESTYLE CHANGES THAT MAKE A BIG DIFFERENCE!

PAGE 300

- Smoking & Fertility: What You Need To Know - Knit Your Way To Better Fertility: Here's Why! - Beer, Wine & Fertility: New Information - How Caffeine Affects Getting Pregnant - Prescription Drugs & Your Fertility - Allergies, Sex & Infertility - Social Drugs & Getting Pregnant

---

CHAPTER FOURTEEN
SAFEGUARDING YOUR FERTILITY -
MAKE YOUR WORLD FERTILITY-FRIENDLY!

PAGE 320

- How The Environment Affects Fertility - The Infertility Chemical: How To Avoid It - 12 Easy Ways To Cut Chemical Exposures - Hand Sanitizers & Infertility: What You Must Know! - Personal Care Products & Fertility - Getting Pregnant In The Digital Age - 10 Things Every Couple Can Do Right Now To Protect Their Fertility & Get Pregnant Faster

---

CHAPTER FIFTEEN
PROTECTING HIS FERTILITY -
WHAT EVERY COUPLE NEEDS TO KNOW

PAGE 348

- Understanding Male Fertility - The Male Fertility Check Up - 5 Super Sperm Assassins & How To Defeat Them - Cell Phones, Laptops & Sperm - Medications That Affect Sperm Count - Make Your Home Sperm-Safe - 6 Sperm-Happy Meals Your Man Will Love - Ancient Chinese & Modern Herbs For Male Fertility - Boxers Vs. Briefs - The New Male Fertility Supplements: What Works, What Doesn't! - Stress & Male Fertility: The Secret You Must Know!

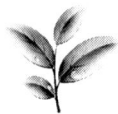

CHAPTER SIXTEEN   PAGE 394
IF YOU HAVE ENDOMETRIOSIS -
SOME SPECIAL FERTILITY ADVICE

- Understanding Endometriosis - How Endometriosis Affects Fertility - Diet, Endometriosis and Your Fertility - The Top Ten Foods For Endometriosis - 3 Must-Have Supplements for Endometriosis - Increase Your Immune Defenses: Here's How - Stress & Endometriosis - Getting Pregnant: Now You Can!

CHAPTER SEVENTEEN   PAGE 414
IF YOU HAVE PCOS -
SPECIAL FERTILITY ADVICE FOR POLY CYSTIC OVARIAN SYNDROME

- PCOS: What It Is, Why It Occurs - Diet, PCOS & Fertility - 7 Key Nutrients For PCOS - The Top Ten Foods For PCOS - PCOS Medications:Important Advice - Exercise, Weight Control, &Acupuncture: The Magic Triad for PCOS - Getting Pregnant: Now You Can Too!

CHAPTER EIGHTEEN   PAGE 439
YOUR PERSONAL FERTILITY GREEN PRINT -
A 6 MONTH COUNTDOWN PLAN FOR GETTING PREGNANT

- Including Green Fertility Goals - Natural Strategies - Mother Nature's Suggestions

CHAPTER NINETEEN   PAGE 452
GETTING PREGNANT -
WHEN SCIENCE & NATURE COMBINE ...MIRACLES HAPPEN!

- Getting Pregnant With Natural Technologies - The New GREEN IVF - Natural Cycle Fertility Treatments - Drug Free IVF -   ACUPUNCTURE: The New-Old Way To Get Pregnant Naturally! All Natural Inseminations - The New At-Home Insemination - Natural Tips For Fertility Treatment Success -

- ABOUT THE AUTHORS -   PAGE 480
- AUTHOR CONTACT INFORMATION   PAGE 482
- INDEX -   PAGE 483

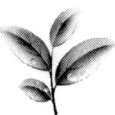

Introduction

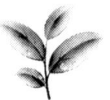

Green Fertility:
How Mother Nature Can Help You Get Pregnant Faster & Easier!

Getting pregnant is one of the most beautiful and natural of all life's activities. It is, in fact, what "boy meets girl" is really all about!

And much like that special chemistry that draws you and your life partner together, so too does a special kind of chemistry draw your egg to his sperm. And when they meet … magic happens, as the most natural of all unions occurs: A baby is created! And it's been happening this way since the beginning of time – and continues to happen every day for millions of couples all over the world.

At the same time, if you and your partner are like many couples trying to conceive today, the pregnancy "magic" seems a bit elusive. While you're sure you're doing everything "right", still, conception just isn't occurring, certainly not as quickly or as easily as you thought it would. In fact, you may even be asking yourselves why, if pregnancy is such a natural event, it doesn't occur as quickly and easily for all couples who try?

And if that is the question that's on your mind, let me reassure you that you are not alone. As a fertility specialist for nearly two decades and an obstetrician for over three decades, I can tell you without hesitation this is a question I have heard over and over, thousands of times.

So what is the answer? For many couples, it's just a matter of patience and time! Indeed, no two couples work on the same pregnancy " time table" – and by that I mean conception is such a unique and individual experience, that no two couples will get pregnant at the exact same moment, even if they "try" on the same schedule. The truth is, that even under the most "normal" circumstances there is only a 25% chance a pregnancy will occur during any given menstrual cycle so certainly it's possible for conception to take up to a year to occur – and still fall within the normal time frame.

At the same time, however, for some couples there are sometimes obstacles which can get in the way of getting pregnant – and in many ways make conception much harder than it has to be.

What kind of obstacles?

Certainly, for a small number of couples these obstacles are rooted in medical problems existing somewhere in their reproductive system. For women it can commonly be a blockage in the fallopian tubes that keep sperm and egg from uniting, or sometimes a problem related to producing or ovulating eggs. In men problems are usually related to sperm that is either defective, slow moving, or in too low a concentration. And in both men and women problems conceiving can be linked to an infection. And if any of these issue turn out to be the reason behind your conception problems, there is a multitude of treatments available to help.

But if you're like most couples having a problem getting pregnant today, research has shown – and my vast experience has proven to me – that there is likely no serious problems standing in your way. Indeed, you may be very surprised to learn that for the majority of couples who visit a fertility clinic - and I believe tens of thousands of those who don't - the diagnosis turns out to be something we call "unexplained infertility ".

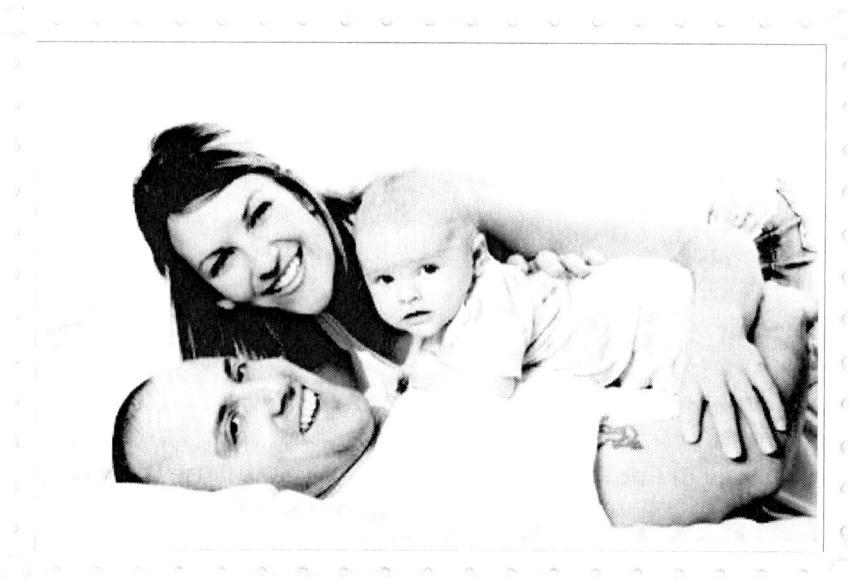

Essentially, this means that although you may be having problems conceiving, tests show both you and your partner are healthy, with no *obvious* signs that something is wrong.

So... now you're probably asking yourself " If you can't find anything wrong – then why can't I get pregnant?"

And that is where Mother Nature comes back into the equation.

Overcoming "Unexplained Infertility" Naturally!

Although the diagnosis of "unexplained infertility" leads us to believe there is, in fact, no reason you can't get pregnant, both common sense and science tells us this cannot be true. When something goes wrong – even in nature – there is always a reason, even if we don't know right off, what that reason is. And the same is true for "unexplained infertility."

Indeed, when this is the case it often means there is "something" some small, sub-clinical problem in one or often both partners - sometimes too small to even measure in a blood test or identify during an exam – that has formed a stumbling block to conception.

In my experience – that "stumbling block", that indefinable "something", can be found in lifestyle factors. Indeed, the latest research – as well as my own personal medical experience – has shown that everything from the foods and nutrients you eat (or miss out on) to the products you use, the environment in which you live, work and play, your daily habits like smoking or drinking alcohol, your exercise routines, and especially, how you deal with the everyday and the big-time stresses in your life – these are the kinds of things that can have not only an important impact on your overall health, but more so on your ability to get pregnant. In fact, nowhere is the power of Mother Nature more evident than when you stop to look at all the ways in which your life and your lifestyle impact your fertility.

What's more, while many couples believe that the only way to "fix " a fertility problem is via expensive medical treatments, I can promise you that this is not so! In fact, some of the most successful "fertility fixes" aren't found in a doctor's office or even a reproductive laboratory. For the vast majority of couples trying to get pregnant, Mother Nature holds the secret to pregnancy success! Moreover, with just a little bit of knowledge and a few small changes in your diet and lifestyle habits, you can unlock those secrets and get pregnant faster and easier than you ever believed was possible. And this is true whether you have just begun to try, or you've been trying for a long time with no success!

And when you think about it, the power of Mother Nature to get you there, is not really so hard to understand – or believe. In the past decade and particularly in the last several years, evidence continues to mount indicating that diet and lifestyle changes can make an enormous positive difference on so many aspects of our health.

From prevention of life threatening illnesses like cancer, heart disease and diabetes, clear down to the common cold, one of the most significant scientific lessons put in place this past decade has been the enormously important role that preventive lifestyle changes can play in not only keeping us from getting sick, but also helping us to heal the problems that plague us.

And nowhere is this tenant truer than when it comes to the world of fertility. In fact, while there have been great strides and tremendous success with some amazing scientific and medical developments in the treatment of infertility, I am happy to tell you there have been an equal number of impressive advances made in identifying important links between lifestyle and fertility as well.

> *The noted Harvard Nurses study of some 18,000 women, validated the idea that women who paid attention to lifestyle factors – including diet – had up an 80 percent lower rate of certain types of infertility, then women who did not pay attention to these factors.*

And certainly, for me, none of this has come as any great surprise. I have been a strong proponent of the importance of diet and lifestyle factors and the valuable role they play in encouraging fertility since I began my medical practice in the 1970's!

Throughout all my many books on pregnancy and reproductive health, including my best selling book " Getting Pregnant: What You Need To Know", I have always emphasized the important role that both diet and lifestyle can and should play in not only getting pregnant, but in insuring the birth of a happy, healthy baby – a baby that also grows forward with superior health and happiness throughout their lifetime.

In fact, I can tell you with all certainty that I helped thousands of couples go from infertile to fertile by doing nothing more than making a few small but significant changes in certain lifestyle habits. I have seen the miracles happen, and I have delivered thousands of these "miracle babies" - so I can tell you not just from the research, but from my first hand experience, that diet and lifestyle issues *do matter* - and they matter a lot. And it's not just in cases of "unexplained infertility."

Indeed, even for those patients who, for one reason or another, come to require medical treatment for their fertility problems, those who also focus on their diet and lifestyle habits no doubt have a much higher rate of conception success – and go on to deliver healthier babies – far more often than those who chose to believe that medicine alone provides all their answers.

Today, I am proud and happy to tell you that the philosophies I have long subscribed to and written about, and the diet and lifestyle changes I have always suggested to my patients as a way of encouraging conception, have come to fruition, having been proven to work in several major and important studies.

Indeed, the noted Harvard Nurses study of some 18,000 women, validated the idea that women who paid attention to lifestyle factors – including diet – had up an 80 percent lower rate of certain types of infertility, then women who did not pay attention to these factors.

In another new study published by researchers from the Department of Nutritional Sciences at Pennsylvania State University it is suggested that diet, particularly one featuring foods high in antioxidant vitamins like C and E, can play a role in not only increasing the opportunity to get pregnant faster, but at the same time help reduce the risk of early miscarriage.

In short, each week my desk is piled high with studies showing that for many women trying to get pregnant, lifestyle factors may be one of the most important factors to consider today. In fact, in many instances, making just a few simple changes could tip the scales from infertile to fertile in just a few months time, without the need for costly fertility testing and treatments!

How This Book Will Help You

Although the research in this area has continued to prove time and again just how effective this "natural" approach to boosting fertility can be, as I traveled the country talking to couples who were having difficulty conceiving, I began to realize how few men and women were actually taking advantage of all we had learned. While some couples would have bits and pieces of information on how lifestyle and infertility could be entwined, time and again I began to see how few really had the "whole picture".

Even more disturbing was how often proven facts about "natural fertility" were being diluted by anecdotal evidence – or confused with totally unproven theories. Unfortunately because the word " natural" still by and large represents "unregulated territory", too often what has never been proven to work gets the same "headline value" as those things that have been scientifically validated.

As time went on I began to see how difficult it can be for many couples to sort through all they hear or read to get to the truly solid *medically proven* evidence concerning what works and what doesn't to boost fertility.

And that is exactly why I decided to write this book – a "green print" to pregnancy success that simply and effortlessly guides you to the most important, proven and up-to-date medical research on the natural lifestyle changes that impact fertility. But it doesn't stop here. Because in this book I will also teach the secrets to using all this new scientific information in a way that will enhance your personal fertility profile.

In fact, my goal for this book is to help you and your partner create your own personal "green print" for healthy conception – a quick and easy way to identify the factors standing the way of your fertility – and the equally quick and easy solutions that can turn your fertility odds around.

And throughout this book, this is what you will find! Not only is it packed with the latest, most important research covering every lifestyle factor known to affect fertility, it's also brimming with my personal, time-tested, proven diet and lifestyle advice, featuring solutions that have already guided thousands of my own fertility patients to successful pregnancies for over two decades!

And the really good news: Once you put these changes into place, most couples can turn their fertility odds around in just 60 to 90 days! Imagine, in less than three months from today, you could be pregnant! Plus, you will feel better, and your overall health will be better so that you can go forward into your pregnancy giving your baby the very best chance in life!

GREEN FERTILITY TREATMENTS: AN EXTRA SECRET SURPRISE

As you read through this book you will no doubt come to see that not only do I believe in the power of Mother Nature to help and heal fertility, but that I am also a great believer in the idea that science and nature can work hand in hand to deliver solutions able to optimize both your overall health and your fertility in ways never before possible.

And to this end I am excited to tell you that in this book also contains the very newest, most cutting edge information on the latest trend in medical fertility care: GREEN Fertility Treatments!

Indeed, one of the most exciting advances in fertility medicine today is that we have "gone back to nature", with a slew of *advanced* reproductive technologies that work hand-in-hand with natural science to give you brand new ways to get pregnant faster and easier.

This includes the exciting new GREEN IVF – a more natural approach to the traditional in vitro fertilization that is not only far less expensive, but also does away with most of the unpleasant side effects and difficulties associated with this procedure, while increasing the success rate! And later in this book you will read about the new GREEN IVF as well as other new and exciting all natural medical treatments for overcoming even the most difficult conception problems.

So, whether you will be among the tens of thousands of couples who will need nothing more than a few small lifestyle changes to get pregnant fast, or those who may need some new "natural" medical help, I can promise that unlocking the secrets in this book will give you the answers you have been seeking – and the baby you have been longing for!

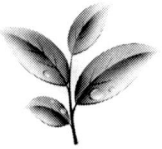

CHAPTER ONE

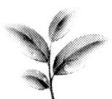

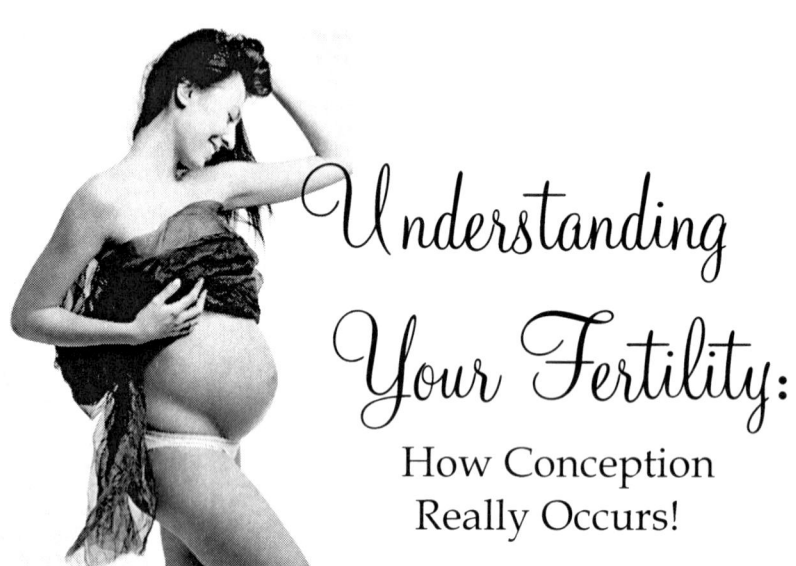

Understanding Your Fertility:
How Conception Really Occurs!

Inside every woman's body lies the basis for all creation. I'm talking about the "egg" - a tiny but miraculous group of cells from which all life springs forth! Every egg contains exactly one-half of the DNA necessary to create a baby - and when combined with the DNA from your partner's sperm it forms the basis of the embryo that will eventually become your beautiful, wonderful child.

But while everything about getting pregnant starts with "the egg", the egg itself must also have a beginning. And while every woman is born with some 400,000 follicles or "egg seeds" inside her ovary, before they can begin to grow a series of biochemical events orchestrated by several key biochemicals must take place.

So what are these "magical" chemicals that put all this activity in motion? It's your hormones! And ironically, it is many of the same ones that formed the "chemistry" which drew you and your partner together – and eventually, put the baby lust in your hearts!

SEX, HORMONES AND GETTING PREGNANT: WHAT YOU NEED TO KNOW

While some of the hormones involved in conception – like estrogen and progesterone – are made in your reproductive organs, what you might not realize is that fertility actually begins in your brain. That's because it is here, in two closely related areas of your brain known as the "pituitary" and the "hypothalamus", where many of the chemical signals that orchestrate reproductive hormonal activity begin. These chemical signals include:

- **Follicle Stimulating Hormone or FSH** - Secreted by the tiny pituitary gland the job of FSH is to send a signal to your ovaries to produce an egg. Indeed, while every woman is born with a lifetime supply of egg follicles (estimates are there are about 400,000 follicles inside your ovaries from the time you are born) without stimulation from FSH, they would never mature into an egg.

- **Luteinizing Hormone or LH** - Also secreted by your pituitary gland, this hormone instructs your matured egg to leave your ovary in a process known as "ovulation". It also directs your egg to travel down your fallopian tube where it can meet with your partner's sperm so that fertilization occurs.

Together these two hormones are known as "gonadotropins". While there is some FSH and LH in your body at all times, a significant amount is released during the first half of your menstrual cycle – when your egg is maturing and developing - followed by a drop in these hormones after ovulation. To help orchestrate the timing of this rise and fall is a third hormone:

- **Gonadotropin Releasing Hormone or GnRH.** Secreted by the hypothalamus (an area of your brain just above the pituitary gland) the function of GnRH is to trigger the release of the proper amounts of FSH and LH into your bloodstream, *at the proper time.*

Finally, there are yet two more hormones that play a critical role in the conception process. They are:

- **Estrogen** – Manufactured primarily by your ovaries, estrogen rises and falls in coordination with brain hormones to help orchestrate egg production and release. It also helps prepare your uterus to receive your fertilized egg. A surge in estrogen around the time of ovulation provides extra vaginal lubrication which in turn can increase your desire for sex, and help your partner's sperm travel more easily through your vagina and cervix.

- **Progesterone** – Manufactured by the corpus luteum (the shell that an ovulated egg leaves behind) progesterone works with estrogen to help prepare your uterus to receive a fertilized egg, and help it to be nourished and grow.

The entire process of growing, releasing and fertilizing an egg goes something like this:

1. At the start of each monthly menstrual cycle, your GnRH messengers sense that your estrogen levels are low – a sign that says you are not pregnant. In response to this signal your body steps up production of FSH - necessary to stimulate the growth of a new egg.

2. As FSH floods your ovaries, many follicles begin to develop. As days pass, however, only one pulls ahead of the rest in growth and development. Eventually it becomes your "egg of the month" – the one that will be released and available for fertilization. At the same time, however, your egg's rapid growth spurt causes your ovaries to produce more estrogen, and the level rises very quickly and dramatically. This serves two purposes: First, it helps stimulate the lining of your uterus to thicken, in anticipation of receiving a fertilized egg. But more importantly, when estrogen levels reach a specific, predetermined level this signals your brain that your egg has matured and is ready to be released. To make that happen, your brain releases LH – which as you remember is the hormone which prompts your newly developed egg to pop from your ovary in the process known as "ovulation".

3. As soon as ovulation occurs the shell which housed your egg turns into a tiny gland known as the corpus luteum, and begins producing progesterone. Together with estrogen – which is still surging – these two hormones work in consort to create a spongy nest of blood vessels inside your uterus.

4. Once your egg is fertilized it develops into an embryo and begins to travel down your fallopian tube where eventually it reaches your uterus, attaches to the lining, and begins to grow. This lining is actually your "womb" – a spongy mass of blood vessels that help "feed" your embryo with important nutrients to stimulate growth and development. To ensure that this nourishment continues throughout your pregnancy both estrogen and progesterone levels remain high. This in turn signals your brain to keep FSH and LH production at a minimum – which also prevents any new egg follicles from being stimulated into growth and development. This is why your menstrual cycle stops and you cannot get pregnant a second time while you are actually pregnant.

If, however fertilization does not occur, estrogen and progesterone drop rapidly. It is this rapid drop that causes the spongy lining inside your uterus to break down and be shed. This shedding process is the basis of your menstrual bleed. Once that bleeding stops – within about seven days – your body is once again ready to start a new cycle; you grow and release a new egg, and another chance for conception occurs.

INTRODUCING SPERM & EGG

Although this finely tuned biochemical and hormonal network is intrinsic to getting pregnant, none of this would matter if your egg could not hook up with your partner's sperm. And the preparation for this very important event begins the moment your egg matures. When it does, petal-like fingers that sit at the far end of your fallopian tube reach up and begin massaging your ovary, creating a kind of suction that gently coaxes your egg to pop from its shell and slide into the top portion of your fallopian tube. This long, narrow corridor is the pathway that leads directly to your uterus – and it's actually the place where his sperm and your egg meet.

In fact, if the timing is right, just as your egg is getting ready to be released from your ovary, your partner's sperm is swimming towards it from the other direction.

Being carried in part by your cervical mucous, sperm swim through your vaginal canal, into your cervix and eventually up into your uterus and then down into your fallopian tube.

How exactly does sperm know where to go? First, cervical mucus offers some guidance. But moreover, the head of each sperm is implanted with a kind of biochemical "radar" capable of picking up hormonal signals from your developing egg. It is this silent communication between developing egg and swimming sperm that ultimately brings the two of them together.

Once sperm and egg do meet there is, however, one more biochemical step that must occur before conception can take place. Namely, your partner's sperm must penetrate and enter your egg – a step that allows your joint DNA to combine and an embryo to form.

To help ensure this happens, all available sperm immediately attach to the outer shell of the egg. This activity initiates the release of a substance located in the head of each sperm that is designed to break down the outside shell of your egg, thus allowing entry.

Although thousands of sperm are simultaneously competing for the chance to be "the one" that gets inside your egg, much like your mate who worked to win your heart, generally one sperm works a little harder and a little faster than all the rest, enabling the entry process to begin.

Then, much like supportive teammates on the football field, once one sperm begins the penetration process, the others step back and begin rooting for the "touch down". To facilitate this, each of the other sperm stops their "drilling" process and pull away from the egg – thus giving the "lead sperm" a chance to gain entry.

Whether fertilization occurs or not, eventually all the other sperm swim away from the egg and within a few days die off and are biochemically dissolved by the body.

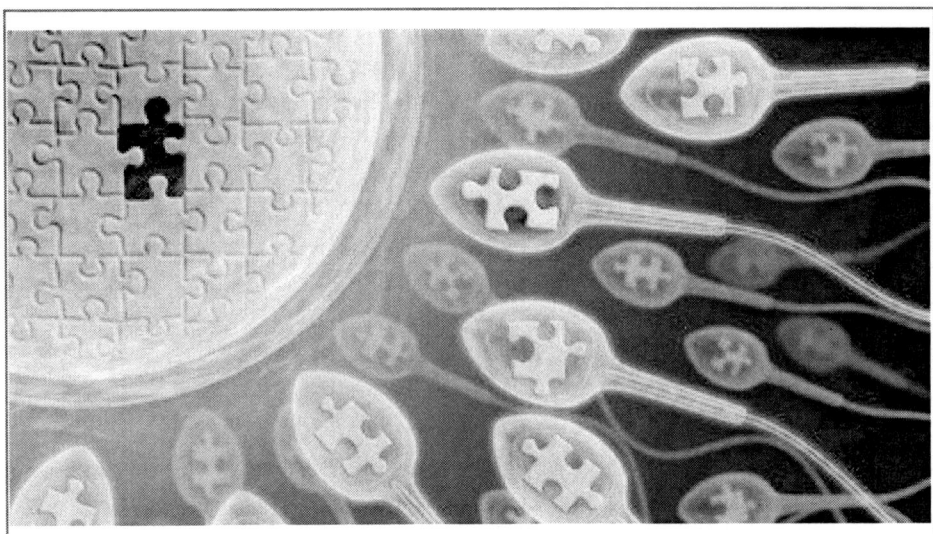

Once your egg matures & grows it sends out a silent signal to your partner's sperm to help guide it through your reproductive system and to your fallopian tube where you newly ovulated egg will be arriving. This helps ensure that fertilization will take place!

TIMING IS EVERYTHING!

While it may seem that all this activity can pretty much happen any time sperm and egg are in the same place at the same time, the truth is, when it comes to getting pregnant, *timing is everything...*

And by this I mean that in order for conception to occur, your partner's sperm must meet up with your egg no later than 24 hours after it leaves your ovary. Why? Because the offer for fertilization is good for a "limited time only"!

While your egg may not carry an obvious expiration date, the truth is, it is only viable – or able to be fertilized – for approximately 12 to 24 hours after ovulation. After that time it begins to break down and disintegrate, so that fertilization cannot occur, or if it does, that "union" usually isn't healthy, and often results in a miscarriage.

Sperm, on the other hand, have a much longer "shelf life". They can remain alive and ready to fertilize an egg for up to five days after they leave a man's body. While this may seem a little unfair, it actually puts the "home court" advantage in your favor! How? Because sperm can live longer, that means they can be in your body, ready and waiting for your egg to be ovulated and arrive!

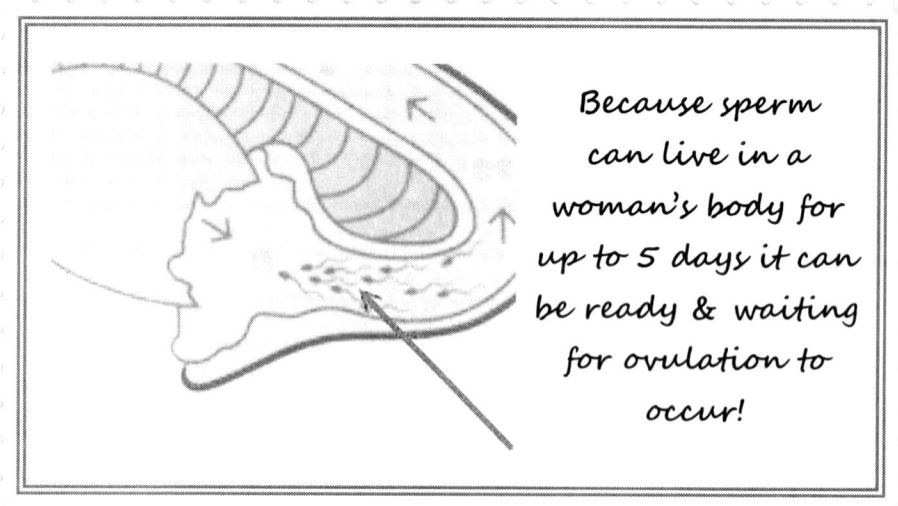

Because sperm can live in a woman's body for up to 5 days it can be ready & waiting for ovulation to occur!

In fact, one of the biggest "conception" mistakes couples make is waiting until ovulation to become intimate and attempt pregnancy. While it's still possible, if his sperm are just a little slow when "swimming" towards your fallopian tube, or if minor biochemical snafus diminish the "guiding" signal from egg-to-sperm, then waiting until ovulation day to have sex will likely mean the egg-sperm "hook up" simply occurs too late in the game for a viable conception to take place.

So in this respect, the number one easiest way to insure conception is to begin making love one or twice daily, up to five days before ovulation is expected to occur (and you will learn how to predict when you will be ovulating in the next chapter). Ultimately this gives your partner's sperm plenty of time to make their way to your fallopian tube and be there, ready and waiting, for your egg to make it's "entrance". This, in turn, allows the fertilization process to begin as quickly as possible, with an egg that is at the "peak" of perfection. Ultimately this creates the optimum circumstance for a quick, easy and healthy pregnancy to occur!

WHEN PREGNANCY DOESN'T HAPPEN: WHAT GOES WRONG

If you're like many couples I speak to almost every day, you may be wondering why making love at the *right time* doesn't automatically lead to pregnancy *every time* – and why it can take so long to get pregnant.

First, remember that no matter how much medical science has learned about the magic of conception there is still some indefinable "magic" involved. Sometimes, even when all conditions are right for pregnancy – a healthy egg is made and ovulated at the right time, and a hearty group of healthy sperm is ready and waiting to pounce – still conception might not happen. It's this indefinable impact of Mother Nature that ultimately reminds those of us in the science world who is really in charge!

But that said, there are also several biological, even medical reasons why conception does not occur each time you have intercourse – *even at the right time of the month.*

The first and easiest explanation is that not every woman ovulates every single month. While regular ovulation is more likely when you are in your teens and early twenties, you may be surprised to learn that by your mid to late twenties, ovulation can be a bit irregular. Moreover, sperm production in men can vary as well – and together these "normal" reproductive irregularities can delay a pregnancy by up to a year.

On the other end of the spectrum, however, there is always the possibility that a potentially serious fertility problem may be behind your conception problems.

In a woman this can involve a problem creating or releasing an egg, or having some type of blockage –usually scar tissue cause by a previous infection somewhere within the fallopian tube. This scar tissue can block or certainly make it more difficult for a sperm and egg to meet. It can also make it more difficult for a fertilized egg to reach the uterus.

Additionally, problems can also be the result of congenital malformations within the uterus itself, or sometimes from menstrual- related conditions such as endometriosis or PCOS (poly cystic ovarian syndrome), both of which you will read more about later in this book.

When it comes to men, the physiologic problems that can block fertility include any condition which hampers the production, maturity, growth, or release of his sperm. These problems can occur in the epididymis (the area of a man's reproductive system where sperm are made) or the vas deferens (where sperm mature, grow and are eventually released). Difficulties can also stem from within the penile system itself, the series of ducts and tubes that help transport sperm from his body into yours. (And you'll learn more about all of this in my chapter on male fertility later in this book).

> **Q:** *I'm not sure I'm ovulating every month – does that mean I can't get pregnant?*
>
> **A:** Not every woman ovulates each and every month - & irregular ovulation can begin as early as your 20's !
> While irregular ovulation will slow down the process of getting pregnant , it certainly doesn't automatically mean that you won't get pregnant. What you might not realize is that oftentimes simple changes in diet and lifestyle habits - including getting more sleep - can help normalize ovulation patterns and get you back on track!

AGE MATTERS!

What's also important to note is the role of advancing age in conception. Although by today's living standards, turning 35 is still considered very young, this is not entirely the case when it comes to fertility.

Indeed by your mid-thirties the reproductive potential of both you and your partner can begin to experience some compromise. While a woman's fertility is much more susceptible to the effects of aging (problems include a reduction in the amount and quality of eggs that are produced) the latest research now shows that, to some degree, age can also impact the quality of sperm, as well as the ability of any sperm that are produced to move through your reproductive system and reach your egg. So, if either you or your partner are over age 35 it's more imperative than ever to do everything you can to optimize your fertility and make the best use of your fertile potential.

Moreover, even if age is not factor, and no obvious medical problems exist for either of you, sometimes small, even medically undetectable issues can still be present capable of forming a stumbling block to conception. Medically known as "unexplained infertility" this is often the diagnosis when no other medical reason can be found for your fertility problems.

THE GREEN SECRET
TO GETTING PREGNANT FAST AND EASY!

As complicated –or even discouraging - as all of this may sound, I have some good news to tell you: As many opportunities as there are for a pregnancy to be delayed, there are equally as many opportunities for you to take control and put your parenting dreams on the fast track! In fact, for the vast majority of you reading this book – in fact for most couples today trying to get pregnant – the key to a faster, easier conception lies totally in Mother Nature's loving hands!

Certainly if you have a physical problem standing in the way, Mother Nature is going to need a little bit of help. And, indeed, if you have been trying to get pregnant for more than 12 months, or, if you are over 35 and have been trying for over six months, it's probably a good idea to see a fertility specialist and have some basic tests to see if there is a physiologic or hormonal problem that needs treatment.

If this turns out to be true, the earlier you seek medical treatment, the faster and easier it will be to get pregnant.

At the same time, however, we now know that the most important key factors involved in the fertility process – particularly the brain chemistry signals that kick off the conception process and the hormonal activity that follows - are very much influenced by lifestyle factors *under your control.*

This factors include :

- Diet
- Vitamin and nutrient status
- Weight
- Fitness level
- Sleep habits
- Environmental exposures
- Personal habits
- Stress responses.

In fact, almost every single aspect of your life and your lifestyle can play a part in how efficiently these essential hormonal signals are transmitted. And while this may seem like a huge "laundry list" of things that you must pay attention to, in reality it really represents a series of opportunities for you to make a huge difference in your fertility, often by making only small changes in *some areas of your life*.

Moreover, if it turns out that you do need some type of medical help conceiving, I can promise that all the solutions and recommendations you find in this book will help you during the course of any fertility treatments, oftentimes increasing the success rate and insuring that they work faster and better. And also ensuring your baby will be healthier right from the very start!

Indeed, studies show that couples who maximize their fertility via natural diet and lifestyle changes before and during fertility treatments, have a much higher pregnancy success rate no matter the treatment that is used.

This is particularly true when it comes to the new "GREEN" medical fertility treatments – such as the new Natural GREEN IVF – a magical new way of combining nature and science that you will read more about later in this book.

In fact, whether you will be among the vast majority of couples who will conceive naturally on your own, or among the small percentage who may ultimately need some "green" medical intervention to help you conceive, I can promise that what you will discover in this book will "level the playing field" and help you not only get pregnant faster and easier today, but also help to improve your overall health and preserve and protect your fertility for the future – *all in the most natural way possible!*

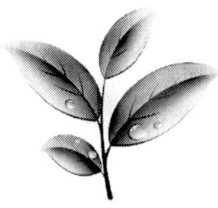

CHAPTER TWO

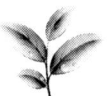

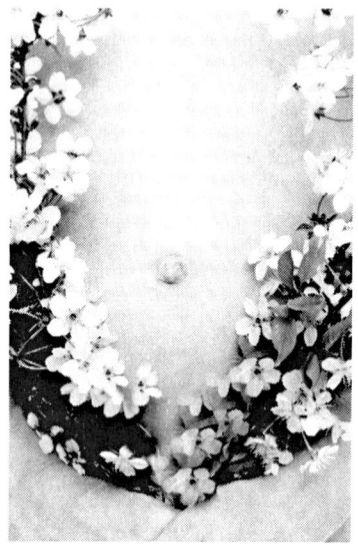

Protecting Your Fertility

With The New Pre-Conception Counseling Exam

Making the decision to begin – or expand - your family is one of the most important and joyous determinations a couple can make. And for many, it can be just that easy: The decision is made to have a baby and within a relatively short amount of time, pregnancy occurs.

But increasingly, however, this *isn't* the case.

Indeed, in the last decade and particularly in the past five years the number of couples for whom getting pregnant is anything but simple, is on the rise.

While some of the problems are due to advancing age – many couples are simply choosing to start their families later in life, when it can naturally take longer to get pregnant - problems are not confined to "older" couples by any means. In fact, I have recently seen an increase in the number of couples in the prime pregnancy age – between 20 and 30 – also having problems conceiving.

Why is this happening?

Well as this book unfolds you will find many of the lifestyle reasons behind today's rising rate of fertility problems – as well as the simple solutions that can help. But before any of these solutions *can* work, it's important that you know a little something about how to increase your chances of getting pregnant *anytime* you try. And among the best ways to do that, is with a pre-conception counseling exam.

Unlike a regular GYN check –up, a preconception counseling exam is a doctor visit that focuses specifically on your reproductive health as it relates to getting pregnant. This is also different – in fact much, much different – than what occurs when you see a fertility specialist . Here, a reproductive endocrinologist looks for reasons why you *can't* get pregnant.

In a pre-conception counseling exam, a gynecologist or fertility expert looks for all the ways in which you can enhance your fertility and give yourself the best possible chance to conceive. It's an exam that focuses entirely on the "positives" and in doing whatever is possible to ensure optimum reproductive health.

But as important as this exam is, I find that not only do many couples skip it , but many doctors don't encourage this important "fertility check up".

In fact, despite how far we have come in our quest for equality health care, some gynecologists still do nothing more than pat their patients on the head and tell them " You're young – just go home and try, try, try!" *Even if they have been trying for quite some time.* Other doctors may perform some perfunctory, outdated tests, and never really give a couple the chance to take full advantage of all we have learned.

For all these reasons I want to take just a few moments out to detail for you what the new pre-conception counseling exam should include. While some doctors may include all these steps, others may include only some – and quite possibly some physicians may have a few "extras" of their own that they add to the list.

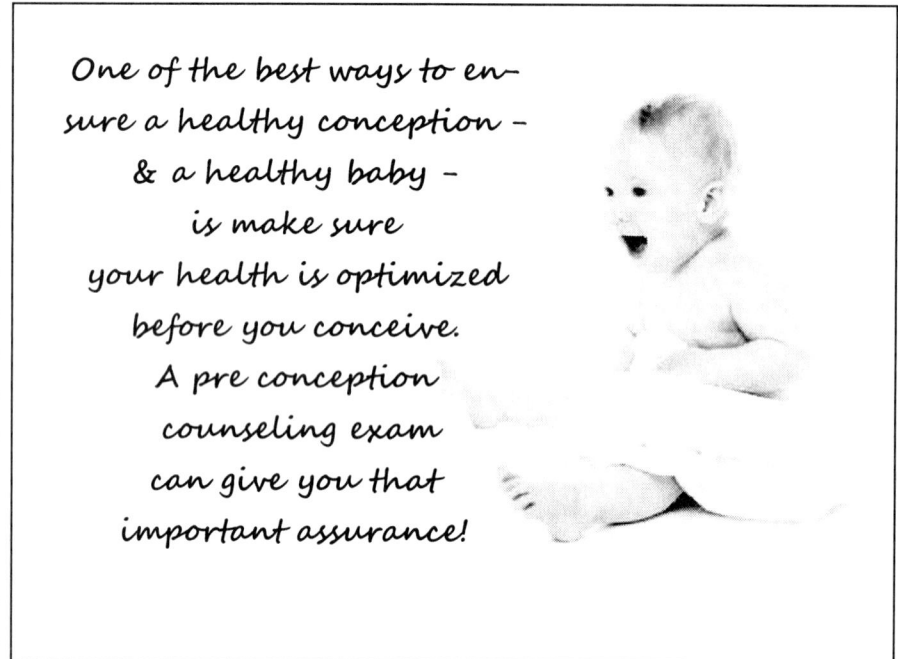

One of the best ways to ensure a healthy conception – & a healthy baby – is make sure your health is optimized before you conceive. A pre conception counseling exam can give you that important assurance!

And if your doctor does deviate, don't automatically think you are getting bad care.

But that said, once you familiarize yourself with the material in this section, you should feel free to discuss with your doctor any of the portions of the exam and get their professional opinion on what they think is most important and relevant to your fertility and your reproductive care.

THE NEW PRE CONCEPTION COUNSELING EXAM: WHAT YOU MUST KNOW

What makes *the new* pre-conception counseling exam so different – and so important – is that it not only includes information about *your* physical health, but it also looks at the life and lifestyle of both you *and* your partner. As such, most Pre Conception Counseling Exams begin with a joint partner history - a time when your doctor will ask both you and your partner a series of questions designed to learn where your reproductive strengths and weaknesses lie. I urge you to be extremely honest and forthcoming with your answers, as this information can definitely help shape and define the quickest ways for you to get pregnant. Some of the more important questions you and your partner should be prepared to answer include:

- **Age**

- **Fitness level and activities** – Including whether either of you participate in regular fitness regimens, and if you do, how often you exercise   (such as three days a week) how much you work out (the length of time you spend exercising during each session) and your fitness routines (running, tennis, aerobics, etc) .

- **Occupation** – This includes where you work, the type of job you perform, the number of hours you work per week, any physical activity your job entails, and any significant exposure to either radiation or toxic chemicals.

- **Weight and Height**

- **Diet** - Approximate number of daily or weekly calories; foods you eat most often ; favorite snack foods; eating patterns (six small meals a day, three meals, one huge meal, etc.)

- **Vitamin and Nutritional Profile** - The number of fruits and vegetables you eat per day and which ones you include on a regular basis; the amount of fiber you consume daily; if you take vitamins (if you do it's a good idea to bring your supplements with you); if you are eating any food supplements such as protein bars or shakes or taking any herbal supplements.

- **Lifestyle** - This should include personal habits such as smoking, alcohol consumption or any recreational drug use, as well as the number of hours you sleep per night,   environmental issues (including exposure to second hand smoke or any regular chemical exposures), general or specific stress levels.

- **General Health** - Note any chronic health conditions such as asthma, allergies, IBS, high blood pressure, high or low blood sugar - and be certain to reveal if any medications used on a regular basis – including herbal preparations or over-the-counter fertility supplements.

MEDICAL QUESTIONS JUST FOR YOU:

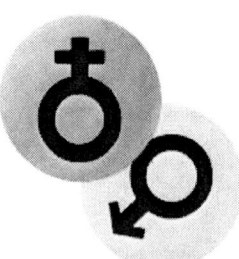

- **Reproductive Health** - This should include your personal history of previous pregnancies and their outcome, including any history of birth defects, premature birth, fetal death or neonatal death; miscarriage; voluntary pregnancy termination; infection (ovarian, tubal, cervical, vaginal or uterine); menstrual history (including cramps, clots, or any irregularities such as irregular cycles, very long or very short cycles) ; abnormal vaginal bleeding. Your history should also include any previous GYN surgeries including D&C, laparoscopy or treatment for ovarian cysts.

- **Family Health History -** This should focus on your mother, grand mother and sisters reproductive history including difficulty getting pregnant, recurrent miscarriages, or history of birth defects. Overall family history should include any incidence of cancer before age 60; history of heart disease, thyroid disorder, diabetes, or any genetic blood disorder.

MEDICAL QUESTIONS FOR YOUR PARTNER :

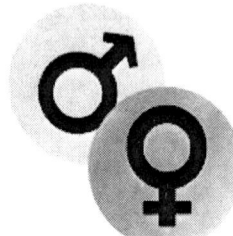

- If he has ever fathered a child.
- If he has ever impregnated a woman and if the pregnancy was terminated.
- Any family or personal history of birth defects, genetic disorders, or infertility.
- History of problems relating to ejaculation or impotence.
- History of sexually transmitted diseases .

Your partner should also make the doctor aware of any outstanding family history of disease, particularly early heart disease, high blood pressure, diabetes, or any genetic blood disorder or family history of birth defects.

YOUR PRECONCEPTION PHYSICAL: WHAT IT MUST INCLUDE

Once your doctor has concluded the history portion of your exam, it's time for the actual physical to begin. Usually this will focus on the woman, with additional care suggested to your partner, in terms of a male fertility exam. Be aware, however that some fertility specialists do include at least a base line fertility exam for men, often done during the same visit as your exam.

A little later in this book you'll learn more about what your partner's fertility exam should include. But for right now, however, I'd like to offer you some detail concerning what your portion of a fertility physical should include.

STEP ONE: THE BODY CHECK

Think of this portion of the exam as a kind of fertility "once over"- a way of checking you from head to toe, looking for symptoms that might indicate a potential problem. The check should include:

- **YOUR NECK** - Your doctor is checking for swollen glands and any growths or other abnormalities indicative of a thyroid condition –a problem which can be symptom-free, but does impact fertility.

- **SKIN AND HAIR** - The texture, color, and general condition can signal any number of conditions related to fertility, including thyroid disorder, hormonal imbalances, ovarian cysts or a nutritional deficiency.

- **WEIGHT AND HEIGHT** –When it comes to getting pregnant, being too thin or being overweight can both interfere with fertility so it's important that your doctor establish a weight baseline.

- **BLOOD PRESSURE** – While there is no direct link between blood pressure and fertility , there is a link once you are pregnant. As such I, and many doctors believe that getting your pressure under control before conception can help ensure a healthier pregnancy overall.

- **ABDOMEN -** Different from a pelvic exam, in an abdomen check your doctor will concentrate on the outside of your pelvic cavity, looking for indications of any tumors or growths or structural abnormalities that could interfere with pregnancy.

- **THE BREAST CHECK -** Again, there is no direct link to getting pregnant, however breast abnormalities, including cysts or fluid retention, can be signs of a hormonal imbalance that might interfere with getting pregnant. Moreover, since the high estrogen levels of pregnancy can encourage the growth of breast cancer, being certain your breasts are in good health before you conceive is one way to help ensure a healthy pregnancy. In truth, no woman with even a suspicion of breast cancer should get pregnant until her breasts are proven to be healthy. If breast cancer is detected, then certainly it's possible to get pregnant after treatment. I have had a number of patients who have conceived and successfully given birth – without harming their own health – following treatment for breast cancer.

STEP TWO : YOUR FERTILITY PELVIC EXAM

Much like a regular GYN check up, the purpose of the fertility pelvic exam is to verify the health of your reproductive organs as they relate to getting pregnant. The exam should include:

- **THE VULVA CHECK -** This is the area outside your vagina and it's the first place you might see signs of any type of infection that could interfere with fertility – including yeast infections or "silent" STDs (sexually transmitted diseases).

- **THE VAGINAL CHECK –** Here your doctor will look for any additional signs of infection, as well as the presence of any abnormal discharges or odors, which can signal potential fertility issues.

- **THE UTERUS CHECK/PAP SMEAR –** This is the "internal" portion of your exam, which will tell your doctor that everything is okay to carry your baby . Specifically your doctor is looking for signs of any benign growths – such as fibroid tumors or polyps – as well as cysts, or any indication of endometriosis (see Chapter 16) which might interfere with fertility.

During this exam your doctor should also check your ovaries and fallopian tubes to ensure they are healthy as well, and you should receive a Pap smear, which checks for cervical cancer. If any problems are suspected during this portion of the exam your doctor may suggest a trans-vaginal ultrasound or TVU. This procedure uses harmless radio waves to create a "visual" picture of the inside of your pelvic cavity and project the image on a computer screen.

STEP THREE: YOUR FERTILITY BLOOD TESTS

These blood tests are designed to help validate that your hormones are working properly and that you have no other "hidden" health problems that might otherwise interfere with your ability to get pregnant quickly. Your fertility blood tests should include:

- **THE CBC –** Also known as the Complete Blood Count, the most important aspect of this test, from a fertility standpoint, is validation that you are not "anemic" – meaning that your iron levels are sufficient to carry red blood cells throughout your body. As you will read in the upcoming chapter on minerals, oftentimes a problem as simple as iron deficiency anemia can temporarily keep a woman from getting pregnant or increase the risk of miscarriage.

- **THE CMP –** The Comprehensive Metabolic Panel is a broad screening tool that is frequently used to help validate that your body is healthy enough for conception. It can also work as an early screening tool to uncover problems such as diabetes, or liver or kidney conditions that could interfere with your overall health and in this way disrupt your fertility. This test also checks your balance of electrolytes (like sodium and potassium) and important acids, all of which work together to promote better hormonal balance.

- **T3, T4, TSH –** These are thyroid hormone tests and vital for every woman to have, particularly if she is planning to get pregnant. Why? Sometimes even small 'glitches' in the production of thyroid hormones (too much or too little) can have a major impact on reproductive hormones. The T4 test measures all levels of active thyroid hormone in the blood; the T3 measures a slightly more active form of thyroid hormone; the TSH measures a hormone that becomes elevated whenever the thyroid gland is overproducing and it falls low when the thyroid gland is under-producing. Remember, if your thyroid function tests have abnormal results, treatment is simple and easy using a variety of medications designed to normalize thyroid gland function – but it should be done before you attempt conception.

- **25-OH Vitamin D Test** - This is among the most accurate ways to test levels of Vitamin D – a nutrient which we now know can play a significant role in getting pregnant.(See Chapter 9). When levels are low you are not only more likely to have a fertility problem, but also other health issues that could keep you from getting pregnant. The most accurate 25-OH test results are achieved in fall and winter, but the test is important to take any time of the year.

Some Additional Blood Tests

If you have highly irregular periods or severe PMS, if you are over age 35, or if you are under age 35 and have been unsuccessfully trying to get pregnant for 12 months or more, then you should talk to your doctor about these additional blood tests.

- **Estrogen, Progesterone, FSH, LH** - These are tests that directly measure levels of the most important hormones involved in reproduction. Testing should be done at specific times of the month for the most accurate results – and your doctor will likely schedule them to coordinate with your monthly menstrual cycle. Of these tests, FSH is among the most important in terms of determining if your body is capable of making eggs and it should be offered to all women over 35 seeking to get pregnant.

- **CA 125** - This is an important test for helping determine the health of your ovaries as well as the presence of other types of inflammation. It is usually given if your ultra sound or gyn exam suggests the possibility of an ovarian cyst. However, it can also be given to help rule out problems when ovulation is irregular, or if you have severe mid-month ovulation pain.

- **AMH** - This blood test is extremely important for every woman over 35 looking to get pregnant. Why? Because it helps determine if you are still ovulating, and your egg making potential. AMH stands for Anti-Mullerian Hormone., which is a biochemical produced by your egg follicle – the "seed" that eventually grows into an egg. Blood levels of AMH can help indicate if your follicles are still active and if you have the potential to make and release eggs. In addition the test can also be used to help gauge how successful an IVF procedure will be and it is also very useful as a test for PCOS – poly cystic ovarian syndrome (See Chapter 17).

Step Four: Fertility Protection Diagnostics

In addition to the tests already mentioned, there are several more "diagnostic" tests that I believe are extremely important for every woman who is seeking to get pregnant. Not only will these tests help uncover problems that could interfere with getting pregnant, they can also help protect your overall health – which is essential for not only a healthy conception, but also a healthy pregnancy. Here are the diagnostics tests you need:

- **The digene HPV Test -** This is the most widely used FDA approved test for detecting the presence of high-risk types of the HPV virus in women over 30. When used along with a Pap to screen women 30 and older, it more accurately identifies who is at risk *of developing* cervical cancer than the Pap alone. The digene HPV Test – which can usually be conducted on the same sample of cells taken for your Pap smear, uses a type of molecular technology that identifies the presence of high-risk types of HPV cells, which is what causes cervical cells to become abnormal in the first place. If you are under age 30 you need this test only if your Pap smear indicates an abnormality or results are considered "borderline".

- **Nucleic acid amplification test for Chlamydia (NAAT)** – This urine test is hands-down the most sensitive and the most accurate way to diagnose the presence of the chlamydia bacteria –a silent sexually transmitted infection that can remain in your system undetected for decades. Why is it important to find and treat chlamydia? Because when untreated it can be a leading cause of infertility in both men and women. Unlike other STDs (sexually transmitted diseases) which have obvious symptoms, Chlamydia can have no symptoms. So, without the test you might never know you have it – until you try to get pregnant and discover that you cannot.

> One of the keys to a successful Pre Conception Counseling Exam is to be totally honest with your doctor. If you feel you can't be honest and open with your physician without being judged then it may be time to find a new doctor

SOME FINAL ADVICE: RELY ON YOUR INTUITION & DON'T HIDE SYMPTOMS!

While each of us would like to believe we are in perfect health – and in fact I'm certain that most of you reading this book are – still, there is one more thing that you can and should do to insure a healthy future – and insure the future health of your fertility.

And that one step is to be totally honest with your doctor and not hide any symptoms – no matter how scared you might feel, or how insignificant you might think your problem might be.

This is particularly vital when you are trying to get pregnant – simply because so many seemingly small, unrelated problems could actually provide your doctor with clues as to what may be compromising your fertility, now or in the future. Even more important, once diagnosed, most of these kinds of problems can be treated quickly and easily - and doing so can usually prevent more serious, long term fertility complications from occurring.

On the other hand, when you ignore those early warning signs and don't talk honestly with your doctor, your fertility can really suffer the consequences. I can't tell you the number of women who came to my clinic seeking help getting pregnant after months or even years of ignoring symptoms that, had they been caught early on, could have allowed them to get pregnant naturally, on their own.

This same kind of honesty is also necessary when discussing lifestyle factors with your doctor. Again, throughout my years of practice I witnessed countless numbers of patients struggling with fertility problems only to discover they had not been honest about lifestyle factors that could have made a difference , such as smoking or drug and alcohol use.

At the same time, if your doctor does not foster the kind of open, honest, non-judgmental communication that would make it easy for you to be honest, then please, find another doctor. Indeed, a doctor-patient relationship is among the most special, sacred and confidential there is, and both the patient and the doctor must have mutual respect and trust in each other in order for the best treatment outcomes to prevail.

And finally do believe in your intuition, particularly when you get a "feeling" that something is wrong. As a firm believer in the power of women's personal inner knowledge and "intuition " I believe that if you have a "feeling" that something is "not quite right" in any one area of your health, you should be able to discuss this with your doctor and he or she should take that seriously – and fully investigate all your concerns. This is particularly true if you are having a problem getting pregnant.

So, whether you have detected symptoms your doctor has not yet picked up on, or if there are no symptoms, but some inner feeling has led you to believe a problem may exist in a certain area of your body or your health, do discuss this with your doctor. At the very least, you can come away reassured that what you are "picking up" is within the realm of normal healthy living.

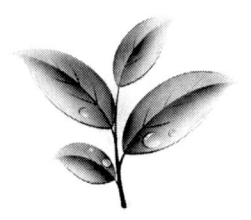

Chapter Three

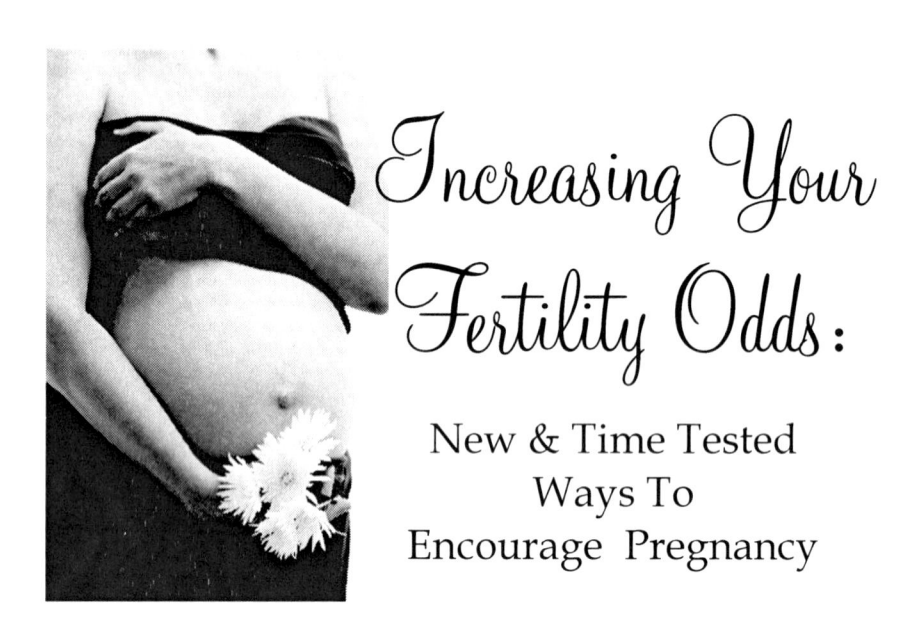

Increasing Your Fertility Odds:

New & Time Tested Ways To Encourage Pregnancy

If you are like most couples trying to make a baby, making love on a "schedule" is the furthest thing from your mind. Indeed, most couples simply become intimate whenever the mood strikes and sooner or later a baby is created!

And while it may all seem like chance, the truth is that no matter how many times you and your partner make love, there is actually only a small window of opportunity each month when pregnancy is possible. And that "window" is the time frame in which you ovulate - the moment within your cycle when your egg pops from its shell, leaves your ovary and travels into your fallopian tube.

As you just read, it's crucial to the success of any conception that sperm and egg meet immediately following ovulation since 24 to 36 hours later, your egg begins to disintegrate. That means conception is not only more difficult to achieve, but when if does it may result in a defective embryo, and usually, miscarriage.

But as critical – and as small - as this window of opportunity may appear to be, you do have a little bit of "breathing room" . And that is thanks to your partner's sperm. Indeed, because sperm can live in a woman's reproductive tract for up to five days, if you begin making love two to four days before ovulation takes place, you can ensure there is a good supply of sperm ready and waiting for your egg to emerge. When it does, fertilization can happen right away, when you egg is the freshest and healthiest. And that means a quick and healthy pregnancy can occur!

But how do you know when ovulation is approaching – and when the time is right to send those sperm on their baby-making mission? Well that's where ovulation prediction technology can help. This is the easy "science" that helps a woman to better understand her body and predict, with some degree of accuracy, when her egg is ready to leave the nest and be fertilized. Having this information – and making love during this time frame - means even if you make no other changes, you will still dramatically increase your chances of getting pregnant fast!

HOW OVULATION PREDICTION WORKS

According to medical text books, a woman's body is on a 28 day cycle - meaning she not only gets a new period every 28 days, but right smack in the middle of each cycle - on day 14 - she ovulates.

Unfortunately, however, I have found that very few women have this *text book cycle* or ovulate exactly on time month in and month out.

In fact, in today's high stress, fast paced world, it is rare that any woman has the exact same menstrual cycle each and every month. Moreover, almost no women ovulate exactly mid-cycle, month in and month out. Indeed, I can tell you from my professional experience, even young, healthy women do not always have completely predictable periods. This is one reason why the rhythm method of birth control - which relies on abstinence during certain times of the cycle – is so unreliable. It's also why couples using this same "rhythm method" to get pregnant, usually have a difficult time doing so.

On the other hand, there are several very reliable ways to predict when your most fertile time will be – no matter how unreliable your cycle may appear to be. That's because each and every cycle is linked to a series of body cues that are in turn linked to hormonal activity that occurs just before ovulation. Learning to read these body cues is, in fact, one way to predict ovulation, even if your period does not occur in "typical" 28 day cycles.

In fact, the science behind *ovulation prediction kits* is based entirely on the ability to harness these hormonal signals and calculate them in various ways to predict when your egg is likely to pop from it's shell - ripe and ready for fertilization.

But while the basis of all ovulation prediction methods may be the same, how each one works to detect and track the information you need can be vastly different. Therefore, I have always believed it is a good idea to use at least two different methods simultaneously, to help ensure the most accurate outcome.

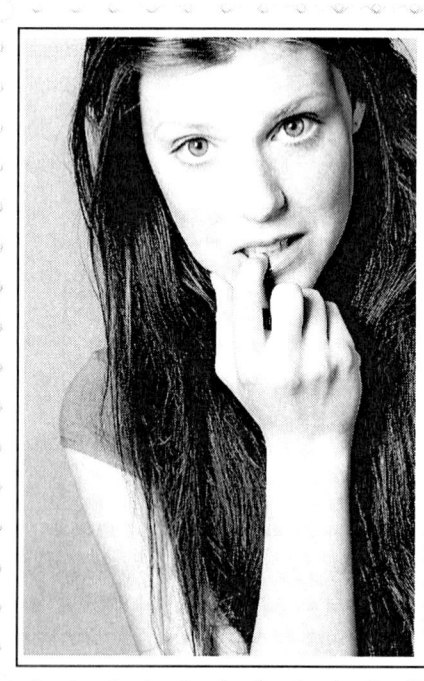

Q: My periods are very irregular – will ovulation prediction work for me?

A: Almost no woman ovulates exactly mid cycle every month. But if you use several prediction methods simultaneously, you can still learn to predict your most fertile time! One tip: Do start calculating several months prior to when you want to get pregnant. This will make it easier to see the pattern and help you navigate around those irregular cycles easier.

FIVE WAYS TO PREDICT OVULATION & GET PREGNANT FAST!

To help you get started in choosing which of the most popular ovulation prediction methods might be right for you, I've put together the following, easy –to-use guide. It features the five methods I have noted as the most successful among my patients, and they are also the ways proven in studies to be the most accurate.

While some of these methods are so tried and true they date back almost to the Bible, others are based on new inventions and discoveries – and some even rely on the latest high tech electronics. That said, don't be fooled into thinking that newer is always better. Most of the time, newer is just, well, *newer*. So in this respect you should simply choose the methods that seem easiest, most convenient and most cost-effective *for you*.

I do, however, want to remind you again that ovulation prediction systems can only reflect what is already going on in your body on a hormonal level. If there is a physical problem within your reproductive system – such as a blocked fallopian tube from endometriosis or a sexually transmitted infection, or some problem that is preventing ovulation - please remember that an ovulation prediction system isn't a cure, and it isn't a way around these problems.

That said, even if a problem does exist, when used correctly many ovulation prediction methods can also provide you with important information about why a pregnancy *might not be happening* - data that together with your doctor you can look at, analyze, and in many instances, do something about. The good news is that for most of you reading this book that "something" involves making the small but significant diet and lifestyle changes detailed in the remainder of this book!

In fact, as you begin to chart your ovulation schedule, it's also important that you simultaneously begin to implement at least some of the suggestions found throughout this book .

Together with knowing the "right" time to get pregnant, you'll give your fertility a "one-two punch" that will boost your odds of getting pregnant significantly!

Ovulation Prediction Method # 1: Using Your Body Temperature To Get Pregnant Faster!

In the classic situation comedy, attempts at getting pregnant are often portrayed by a wife making a frantic call to her hubby whispering that her temperature is "up" – and it's time to make love! Inevitably he's at the gym, in a business meeting, or about to board a plane when the call comes – and the comedy takes flight as he jumps through hoops to make it home "in time".

And while this scenario is rooted in some truth – body temperature does rise and fall relative to ovulation – the fact is that once your body temperature rises, ovulation has already passed! So unless your partner is ready, willing and able at the exact moment your temperature goes up, this is not the signal you should be looking for!

So what temperature related sign should you be watching for? Before I tell you that I want to fill you in on just a little bit of background about how and why body temperature is related to getting pregnant.

How Your Body Temperature Predicts Ovulation

The method that uses body temperature to help you get pregnant is called the Basal Body Temperature guide or BBT. The system is based on the principle that your body temperature rises and falls in distinct patterns that are connected to the rise and fall of reproductive hormones. Why is this important?

Because it is the rise and fall of these hormones that orchestrate not just the growth and development of your egg, but also ovulation. As such, having as much information as you can about the specific timing of these processes can give you a real edge when it comes to knowing the "right" time to make love. So where does body temperature fit in?

Right before ovulation is about to occur, your body temperature takes a subtle but important drop, by about one-half of a degree. And therein lies the secret to using your BBT or basal body temperature as a guide to getting pregnant. Indeed, when you take your temperature every day, you will be able to see

INCREASING YOUR FERTILITY ODDS

instantly when the drop occurs – and when it does you know ovulation is likely to follow, usually within 12 to 24 hours. Once ovulation does take place, you'll see a subtle rise in body temperature – usually by that same one-half degree.

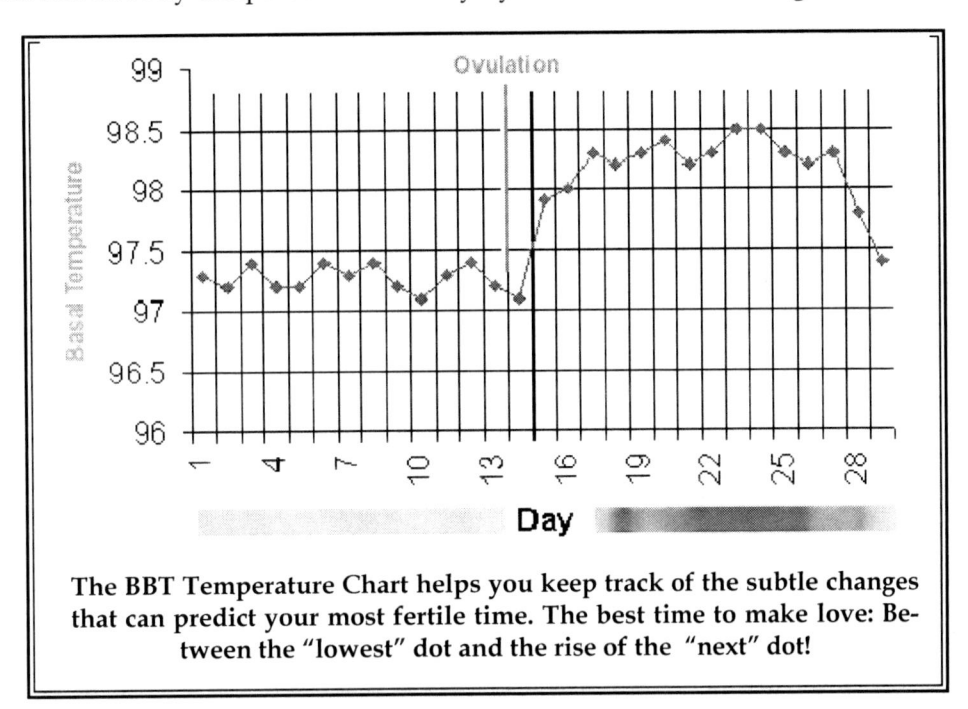

The BBT Temperature Chart helps you keep track of the subtle changes that can predict your most fertile time. The best time to make love: Between the "lowest" dot and the rise of the "next" dot!

TO GET PREGNANT FAST: Make love between the time your temperature drops and before it rises- a period of about 12 to 24 hours that usually occurs about 13 to 15 days after the start of your period.

An Alternate Method: If you chart your BBT everyday for two to three months, you will begin to see a pattern emerge – one that allows you to "predict" when the drop in temperature is going to occur. With this information you and your partner can begin to make love every day, beginning three to five days before you expect the temperature drop.

You should continue making love until your temperature rises again. Because sperm can live in a woman's body for up to five days, making love before ovulation means there will be plenty of sperm ready and waiting in your fallopian tube the minute your egg "arrives.

SOME EXTRA BBT SUCCESS TIPS

1. ESTABLISH A BBT SCHEDULE

As easy as the BBT method is to use, it's important to note that other factors beside ovulation can alter body temperature. A lack of sleep, for example, as well as stress, diet, even a slight cold or virus can all force changes in your BBT. For this reason you should begin to chart your BBT at least two to three months prior to when you want to get pregnant and again, look for the pattern to emerge.

2. BE TIMELY!

To get the most reliable BBT readings possible – and to predict accurately when ovulation is about to occur – take your temperature at the same time every day. The best time is first thing in the morning, before getting out of bed, eating, drinking or smoking. This will help ensure it is your true BBT – and that in turn will make it easier to predict ovulation.

3. USE A BBT THERMOMETER

While it's not critical that you use a specialized BBT thermometer, doing so can help ensure a more accurate temperature reading. Why? A basal body thermometer is more sensitive than a regular fever thermometer, so it is capable of alerting you to small changes in your temperature that might otherwise go unnoticed.

Indeed, while some women see an obvious change in temperature right before ovulation – one-half to one degree drop – for some the change can be more subtle, and might easily go unregistered on a regular thermometer. While a good BBT thermometer can cost a bit more, if you shop around you should be able to get one at a reasonable price – and I believe it's well worth a few extra dollars.

4. WRITE IT DOWN!

While you might think it's simple to remember temperature changes – and that it's easy to note when the drop occurs – still, it's very helpful to keep a written daily record. Moreover, remember that part of your goal should be to establish a temperature *pattern*, which is far easier to see when you are looking at a written chart. While you certainly can keep track of your temperature in any notebook, most of my patients found it much easier to use a pre-made BBT chart – like the one pictured in this chapter. As you can see the chart not only makes it easy to record numbers, but when you "connect the dots" it also gives you an excellent graphic interpretation of when your body temperature changes. A side-by-side comparison of your monthly charts can also make it super easy to track ovulation and predict when the time is right to make love. You can get a free BBT blank chart which you can download and print out by visiting GettingPregnantNow.org or GreenFertility.com

---

Q: Lots of times my temperature can go as high as 101 degrees right before I ovulate and stays up for a few days. Is this normal?

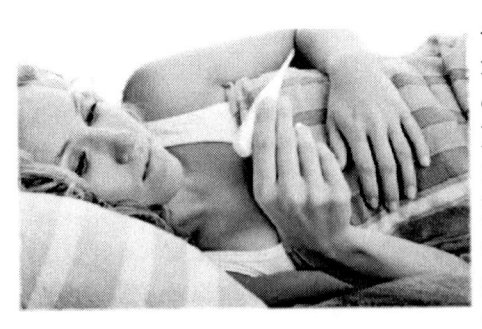

A: No, it is not normal to run a fever around the time of ovulation unless you have a cold or flu. If your temperature is rising this high right before every ovulation then you need to speak to your doctor. It's possible you may have a cyst on your ovary or a V zone infection.

Ovulation Prediction Method # 2: Listen To Your Body

In addition to temperature changes, there is another way your body lets you know that ovulation is approaching. And it's through changes in your cervical mucous and in the shape of your cervix. While this may sound like signs only your doctor could recognize, it's actually quite easy for you to determine on your own.

What can make it even easier is to do your first "cervical check up" as soon as your menstrual cycle ends. Because this is a time when we know for certain you cannot get pregnant, it will allow you to establish an important "base line" reading. Then, later on in your cycle you can compare changes to this baseline. Ultimately this makes it easier to recognize when your most fertile time is approaching.

So, *what are* you looking for ?

Changes in both the look and feel of your cervical mucous and the shape and feel of your cervix. And doing so takes just three easy steps.

1. Begin by washing your hands thoroughly with soap and warm water.

2. Separate the outside lips of your vulva and gently insert your finger into your vagina. You should be able to feel your cervical mucous on contact.

3. Insert your finger just a little farther in, until you feel resistance. This is your cervix.

Now that you know where to look, use the following guide to help you find the specific information you need to help determine your ovulation status.

Remember, the timing of every woman's cycle is slightly different, so if these events don't happen exactly the same for you, not to worry ! The most important thing is to keep track of the changes.

Stage One: As A Menstrual Cycle Ends

Mucous: At the end of your cycle, your vagina should feel somewhat dry – in fact, for some of you it may feel so dry that you don't feel any mucous at all!

Corresponding Cervical Changes: During and right after menstruation your cervix will be in a low position. It will be easy to touch, and it will feel firm and have a somewhat pointy shape. You should have no problems locating or feeling it.

Stage Two: One-Third Into A New Cycle

Mucous: About a third of the way into a new cycle – about the 9th or 10th day after your last period ended, your mucous will take on a creamy wet look and feel. It will seem somewhat thicker than before – and should be abundant.

Corresponding Cervical Changes: Your cervix may feel as if it's "receding" a bit – pulling up inside your body, which, in fact, is the case. You may have to reach a little deeper inside to touch it, but when you do it will still feel somewhat firm.

Stage Three: Mid-Cycle, Approaching Ovulation

Mucous: If your cycle is on a 28 days schedule , somewhere between days 12 and 14 your mucous will start to feel very thin and slippery and have a somewhat "stretchy" consistency. By the time you actually reach ovulation, your mucous will resemble raw egg white – it will be almost translucent, and have a runny look and feel. This occurs to ease the transport of sperm through your vaginal canal and into your fallopian tube.

Corresponding Cervical Changes: As your body responds to an increase in estrogen, your cervix pulls up slightly, and rotates forward, making it easier for your partner's sperm to swim in and reach your egg. At the same time, however, it makes it a little more difficult for you to touch your cervix – which is actually a sign that ovulation is approaching. If you do feel it, you'll notice that it seems softer to the touch and somewhat wetter. This is because at this point in your cycle your mucous is very abundant, creating a soft "wet" feeling inside.

STAGE FOUR: AFTER OVULATION OCCURS

Mucous: Unless fertilization occurs, within hours after you ovulate, your estrogen levels begin to drop, and your mucous supply begins to dwindle. Within 24 to 36 hours after ovulation, your mucous production takes a sharp decline. Whatever is left becomes extremely thick and sticky, with an almost glue-like consistency. Many women have reported it looks and feels somewhat like rubber cement! Generally speaking, your mucous remains this way for two to three days, after which time it can become so dry you will barely feel it.

Corresponding Cervical Changes: As your mucous is drying, your cervix responds by dropping back down, once again making it easier to touch. It will also feel harder and firmer again, much like it did at the start of your cycle. This is caused by a drop in estrogen levels.

TO GET PREGNANT FAST: Using your mucous production and cervical changes as a guide, **the easiest way to insure a quick pregnancy is to begin making love at *Stage Two* when your mucous is creamy and wet - starting three to four days before ovulation.** Remember, your partner's sperm can live in your body for up to five days, so starting early will insure that you won't miss the chance to have sperm ready and waiting when ovulation does occur.

To ensure your chances even more, continue being intimate with your partner until you see a noticeable decline in mucous production. This, of course, signals that ovulation has occurred, meaning your fertile window for this cycle has ended.

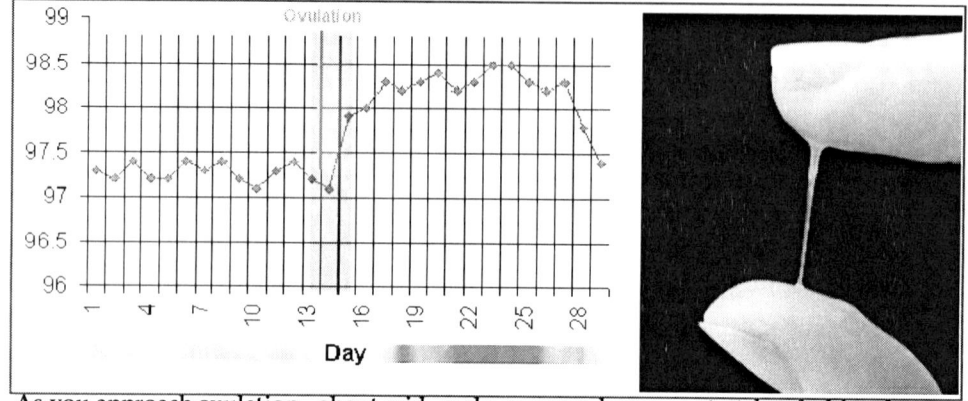

As you approach ovulation - about mid-cycle, mucous becomes stretchy, & thin, almost the consistency of raw egg white.

Q: *I've heard that Robitussin Cough medicine helps you get pregnant. Is this true?*

A: One very common cause of infertility is mucous that does not become thin enough at the time of ovulation. When this is the case, sperm can get "stuck" midstream and not be able to swim fast enough to reach the egg. So, taking steps to thin the mucous will help sperm move more freely and reach the egg faster and easier.

One of the best ways to thin mucous is by taking a cough medicine containing the ingredient guaifenesin . Much the way it thins the mucous in your lungs when you have a congestion it will also thin the mucous in your reproductive system.

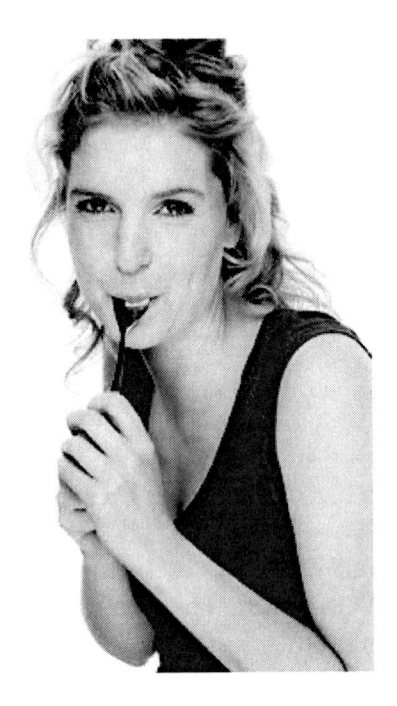

Be certain however the cough medicine contains only guaifenesin – such as **Robitussin For Chest Congestion.** If the cough medicine also contains the cough suppressant dextromethorphan *don't use it.* There are some reports this ingredient may interfere with a healthy conception.

Sex, Desire, & Fertility

Did you know that for many women the "sexiest" time of the of month is just before ovulation? It's true!

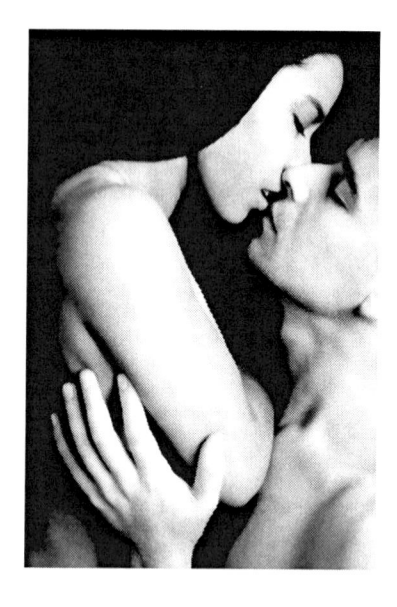

That's because this is the time when cervical mucus is most abundant - which in turn makes intercourse feel much more pleasurable and even exciting.

Not coincidentally, studies show that men find women more attractive during the time when they are ovulating.

Researchers believe this is because the increase in female hormonal activity gives off a subtle scent usually only perceived by men – and it helps increase their libido, and their desire for sex.

All of this is just Mother Nature's way of bringing men and women together – and increasing their attractiveness to each other – in order to make a baby, and keep the world going round!

Ovulation Prediction Method # 3: Ovulation Predictor Kits

If you're like most of my patients, then you probably associate the hormones estrogen and progesterone with getting pregnant. And indeed, as the main hormones produced in your reproductive system, they are indeed important to the entire fertility process.

But that said, as you read earlier, both estrogen and progesterone don't really begin to play their respective roles until well after two other hormones are in full swing. They are, FSH (short for follicle stimulating hormone) and LH (short for luteinizing hormone). Both are secreted by your brain, and without them your eggs would not grow and develop and ovulation could not take place.

Let me also remind you that FSH jump starts the baby-making process by sending a chemical message to your ovaries to start the process that turns egg follicles into actual eggs. As one of those follicles reaches maturity, estrogen levels peak, which in turn tells your brain it's time to release LH, the hormone which prompts ovulation. In fact, normally within 24 hours after the surge of LH, your egg will pop from its shell and swim into your fallopian tube where it can meet your partner's sperm.

So how can this information help you get pregnant faster? That's where ovulation predictor kits can help! Once your LH surges, it's quickly processed by your body, causing the natural chemical residues to be discharged into your urine. And this, in fact, is the basis of how ovulation predictor kits work. Indeed, all kits consist of test strips chemically treated to register the presence of LH in the urine – usually by turning a specific color when the hormone is present.

To Get Pregnant Fast:
By urinating on the test strips once daily, beginning around the 9th day of your cycle, you can watch for your LH surge color change. Once you see it, you know ovulation is imminent , and will usually occur within 24 hours or less. So, you should begin making love as soon as the test strip indicates the presence of LH. Continue making love any time the mood strikes you, for up to 48 hours afterwards.

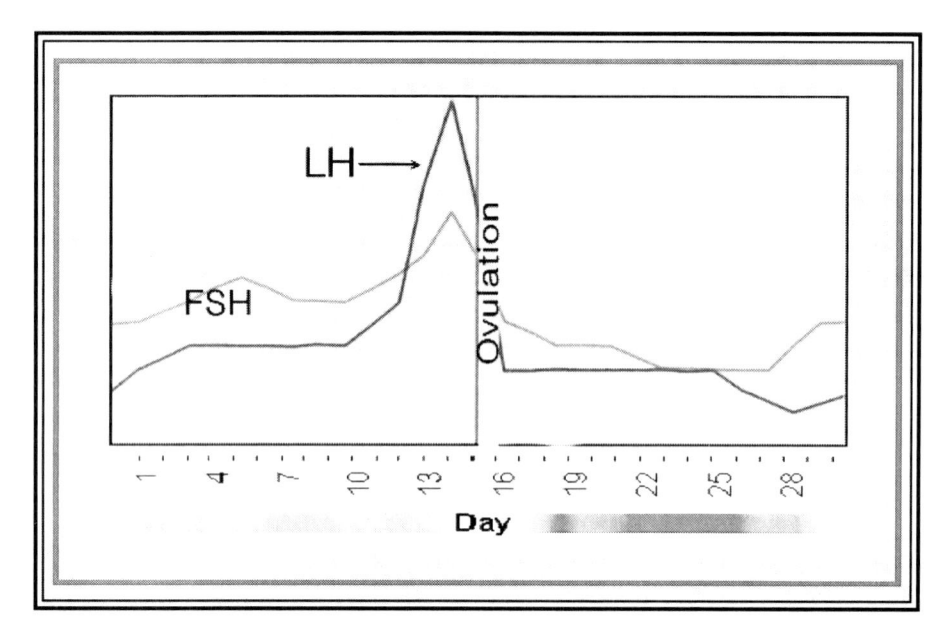

*An ovulation prediction kit can help you to know when your
LH surges - which means you are about to ovulate!*

To Dramatically Increase Your Success: Begin using the ovulation prediction kit two to three months prior to when you want to get pregnant . Using the blank chart from the Basal Body Temperature or BBT guide, indicate the start of your cycle, when you start testing, and when the LH surge appears on your test strip. Do this every month for two or three months, after which time you will see a pattern start to emerge indicating when you are the most fertile. This is the time frame in which pregnancy can occur.

The Month You Want To Conceive: Begin making love three to five days prior to when you expect ovulation to occur. Use the test strip during this time, and continue being intimate with your partner as long as it shows ovulation is approaching. This will help ensure there is sperm ready and waiting when ovulation does occur.

If you use an ovulation predictor kit in conjunction with either your BBT or your body signs, then your chances of getting pregnant will increase even more.

Ovulation Prediction Method # 4:
The Saliva Test

One of the newer – and some say more reliable – ways to predict not only ovulation, but a variety of hormonal activity linked to conception, is through the analysis of saliva. How is this possible?

Research shows that many of the hormonal changes that occur just prior to ovulation yield corresponding changes in saliva! And while tracking those changes may seem difficult or even impossible, the method is actually quite simple and the test kits are quick and easy to use.

What makes the test possible: When saliva dries, the liquid portion crystallizes into various patterns. While you can't see them with the naked eye, much like snowflakes, there is a pattern - and it changes in response to various hormones, particularly estrogen.

In fact, studies show that when estrogen rises, the liquid crystals in your saliva take on a very distinct and identifiable pattern – one that very much resembles a fern. In fact, the pattern looks so much like a fern that the activity leading up to ovulation is known as "ferning."

So, how can you can you make use of this information? Since you can't see the crystal changes with your naked eye, simply looking at your saliva won't give you any clues. What can help is viewing your saliva under a microscope – and this is where the new salvia testing kits can help. Each kit comes with an inexpensive but powerful portable microscope with a lens that is specifically designed to not just magnify but actually enhance and define the crystallization process. This enables you to watch for and identify the changes throughout each menstrual cycle.

How The Saliva Test Works

You begin by placing a drop of saliva on a glass slide (included with the test kit), and letting it dry – which should happen in ten minutes or less. You then place the hand held microscope over the glass slide (it resembles the size and shape of a lipstick tube so it's super easy to handle) and you view the crystallized saliva patterns.

If you begin viewing your saliva at the start of your cycle, and you continue to view it every day, somewhere around the 9th day you will see the fern pattern begins to take shape. This is an indication that ovulation is three to five days away.

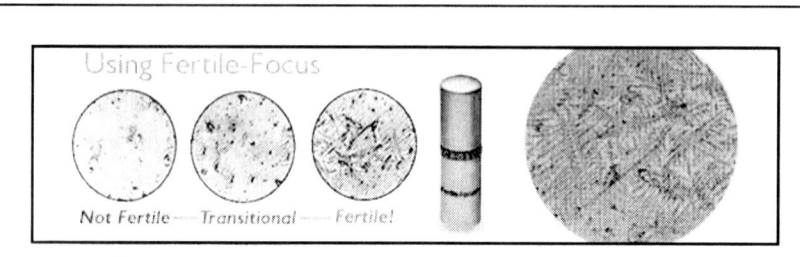

Fertile Focus is one of several new fertility saliva tests. It's easy to see the changes - and know your fertile time!

TO GET PREGNANT FAST: Begin making love as soon as you notice a change in your saliva crystal pattern. While you should see the "fern" shape start to form beginning around day nine of your cycle, sometimes it isn't always so easy to identify. If this is the case, just look for any change in shape. Usually this will indicate the hormonal activity that signals ovulation time is near. You should continue making love daily for up to seven days after you see the change.

The Ova Cue: Saliva Testing PLUS!

If you want to take your ovulation prediction into the computer age, then the OvaCue is for you! This ingenious little hand-held computer uses a spoon-sized electronic sensor to "read" the hormonal changes in saliva. You simply place the sensor on your tongue for five seconds every morning, and OvaCue will automatically display your "fertility status" for that day.

But how reliable is the Ova-Cue? Independent studies published in over ten top medical journals have not only proven that OvaCue works, but that it is among the most effective ways available to predict ovulation up to a full seven days before it happens!

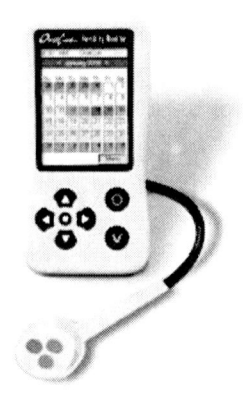

OVULATION PREDICTION METHOD # 5: FERTILITY MONITORS

In many respects, every type of ovulation prediction mentioned in this chapter thus far has been a type of "fertility monitor". In fact, any test which helps alert you to the time frame that just precedes ovulation is, in a sense, monitoring your fertility.

But that said, in recent years a bumper crop of new test kits known specifically as "fertility monitors" have burst on the scene. Although each one functions slightly differently, they all have one goal in common: To help determine when you are going to ovulate.

So, how is this different from other types of ovulation predictor kits or methods? Primarily the difference is in the time frame and the amount of advance notification these kits can provide. How do they do it? Much like ovulation predictor kits, fertility monitors rely on hormone levels found in urine. But where they differ is in the hormones that are measured.

Remember I told you earlier that an ovulation prediction kit measures LH – the hormone that is secreted 12 to 14 hours before ovulation occurs? Well a fertility monitor measures not only LH, but also estrogen levels leading up to the surge in LH – and that in turn gives you the opportunity to "predict" ovulation with advance notice of up to seven days.

In the *Clear-Blue Easy Fertility Monitor* – arguably the most popular brand sold today – testing is actually a two step process. It begins by entering personal information about your cycle into a hand held computerized monitoring device. Using that information as a guide the monitor alerts you to when it's time to begin step two, which is when the actual hormonal monitoring takes place. This step uses chemically sensitive strips designed to measure both estrogen and LH residues in urine. The result of each test strip reading is also entered into the monitoring device which then calculates three sub-cycles within each menstrual cycle.

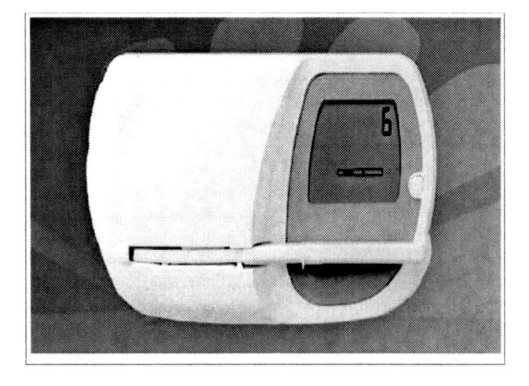

The three sub-cycles are as follows:

> **Low -** The chance of conception is very small – not quite impossible, but almost!
>
> **High -** There is an increased chance for conception, with this phase typically representing about five days prior to ovulation.
>
> **PEAK -** This is the time frame just before ovulation and represents the highest chance of immediate conception following intercourse.

TO GET PREGNANT FAST:
Begin making love when your fertility monitor indicates "high" conception status. Continue having regular intercourse, at least once a day, until you are 24 hours passed the time when your fertility monitor registers "peak" conception status.

OVULATION PREDICTION: SOME FINAL ADVICE

Certainly the "science " of ovulation prediction is not as precise as we would like it to be. In addition to the factors that can influence the tests themselves, many more factors can influence ovulation – to the point where month to month changes can make it difficult and frustrating for some women to predict their most fertile time.

If this turns out to be the case for you, don't stress over it – and don't worry. Use these methods to the best of your ability. If you pay attention to the signs I promise you will garner some important information that will help you get pregnant – or at least better understand the reasons why you are having difficulty.

Moreover when you combine the information you glean from ovulation prediction, with the additional hints and tips found in this chapter and throughout the book, all the pieces will fit together and the picture of your fertility will be much clearer and easier to see. For most of you this will be enough to help you get pregnant – and to do so faster and easier. For the few who may still have problems, understanding how your body functions will ultimately help you to work with your doctor in selecting the best treatment options.

MAKING LOVE AND MAKING BABIES: WHAT YOU MUST KNOW

When it comes to natural conception, one fact is undeniably clear: The act of making love is the optimum way of getting sperm to egg! But what many couples don't realize is that the physical chemistry involved in making love, even the mysterious mind-body interactions related to being "turned on" also play a role in how quickly and how easily you conceive. This is particularly true for women, since the hormonal balance necessary for conception initially takes place in the brain - which, not coincidentally just happens to be where the desire to make love is first felt by a woman.

In fact, unlike men, who usually require nothing more than physical stimulation to have an erection and an ejaculation of sperm, a woman's sexuality is much more complex, requiring both mental and physical stimulation in order for the intimate connection that stimulates desire is made. Not surprisingly all this activity is also related to her fertility.

Indeed studies show women who have a regular, satisfying sex life with intercourse at least once weekly, have more regular menstrual cycles and fewer ovulatory - related fertility problems than women who don't. Research also shows women often feel their sexiest – i.e., the most turned on to the thoughts of making love – in the middle of their menstrual cycle, a time when hormones are soaring, ovulation is nearing, and fertility is peaking.

Not coincidentally, studies also show men frequently find women more sexually attractive during the time they are ovulating – turned on by subtle smells that are released by her body when an egg is getting ready to be ovulated! But chemistry aside, it's not just hormonal activity that aligns our fertility with our sexual desires. For many couples it is also the emotional side of their relationship that can impact not just the quality of their lovemaking, but also their ability to get pregnant.

SEX, FERTILITY AND RELATIONSHIPS

Throughout more than three decades of counseling patients on getting pregnant I never ceased to be amazed at just how big a role a loving, caring, emotionally supportive relationship can play in a couples quest to have a baby.

In fact you may be surprised to learn that women who have not had a menstrual cycle for years can go into spontaneous ovulation when they fall in love! In fact, sometimes simply meeting " Mr. Right" can have enough of a biochemical impact to jump start hormone production and kick off ovulation in women who had met the clinical definition of "infertile" before.

Certainly there are instances where women get pregnant as a result of rape, or even at the hands of an abusive partner - situations where there is obviously no love or support involved. And there are also times when sperm and egg just meet – accidentally or not – and nothing will stand in the way of conception taking place.

But for the vast majority of couples – and in particular women – emotions *are* intimately entwined with reproductive biochemistry, often to the point where a couples love life and the quality of their relationship can physically impact their ability to get pregnant. How does this occur?

As you learned in an earlier chapter, your hypothalamus gland – located in your brain – is the command central for all hormonal activity linked to ovulation. But what you might not know is that your hypothalamus is also an extremely sensitive barometer of your emotional life. When you feel good, when you are happy, contented, and yes, sexually satisfied, your hypothalamus "knows" – and the subsequent production and release of the compounds that encourage fertility are released on a regular basis.

When, however, you are severely troubled, unhappy, depressed, anxious or even stressed, your hypothalamus gland perceives this as well and activity can dramatically slow down. Perhaps due to natural instincts which signal it's not the best time to have a baby, the activity of the hypothalamus gland decreases, sometimes to the point where there is a complete shutdown of the hormones necessary for egg production and release. The result is often "unexplained infertility".

And in fact if you have ever skipped a menstrual cycle or experienced periods that arrive early or late during times when you are stressed, you may have already experienced a temporary bout of "unexplained infertility." While most women bounce back quickly, some – particularly those who continue to endure emotional upset in their lives - do not, and the fertility problems linger. In this respect, one of the best things you and your partner can do to increase your chances for conception is to cultivate a warm, loving supportive relationship.

If there are some problems cropping up now and again – and I've never known a couple who does not have ups and downs in the course of a serious, intimate relationship - don't let resentments and anger build. Talk to each other and share your feelings, working together to create a loving, *safe* environment where each of you are encouraged to share your feelings in a non-judgmental and honest way. This is particularly important if you have been trying to conceive for a while and have not been successful.

Indeed, I have seen many couples who, rather than turn towards each other when things go wrong, instead turn away, blaming each other, as well as themselves when a pregnancy does not occur as planned. Too often partners can hold feelings of resentment and anger, as well as fears of inadequacy inside. This causes the negativity to fester and the resent to grow, ultimately causing it to be released on each other in various ways. Short tempers, harsh words, angry glances or those "deep sighs" of discontent all send subtle (or sometimes not so subtle) messages that emotionally, things are not quite right.

Sooner or later a wall of miscommunication is erected that can be so high, you can no longer see the love in each other's eyes – even when standing toe to toe. And this often means that getting pregnant becomes next to impossible.

At the same time, if you and your partner make a pact to keep the lines of communication open, if you learn to share with each other your doubts and fears, and to keep talking to each other about how you feel - even when you aren't feeling so great - I can promise that not only will your relationship grow stronger and healthier, so will your fertility!

HAVING SEX – MAKING BABIES : SOME PRACTICAL ADVICE

As I mentioned to you when this chapter started, for many couples simply making love when the mood strikes can be enough to insure a pregnancy. But what many couples who aren't getting pregnant might not know is that when it comes to conception, *how* you make love can be as important as *when you do it!*

Indeed, the operative function here is getting sperm to egg – so in many respects as long as intercourse occurs within five days prior to ovulation, there's a good possibility this is going to happen. That said, there are also a number of what I like to call "intimacy variables" – ways of making love that can definitely influence how quickly you get pregnant!

So what are the best ways to make love – and have a baby?

1. **MALE DOMINANT OR "MISSIONARY" POSITION** - While it may not be the most exciting way to make love, when it comes to getting pregnant, " man on top" has some definite advantages – not the least of which is a clear path to *shooting* sperm deep into the vagina. This position can be made even more effective if you place a pillow under your pelvic region, causing your vagina to be tilted slightly backwards. Again, this will facilitate the flow of sperm into your reproductive tract, and also help avoid "back ward flow " – a situation where sperm which may not be the best swimmers actually take a retrograde path out of the vagina.

2. **KNEE-TO-CHEST OR "REAR ENTRY" POSITION** - Using this technique you bring your knees very close to your chest while your partner slips inside your vagina from underneath. This position allows your partner to deposit his sperm much deeper, and much closer to your cervix, meaning more sperm are likely to make their way inside. This can be an especially good position if your partner has a marginally low or even very low sperm count. The increase in pregnancy success can be dramatic!

3. **LYING ON YOUR SIDE** - This position can very conducive to pregnancy if either you or your partner suffers from any back pain , or if either of you is overweight. By taking pressure off the nerves in the lower portion of your pelvis you may be able to relax more and that could influence how quickly and easily sperm will make their way to your fallopian tube.

INCREASING YOUR FERTILITY ODDS

The Worst Love Making Positions for Getting Pregnant:

- Sitting

- Standing

- Female dominant (woman on top)

- Bending over

All these positions slow down the transport of sperm and can make conception more difficult.

Q: *Is it easier to get pregnant if you make love in the morning ?*

A: Many couples have asked me whether or not the time of day they make love can influence the ease with which they conceive. And the answer is "No" – with some qualifying information. While there are no studies to show that the rate of pregnancy is influenced by the time of day a couple makes love, that could change if your partner has even a marginally low sperm count. Why? Generally speaking, a man's hormones are at their peak in the morning upon waking – one reason why many men are more sexually stimulated at this time then they are at night. But besides the issue of desire, there is also evidence that sperm count may be higher in the mornings as well. So, to maximize his sperm potential, making love after a good night's rest just might help you get pregnant faster!

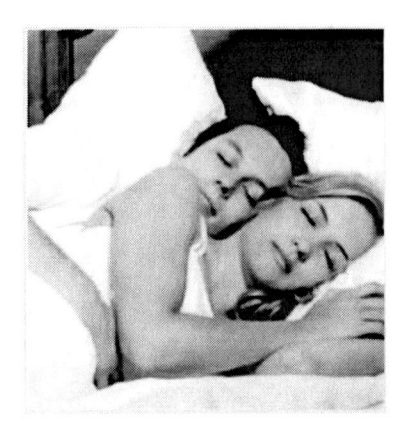

Sex Dos and Don'ts : How To Increase Your Fertility

In addition to the positions that increase your chance of getting pregnant there are also a few sexual "Dos and Don't's" that, for some couples might make a difference in how quickly they conceive. By no means am I saying that these practices are wrong or that they should not be enjoyed. But if you are trying to get pregnant it's important to understand the impact of certain activities as they relate to getting pregnant quick and easy.

Oral Sex and Fertility
If you and your partner regularly practice oral sex it should have no adverse affects of any kind on your fertility. However, that said, you might want to hold off on this practice during the specific love making sessions during which you are actively trying to conceive. Why? Bacteria normally found in saliva can sometimes have some degrading affects on sperm, reducing their ability to fertilize an egg. So if your saliva is present on your partner's penis just before he ejaculates or, more likely, if his saliva is present in your vagina just prior to him ejaculating inside your body, problems could result. So to increase your chances for getting pregnant, skip the oral sex while trying to make a baby!

Anal Sex and Fertility
When done properly, with mutual consent, anal sex can be highly erotic and pleasurable for both partners. However, this activity does come with an important precaution : A man must wash his penis with hot water and soap between acts of anal and vaginal penetration. This must be the case whether you are trying to conceive or not, since bacteria which live harmlessly in the rectum can turn deadly if they enter the vagina. This can not only cause a whopper of a reproductive tract infection in you, should conception occur when bacteria is present in your reproductive tract, any resulting conception may be negatively affected. The most common problem is early miscarriage.

Sex Toys and Fertility
I whole heartedly agree with the idea that getting pregnant should be fun! In fact, I often counsel couples to pay less attention to time tables and temperature charts and put some honest-to-goodness play time back into their love making as way to help encourage fertility. Indeed, the stress of "trying too hard", and the mind set

| Increasing Your Fertility Odds

that turns making love into "serious business" can definitely put a damper on the biochemistry that is necessary for conception.

At the same time, if sex toys, lubricants and other love making aids are a part of your fun there are just a few guidelines to follow. While many of these items are safe to use during baby-making sex, here are a few precautions you should not ignore.

LUBRICANTS

Many women find that using a lubricant intensifies sexual pleasure - and in this respect they may even subtly encourage fertility. However, your choice of lubricants is critical, since some can have a degrading affect on sperm – and some may even kill sperm on contact!

What to avoid: Oil based lubricants such as petroleum jelly or massage oils, both of which can upset the natural acid balance inside your vagina, which in turn can destroy sperm. Moreover some oil-based lubricants can also slow sperm down, making it harder for them to swim and sometimes even block the passage to your egg. Just think of all the poor marine life affected by the Gulf oil spill of 2010 and you get an idea of how sperm reacts when smothered in a heavy lubricant!

Also be absolutely certain to avoid any lubricant containing non-noxyol 9. This is a spermicide developed to kill sperm and used as form of back up birth control. Since many lubricants automatically contain this ingredient be sure to check the label!

What to use: Water based lubricants or those suspended in a light gel formulation. Look for the words "Safe to Use With Condoms" on the package. If it won't break down the latex in a condom it's not likely to harm sperm.

VIBRATORS

Generally speaking a vibrator, in and of itself, is not going to harm your fertility. That said, it can harbor bacteria that can affect your ability to get pregnant. To make sure it doesn't, always wash your vibrator with soap and hot water before using - even if you washed it before you put it away. Taking this one step helps insure your fertility won't be affected.

HOT TUBS

Though not technically a sex aid many couples find a relaxing soak in a hot tub is a great prelude to sex – and it really can work! In terms of your fertility however, it may not be worth the price. First, the high temperatures of the water can cause some immediate harm, affecting not just your egg, but possibly your ability to ovulate. While the affect on sperm is not immediate, as you will learn later in this book, anything that raises the temperature of the testicles by even a few degrees can harm sperm production. While this won't affect the sperm he about to ejaculate (it's made weeks in advance) if you are accustomed to soaking in a hot tub on a regular basis, eventually his sperm will be affected. So while you are trying to get pregnant – no hot tubs!

DOUCHING & YOUR FERTILITY

While many patients always report feeling "cleaner" after douching, this is not a practice I routinely recommend. The reason? First, your vagina is self-cleaning – meaning that normal regular secretions help keep the interior clean with a system of natural hygiene.

More importantly, there is good evidence to show that douching can dampen your fertility. How? Much like the skin on the outside of your body, the cells lining your vagina have a certain pH or acid balance. Normally, that should be between 4.5 and 5.0. – which, not coincidentally is also the acid balance that sperm just love!

Douching, however, changes that acid balance, causing your vagina to become either too acid or too alkaline – and either extreme can impact sperm motility and even survival. Unless your doctor diagnoses an abnormal vaginal pH – in which case a douche may be recommended to correct the problem – you should never use any douching product on your own.

In fact, you should not only avoid douching before intercourse, but if you are trying to get pregnant, you should avoid douching directly following intercourse. Why? Sometimes sperm can be a bit slow and linger for a while in the upper portion of your vagina before heading to your uterus. Douching drenches and drowns these sperm – which means fewer are available for conception. And that, in turn, cuts your chances of getting pregnant at that particular moment. If your partner has even a marginally low sperm count, or if his sperm are poor swimmers, douching after intercourse can keep pregnancy from occurring.

Finally, be aware that any time you douche you increase the risk of developing a reproductive tract infection- one that may ultimately steal your fertility! How? If there is an infection present in your vagina, or if there is any bacteria lingering on the outside of your vaginal "lips" (called the labia) douching can push those germs deeper into your reproductive tract, resulting in a much more serious pelvic inflammatory infection and an increased risk of ectopic pregnancy – a condition whereby a fertilized egg gets stuck inside the fallopian tube causing life threatening risks to the mother.

> If you have a vaginal odor that is really bothersome, don't try to "douche" it away. Instead, see your doctor right away. An V zone odor is often the sign of an infection that could interfere with your fertility. Treatment is fast & easy so don't wait!

If you do happen to smell an odor "down there" that doesn't seem right, often it can be the result of bacteria on the outside "lips" of your vagina, occasionally even from urine which comes in contact with this area. When this is the case, washing the outside of your "V" zone with soap and warm water will usually take care of the problem. If it doesn't, or if the odors persist and/or are extremely unpleasant, or if you develop an abnormal or odorous discharge following intercourse – or any time – this may be a sign of a infection requiring antibiotics, so be sure to see your doctor.

Ultimately , if you find you must douche, a natural solution is best.

To reduce vaginal acid: Use two tablespoons of baking soda in one quart of water.
To increase vaginal acid : Use two tablespoons of vinegar in one quart of water.

Under no circumstances should you ever use a commercial douche labeled "unsafe for use during pregnancy." Any douche that is harmful during pregnancy should never be used when trying to conceive.

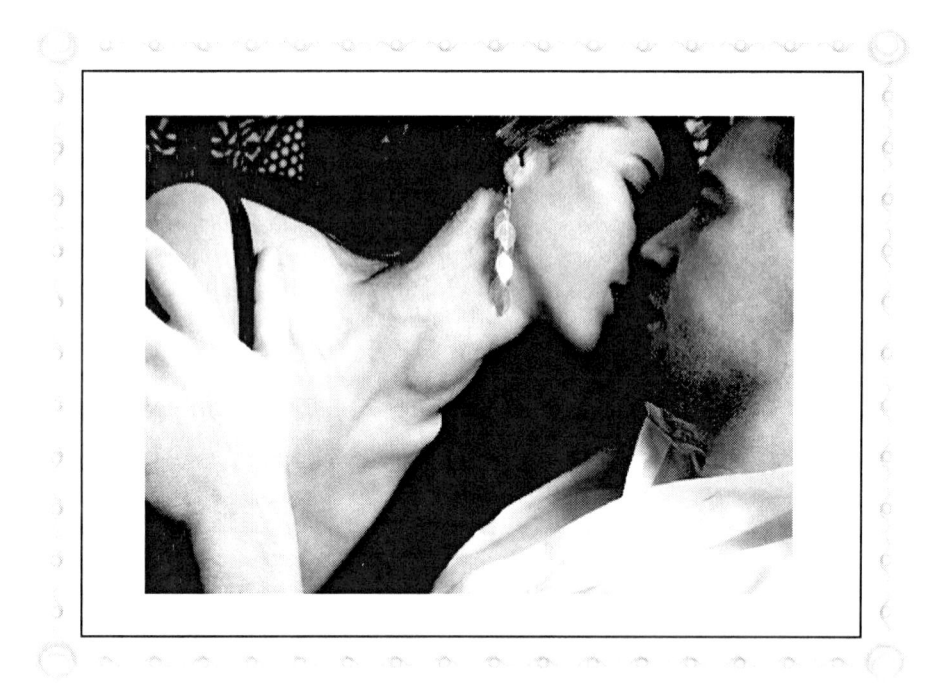

THE SCENT OF FERTILITY

Have you ever noticed that you like the way your partner smells? I don't mean his aftershave or cologne or shower gel – I mean the way *he* smells when he isn't wearing any fragrance of any kind. Or maybe you simply like being around him – and never even noticed that it's his personal fragrance which makes being with him feel so good.

Whether you have noticed his scent – or you haven't - the truth is that both you and your partner give off a subtle unique odor based on the production of what are known as "pheromones" – hormones that, among other things, are designed to give off silent signals that attract us to our mate. In fact, some research shows that using our sense of smell we unconsciously seek out someone with whom our DNA will be a perfect blend so that we *can* make healthy babies!

Moreover studies published in the journal *Nature* and other publications have shown that certain partner scents can encourage ovulation even in women who are having problems making eggs! Indeed, studies show that the scent of a man's perspiration when he is turned on can not only turn on a woman, but, over time, increase her fertility by helping to regulate her menstrual cycles. In reports presented to the American Chemical Society by the Monsell Chemical Senses Center in Philadelphia, it has been suggested that these natural odors influence the secretion of a variety of hormones linked to fertility.

In addition, as I mentioned briefly earlier, studies show many men can actually "smell" when a woman is ovulating, and feel more sexually attracted to her during this time. In studies conducted at Florida State University researchers found that men who smelled the T-shirts of women who were ovulating experienced a wild surge in testosterone – which as you probably know is the hormone responsible for a man's sex drive as well as his production of sperm.

So, is there a "scent of fertility"? No one can say for sure. But, if you do love the way your partner smells – and he likely feels the same about you – spending time with each other when these 'natural' scents prevail might end up helping you get pregnant faster!

> **Q:** *Are intimate feminine deodorants harmful to my fertility?*
>
> **A:** While there are no studies linking the chemicals in these products to infertility *directly*, there is lots of evidence to show that many of the chemicals and preservatives and even the fragrances used in these products can have endocrine disrupting properties. While occasional use won't harm you, regular and continued use might have some effects. If you can skip these products, do so and instead try baby powder made with cornstarch to absorb natural odors.

SEX AND THE SEX OF YOUR BABY

There is no question that virtually every couple trying to get pregnant would be equally happy to conceive a boy or a girl. This is particularly true if you've been struggling to get pregnant for quite some time.

Still, for some couples there remains an overwhelming desire to conceive either a boy or girl. This may be especially true if this is your second or third child, or perhaps the child of a second marriage.

Although there are clearly some proven high tech methods that many fertility clinics offer, there are also a few tried and true natural approaches that, at least anecdotally appear to work! Of course, simply by the rules of chance you are 50% likely to have a boy and 50% likely to have a girl – if it is your first pregnancy. So in this respect it's a bit harder to determine if these natural sex selection methods work. That said, the more times you give birth to children of the same sex – for example three boys in a row – the more likely you are to have another boy during the fourth try. And in these instances I have seen couples use these natural sex selection methods to change their gender pregnancy profile and finally have that little girl – or little boy – they wanted to make their family complete.

If you are interested in giving natural sex selection a try what follows are a few tips on what you can do. Remember, however, your goal should always be to have a healthy, happy baby and to love and cherish every child you conceive, regardless of their gender.

NATURAL GENDER SELECTION: WHAT YOU NEED TO KNOW

Every child that is conceived is a combination of the genetic material inside the mother's egg and the father's sperm. The genes which determine a baby's gender are known as the "x" and the "y" chromosomes. An embryo which carries two "x" chromosomes will produce a girl, while an embryo that carries an "x" and a "y" chromosome will produce a boy.

Because a woman's egg always contributes the "x" chromosome, gender determination is always the responsibility of the sperm. That's because there are sperm which carry the "x" chromosome and sperm which carry the "y". If your partner's sperm carrying the "x" chromosome fertilizes your egg, then you will give birth to a girl. Likewise if it's his "y" chromosome that reaches your egg first, then it will combine with your "x" chromosome and you will give birth to a boy.

And this is really the key to what natural gender selection is all about: If your partner can get either his "x" or his "y" chromosome to your egg first, then there's a good chance you can influence the gender of the child you will conceive.

So, how do you do that? According to at least some scientific research, how you have sex holds the key!

SEX AND YOUR BABY'S GENDER

Among the first theories linking sex to a baby's gender was developed by Dr. Landrum Shettles. The basis of his theory is that sperm which carries the "X" chromosome (the one that makes a girl) swim slower but are heartier and live longer than sperm which carry the "Y" chromosome, that makes a boy. Since we know that sperm can live inside a woman's reproductive tract for up to five days, Dr. Shettles theorized that manipulating the timing of when you have intercourse could control whether the "X" toting sperm or the "Y" toting sperm reaches your egg first.

But there's a bit more to this theory than just making love at the right time. You can further influence which sperm gets there first via specific love-making techniques, with certain ways of being intimate more likely to encourage either the "x" or the "y" sperm to get to your egg first.

And finally, there is some research to show that eating certain foods in the days just prior to attempting conception can also make a difference. The theory here is that gender is influenced, at least in part, by what scientists call the "ionic" factor. Simply put this is a type of biochemical "electric" charge that attracts his sperm to your egg. The theory is that by eating certain foods which contain high levels of minerals with these "ionic" charges – including calcium, magnesium, potassium and sodium - a woman can manipulate whether her egg attracts the "X" or the "Y" sperm.

In research on 49 French couples conducted by a European physician named Dr. Joseph Stolkowski, 39 of the couples were able to influence the gender of their baby by manipulating their diet.

So with all this information in mind, here is your formula for natural gender selection:

- **To make a girl:** Have sex three to five days before ovulation using shallow penetration in the "missionary" position. This allows sperm to be deposited at the mouth of your cervix – which favors the slower-moving female sperm. Try to avoid orgasm which will keep your vaginal environment acidic, which helps to kill off the "Y" sperm before they reach your fallopian tube, allowing the "X" sperm to fertilize your egg.

  To increase your chances further: Eat foods high in calcium and magnesium such as milk, cheese, nuts, beans and cereal.

- **To make a boy:** Have sex as close to ovulation as possible, using deep penetration and the "rear entry" position. This allows sperm to be deposited above the top of your cervix for fastest entry into your uterus. In addition, this area of your V zone is generally more alkaline, thus favoring the survival of male sperm. If you can achieve orgasm, this helps foster an even more alkaline environment and further increase the likelihood a "Y" sperm will fertilize your egg.

  To increase your chances further: Eat foods rich in potassium and sodium such as meat, fish, vegetables, chocolate and salty snacks.

While there are only a few small studies to show that these methods work, there are undoubtedly tens of thousands of anecdotal stories from couples who say that they do. In my own practice I have seen all these methods work more times than would be allowed by chance. And following the publication of our best selling fertility book "Getting Pregnant: What You Need To Know Now" where I also discussed these and high tech ways of performing gender selection, we heard from thousands of couples who used these simple methods and succeeded!

That said, if you do decide to give it a try I want once again to remind you that first you should have fun, enjoy the sex and the baby making process and don't turn conception into a chore; and second, always remember that what is most important is conceiving and giving birth to a healthy, happy baby – regardless of their gender.

Some Final Advice:

If there is one thing I can tell you from decades of helping couples get pregnant, making love at the "right time" is certainly one important way to ensure you will not only conceive, but do so quickly! And for some lucky couples, "good timing" is the only factor necessary to get pregnant fast.

But increasingly, I've seen that this isn't the case – even for young men and women. Indeed, more and more I see couples who, no matter how exquisite their timing, just can't seem to get pregnant – even when tests show nothing medically is wrong.

So if you find yourself among this group, take heart: There is much you can do to boost your fertility so that making love at the "right time" *really does work*. And that is what you will find in the remainder of this book – simple, easy ways to encourage and boost your fertility with methods and advice that will have both an immediate and a long term impact on your ability to conceive. Together with the information from these first few chapters, I remain certain that you will not only get pregnant faster, but also have a healthier pregnancy, and even a healthier, smarter baby!

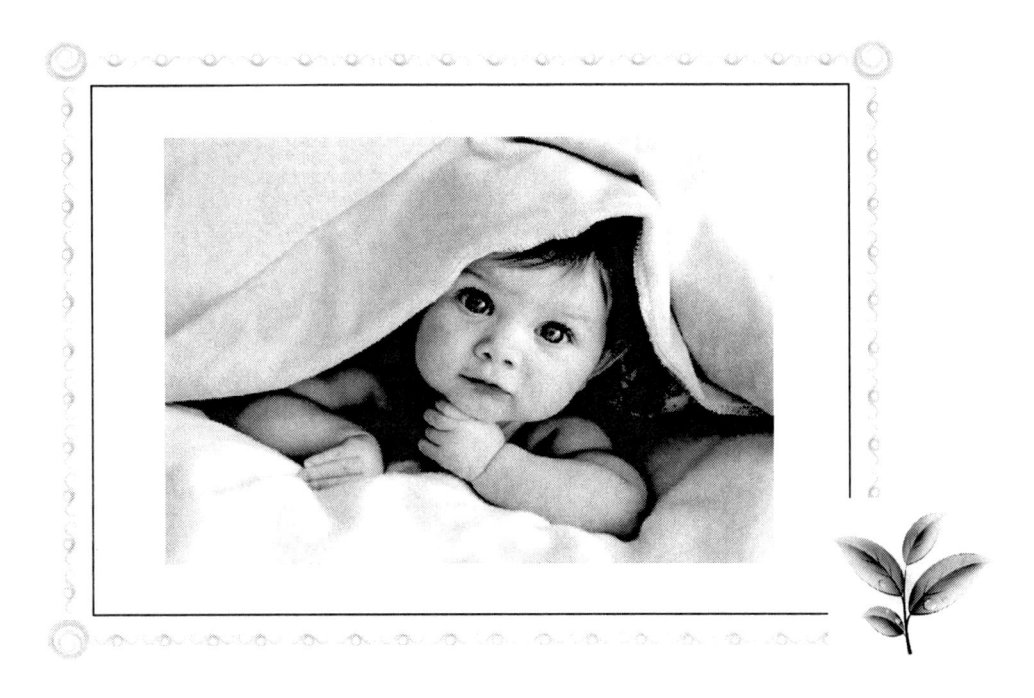

Chapter Four

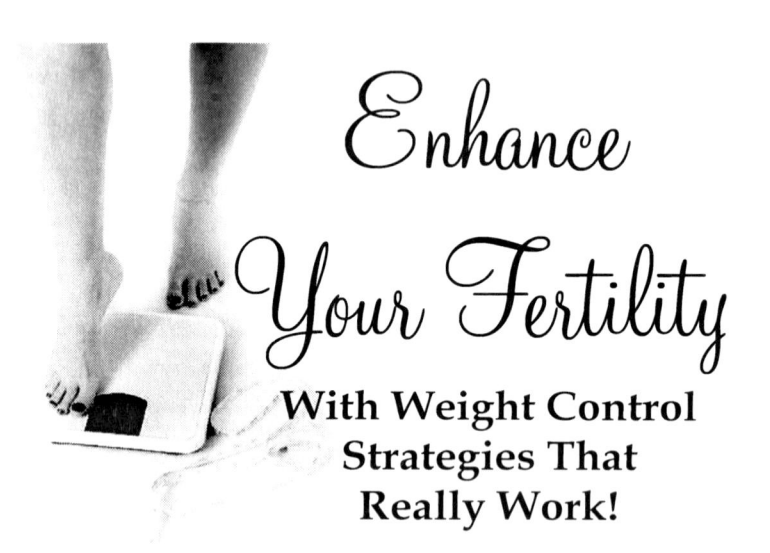

Enhance Your Fertility
With Weight Control Strategies That Really Work!

If I asked you to name which part of the pre-conception exam that nearly all my patients *dreaded,* do you think you'd guess? If you're thinking "stepping on the scale", then you are right!

Indeed, for many women the dreaded "weigh in" was in fact a bigger deal than even some complex testing procedures ... and most tried every reason you can think of to avoid it!

But the truth is, increasingly we are discovering that weight plays an enormous role in our health, affecting everything from our risk of heart disease, high blood pressure and stroke, to insulin, resistance, type 2 diabetes, and, of course, fertility.

Now if you're thinking that it's only excess weight that causes problems, guess again. Studies show that for many women being underweight can be just as harmful to fertility as being overweight - both can make getting pregnant more difficult than it has to be.

The good news is that often it only takes a small shift in weight to make a huge difference. According to the American Society of Reproductive Medicine, losing or gaining as little as 10% of your body weight (around 10 to 15 pounds) can kick start your fertility and put you on the fast track for getting pregnant!

Indeed, I have seen many patients turn their fertility odds completely around and get pregnant by simply losing or gaining as little as 10 pounds!

Moreover, it's not just *your* fertility that's affected by weight. Your partner's fertility is also affected by *his* weight. Indeed, studies show that everything from sperm production to motility (how fast those little guys swim to meet your egg) can suffer when a man is overweight. Later in my chapter on male fertility you'll learn about what happens and why.

But for right now I want to concentrate on you, filling you in on all the details you need to know to maximize *your* preconception weight so that you can get pregnant faster and easier!

HOW OVERWEIGHT AFFECTS FERTILITY

Although a link between weight and fertility has long been known, it wasn't until very recently that we began to understand what that link is really all about. Among the theories quickly proving true involves a specific and distinct association between fat cells – medically known as "adipocytes" - and hormone production, particularly estrogen, which you know is the basis for all egg production.

While most of the estrogen necessary for conception is manufactured by your ovaries, what you may not know is that fat cells *also produce estrogen*. So, the more fat cells you have, the more estrogen your body makes. This is one reason why overweight women often experience a later menopause and milder change-of-life symptoms – they simply don't experience the impact of estrogen deprivation as intensely as do thin women. At the same time however, it's also why being overweight is a risk factor for estrogen – related cancers, including breast and uterine cancer – and why thin women are so much less likely to get these diseases.

> *The more fat cells you have, the more estrogen your body produces ...and that can lead to a hormone imbalance that disrupts your menstrual cycle and ultimately contributes to infertility.*

But getting back to your fertility, when estrogen levels fall too much outside the norm – either too high or too low - it can create a hormone imbalance that ultimately throws your menstrual cycle into a tailspin. What happens?

As you read earlier, in order for your ovaries to begin manufacturing and releasing eggs, your brain must produce FSH (follicle stimulating hormone). What's key, however, is that the FSH signal gets "turned on" by estrogen. So, when estrogen levels are low, as they are at the conclusion of each month's menstrual cycle, those low levels signal the brain that it's time for a new cycle to begin. As such, FSH kicks in and starts the process rolling.

But what happens when, due to an increased number of fat cells, you have an excess of estrogen in your bloodstream? Your brain responds by thinking you don't need any FSH stimulation – so production of this hormone is turned off. When this occurs, your ovaries don't receive the "egg making" message at all – and suddenly the entire ovulation - reproductive cycle is disrupted.

In fact, many women who are overweight frequently report irregular cycles, which are usually caused, at least in part, by a lack of FSH stimulation. But it's not just irregular cycles that cause problems. In general, women who are overweight have a more difficult time getting pregnant – and he amount of extra weight you carry correlates to the amount of difficulty you can experience. Indeed, in one Dutch study of some 3,000 women doctors found for every extra unit of body mass or BMI (a measurement of total body fat) there is a 4% drop in the chance of getting pregnant. Writing in the journal *Human Reproduction*, the researchers suggest that the more overweight a woman is, the more likely she is to have problems conceiving.

INFLAMMATION: THE NEW LINK TO INFERTILITY

In addition to producing estrogen, each fat cell in your body is also a tiny chemical factory, producing and excreting several compounds capable of affecting your health. These include hormones and proteins such as tumor necrosis factor and interleukin, both of which are linked to cancer.

But perhaps most important, from a fertility standpoint, fat cells also appear to produce a series of inflammatory compounds - chemicals which work to increase inflammation body wide. How does this affect fertility?

First, inflammation of any kind worsens two of the most important fertility robbing conditions in young women – endometriosis and PCOS (poly cystic ovarian syndrome). If you have either of these conditions (which you'll learn more about later in this book) inflammation cannot only worsen your symptoms, but also make it much harder for you to get pregnant.

But what if you don't endometriosis or PCOS – can body fat still be harmful to your fertility? Indeed, it can.

We now know, for example, that even low levels of chronic inflammation can exert subtle but important influences on fertility.

In some instances the inflammation may impact ovulation; other times it can cause problems within the fallopian tubes which in turn may keep a fertilized egg from traveling to the uterus in the correct time frame necessary to ensure a healthy conception. For still other women inflammation within the uterus itself may compromise a healthy implantation, thus increasing their risk of early miscarriage.

As grim as this sounds, it's important to remember that losing even a few pounds means you will dramatically reduce the amount of fat cells able to produce these harmful chemicals – and yes, when it comes to getting pregnant, reducing levels of inflammation by even a small amount can make a huge difference!

BELLY FAT : WHY IT'S ESPECIALLY BAD FOR FERTILITY

Although fat cells located anywhere in the body can produce these harmful, inflammatory compounds, it is fat cells located in the stomach - creating what is medically known as "belly fat" - that may, in fact, do your fertility the most harm.

Indeed, when we use the term "belly fat" we don't just mean that outer layer of skin you can "pinch" between your fingers – the way you might do on your hips or your thighs. Because true belly fat lies deep within your abdomen in a structure known as the "omentum". Normally, this is a thin layer of fat meant to surround and cushion your internal organs. But what happens when the "omentum" begins to accumulate too many fat cells?

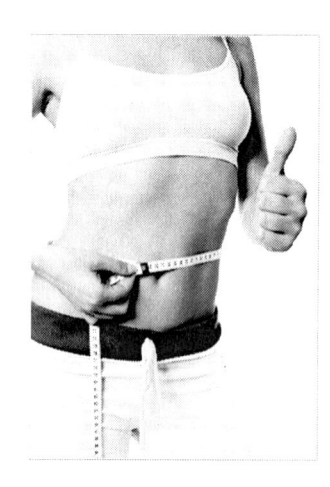

First, that fat presses against, and eventually entwines into, your internal organs, so nothing works the way it should. But more importantly, this fatty layer begins to produce an enormous amount of inflammatory compounds - much more so than fat found anywhere else in your body. In fact, while you may think that a little bit of excess fat on your hips and thighs is unattractive, in reality, history shows that carrying extra weight in this area is often associated with *increased* fertility!

Unfortunately the same cannot be said of belly fat. When loaded down with an excess of fat cells, the omentum can produce so many harmful compounds, it not only increases your risk of infertility, but also your risk of heart disease, high blood pressure, diabetes, even some cancers. This is true even if you are not considered overweight, but still carry extra pounds in the way of true "belly fat".

IS YOUR BELLY JUST PLUMP – OR DANGEROUSLY FAT:

Most women – particularly those who have given birth to a child in the past - have that all-too-familiar "pooch" characterized by a little bit of a chubby belly that may even have a "jiggly" look and feel. While this may make it difficult to wear the bikini of your dreams, generally speaking, this is probably not true "belly fat" - but instead a little bit of outer fat mixed with some loose skin.

THE BLOOD TEST THAT MEASURES PREGNANCY POTENTIAL

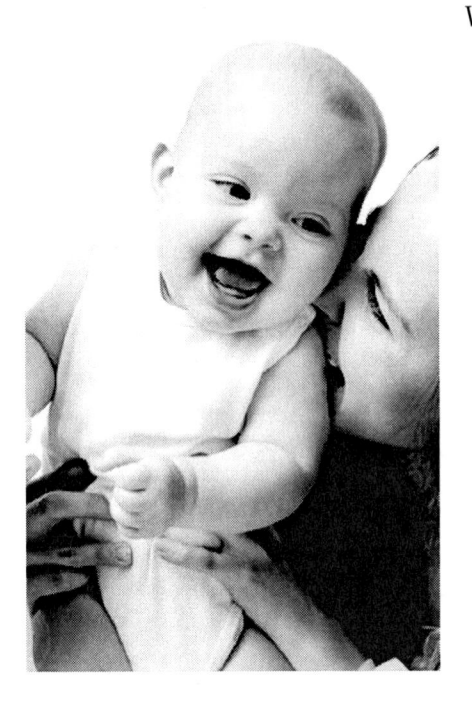

While being overweight automatically increases your risk of inflammatory compounds, just how much your body is being affected can now be measured via a simple blood test that checks for levels of a compound known as CRP – short for C-reactive protein.

This blood protein rises in relation to how much inflammation is present in your body – and generally speaking, the more overweight you are, the higher your level of CRP.

Although inflammation can be caused by any number of factors, studies conducted at the University of Texas MD Anderson Cancer Center found that compounds produced by fat cells are powerful enough to cause a spike in CRP.

If in fact, you are overweight and having problems getting pregnant, talk to your doctor about a CRP blood test. If levels are high – indicating an increased level of inflammation in the body - then you can be fairly sure that your weight may be harming your fertility.

One way to know for certain, however, is to check your BMI or body mass index. This is a type of calculation that uses your weight and height to determine what the healthiest level of body fat should be. (See the BMI Calculator on the facing page). For most women, a BMI of 25 is considered *overweight* while a BMI of 30 or more is considered *obese*. When either of these conditions exist it's very likely there is at least some "belly fat" involved.

But another way to tell if you are harboring dangerous belly fat is simply to look in the mirror and check your shape. If see an "apple" - a rounded shape through the middle, with little or no definition to your waist, usually paired with thinner legs and arms - then it's highly likely you do have enough belly fat to interfere with your fertility, even if you are only a bit overweight.

If you are pear shaped - holding most of your weight in your thighs and rump – then you might also be holding significant belly fat as well. This is particularly true if your waist measurement is over 35 inches, or if your waist-to-hip ratio is less than 0.8.

In fact, even if you are of normal weight, but there is less than 8 inches of difference between your hips and your waist then you may also be harboring some of this dangerous belly fat.

The good news: Any program that helps you to cut calories and lose overall body fat will also help you to lose dangerous belly fat!

USING BODY MASS INDEX
TO CHART YOUR FERTILITY

Body Mass Index or BMI is way of using a person's height and weight to calculate their level of body fat.

While a BMI calculation does not measure body fat directly, research shows the results correlate with those tests that do – such as underwater weighing, or a type of special x-ray known as a Dual Energy X-ray Absorptiometry or DEXA scan. Since however, both these tests can be expensive – and the BMI is free for anyone to use – it's easy to see why it's become one of the most popular forms of fat measurement.

ENHANCE YOUR FERTILITY WITH WEIGHT CONTROL

Today, most doctors use a BMI measurement as a screening tool to help identify your risk for certain weight-related diseases. As a fertility doctor I have also found the BMI helpful in identifying those women at risk for some specific weight - related fertility problems.

If you are actively trying to get pregnant, or if you're already having a problem conceiving, then you too can use your own personal BMI calculation to do the same.

The first step in the process is to find your BMI. While there is a mathematical formula you can use to calculate it out, I've gone ahead and done most of the work for you – and put the results in the table that follows.

To use it, all you need do is find your height (in inches) in the column to the left, then move your finger across the chart until you hit the weight (in pounds) that comes closest to what you weigh, rounding numbers up rather than down. Once your finger hits that number, follow that column straight up to the top column labeled BMI. This will be your approximate BMI or body mass index.

Example: If your height is 64" (5'4") and your weight is 143 pounds, your BMI would be approximately 25.

production of hormones necessary to build a strong uterine lining. Without that, your fertilized egg – or embryo –may fail to attach and grow. This is one reason why very thin women are at greater risk for early miscarriage.

BMI	19	20	21	22	23	24	25	26	27	28	29	30	35	40
							WEIGHT IN POUNDS							
5'0"	97	102	107	112	118	123	128	133	138	143	148	153	179	204
5'1"	100	106	111	116	122	127	132	137	143	148	153	158	185	211
5'2"	104	109	115	120	126	131	136	142	147	153	158	164	191	218
5'3"	107	113	118	124	130	135	141	146	152	158	163	169	197	225
5'4"	110	116	122	128	134	140	145	151	157	163	169	174	204	232
5'5"	114	120	126	132	138	144	150	156	162	168	174	180	210	240
5'6"	118	124	130	136	142	148	155	161	167	173	179	186	216	247
5'7"	121	127	134	140	146	153	159	166	172	178	185	191	223	255
5'8"	125	131	138	144	151	158	164	171	177	184	190	197	230	262
5'9"	128	135	142	149	155	162	169	176	182	189	196	203	236	270
5'10"	132	139	146	153	160	167	174	181	188	195	202	207	243	278
5'11"	136	143	150	157	165	172	179	186	193	200	208	215	250	286
6'0"	140	147	154	162	169	177	184	191	199	206	213	221	258	294
6'1"	144	151	159	166	174	182	189	197	204	212	219	227	265	302
			N O R M A L				O V E R W E I G H T					O B E S E		

HEIGHT (leftmost label)

USING YOUR BMI TO DETERMINE YOUR RISK OF FERTILITY PROBLEMS

Now that you know what your BMI is, it's time to use this information to access your weight-related fertility risks. To help you do that, all BMI results fall in to one of these 6 categories: Underweight; Normal Weight; Overweight; Obese 1; Obese 2, and Extremely Obese. Remember, however, these are just terms used to differentiate the different levels of risk, so don't let the "labels" upset you.

The first step in determining your risks is to use the chart below to determine in which of these categories your BMI measurement falls. Because, however, it's not just your level of body fat that is important – but where that fat is concentrated that also matters - the next step requires you to take one more measurement. Indeed, as you just read, body fat that is located in the belly region is particularly bad for your fertility, so I'm going to ask that you grab a tape measure and determine is your waist is greater than, equal to, or less than 35" (For men, by the way, the target measurement is 40").

TO DETERMINE YOUR WEIGHT RELATED FERTILITY RISK:

Using the chart to the right, find your BMI in the column on the left, then follow across that line to determine your level of risk. If your waist is 35" or less, stop at column number 3; if your waist is greater than 35", follow over to column 4.

Example: If your BMI is 26 and your waist is 33", your risk of a fertility problem is "increased". If your waist is 37" then your risk of fertility related problems is "high".

Definition of probability odds:

Increased Risk: 50% or more likely to have a problem getting pregnant.
High Risk: 50-75% likely to have a problem getting pregnant.
Very High Risk: 80% likely to have a problem getting pregnant.
Extremely High Risk: 90-100% likely to have a problem getting pregnant.

ENHANCE YOUR FERTILITY WITH WEIGHT CONTROL

Risk of Weight -Related Fertility Problems

BMI	Weight Category	Waist less than or equal to 35 "	Waist greater than 35"
18.5 or less	Underweight	Increased	N/A
18.5 - 24.9	Normal	***	N/A
25.0 - 29.9	Overweight	Increased	High
30.0-34.9	Obese	High	Very High
35.9 - 39.9	Obese	Very High	Very High
40.0 or greater	Extremely Obese	Extremely high	Extremely high

Q: My husband is convinced the only way to get rid of belly fat is a gazillion sit ups every day. I say you can get rid of belly fat just as well by running. Who's right?

A: The fact is, there is no such thing as "Spot reducing" - which means no single exercise is going to reduce fat in any one area of the body. The key to losing belly fat is the same as losing weight anywhere else - you have to take in fewer calories than you burn up. And when you do you will lose weight - with the area that carries the most fat cells usually the first to reduce in size. What exercises like sit ups can do is tone, tighten and build muscles in the stomach area and that can make your overall shape look better. Plus, the more lean muscle mass you have the more calories your body will burn and the easier it will be to control weight!

TOO SKINNY TO GET PREGNANT?

Once upon a time having a "model figure" meant you were curvy in "all the right places" - including your hips. Not coincidentally, these same curves also represented fertility - and they were something that made a woman very attractive to a man, both on a visual and hormonal level. Indeed, studies have often revealed that men are frequently attracted – on an unconscious hormonally driven level – to women that they view as "fertile". And part of that fertility picture is the classic "Goddess" curvy body.

Today, however, our definition of "model perfect" has changed. Indeed, in many areas of the world being extremely underweight is now considered the " ideal" body type – and one we have come to culturally worship and even idolize.

Unfortunately, however, this is a very dangerous ideal - dangerous not only for your overall health, but in particular for your fertility. Why? Simply put, you can be too skinny to get pregnant! Indeed, while we often associate weight-fertility problems with carrying too many pounds, the truth is, that when you don't weigh enough just as many fertility problems can occur!

In fact, doctors have long known that women who have almost no body fat – such as marathon runners or professional dancers - are frequently diagnosed with anovulation , a condition where no eggs are being made or ovulated. Certainly in my professional experience I have found this to be true time and again.

Indeed, many days my office was packed with models, athletes and dancers in a panic because their menstrual cycle had completely shut down - all due to their low weight. In fact, studies show complete hormonal shutdown can occur if your body fat dips just 10 to 15 percent below the normal 29% (a BMI of around 25). Sometimes, even a slight drop below normal to a body fat level of 22% (a BMI of 19 to 20), can disrupt hormonal production enough to make it more difficult to get pregnant. Depending on what degree to which this disruption occurs, any number of problems can result , including those that impact egg production and ovulation.

Moreover, even if ovulation does occur, being underweight can dampen the production of hormones necessary to build a strong uterine lining - one reason very thin women are at greater risk for early miscarriage.

The good news is that restoring your weight to a normal level is usually all you will need to to restore your fertility and get pregnant.

However, I caution you not to put off gaining back some weight for too long a time. Indeed, if you remain severely underweight for a significant period of time, it sends a signal to your brain that your body is unable to sustain and nourish a new life. And that in turn completely shuts down your reproductive brain chemistry, making it virtually impossible to get pregnant naturally. If left to go on long enough, your infertility problems may be irreversible.

BODY WEIGHT, HORMONES AND FERTILITY: THE BREAKTHROUGH DISCOVERY THAT CAN CHANGE YOUR LIFE!

While we have long known that being either overweight or underweight can have a detrimental impact on fertility , recent studies have begun to shed some light on exactly why. And that, in turn, has helped us to understand a little more about what we can do to prevent problems from occurring.

The basis of all this new research revolves around a relatively new hormone called "leptin". From the Greek word Leptos – which actually means "thin" - leptin is a protein hormone that produced by fat tissue.

In fact, you may have already heard about leptin (as well as another newly discovered hormone known as ghrelin) in relation to studies on weight loss. Here doctors learned fluctuations in both leptin and ghrelin can influence not only weight gain and loss, but also how well our metabolism works. And here is where the interesting link to fertility also came to light.

In studies conducted at both Brown University in Rhode Island and Harvard Medical School in Massachusetts doctors discovered that once leptin leaves your fat cells it travels through your blood stream to an area of your brain known as the hypothalamus. You may remember from an earlier chapter this is "hormone central" – the area of your brain that secretes chemicals that put the entire egg production and ovulation process in motion.

More specifically the researchers discovered that when leptin hits the hypothalamus, it acts like a switch, turning on a chemical chain reaction that stimulates your pituitary gland, then your thyroid. This in turn sends out a body-wide message to increase energy production necessary for a wide variety of bodily functions, including not only calorie burning, but also reproduction.

But what happens when body fat is too low? Not enough leptin is produced. And this in turn signals the hypothalamus that there is an energy crisis. Your hypothalamus responds with efforts to conserve energy, which it does by shutting down all "non-essential" body functions. One of the first of those functions to go is reproduction. Indeed, there is now research documenting that when leptin levels drop low enough, the brain fails to produce either FSH or LH – without which egg production and ovulation cannot occur.

And while this might seem as if only underweight women would be affected by a leptin snafu, the truth is, women who are overweight are affected as well. How?

When the brain is continually bombarded with an oversupply of leptin – as it is when we have too many fat cells - it becomes desensitized to its effects, and begins to act almost as if no leptin is being produced at all! This not only interferes with the chemical chain reaction necessary to burn calories, it also interferes with the chemical chain reaction necessary for reproduction.

The result : You gain even more weight, you produce even more leptin, and it becomes increasingly harder to get pregnant.

But there is some hope - and some help for the future of those battling leptin issues. Currently, the FDA has approved two drugs - 4-PBA and TUDCA are helping to increase the sensitivity of leptin receptors in the brain.

While it's still to early to know if, in fact, these drugs will be the answer for those with overweight women who are infertile, it's certainly an important advance worth watching.

But what's really exciting about all this new research is that it has given new credence to the idea that controlling your weight is really a major way to improve

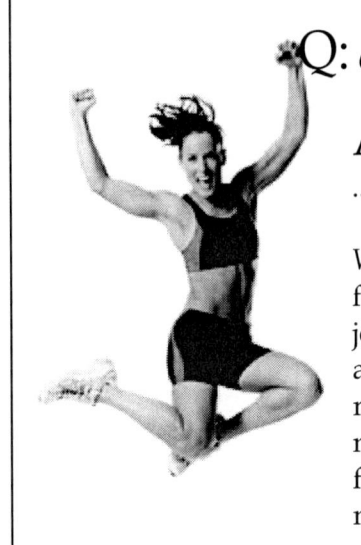

> **Q: Can exercise ever harm my fertility?**
>
> **A:** In general, exercise is great for fertility ...but there can too much of a good thing!
>
> When exercise causes your percentage of body fat to drop too low it can put your fertility in jeopardy. Moreover certain exercises can work against fertility by actually encouraging hormonal snafus that make it harder to get pregnant (see Chapter 5). But as long as your body fat is within normal limits, exercise can definitely boost your fertility!

your fertility profile since it appears as if leptin resistance responds favorably to even a small weight loss or weight gain – depending on your specific needs.

What we have also learned, is that reproductive hormones can be affected by the way in which you gain or lose weight, with any sudden changes up or down having negative effects. This means that any kind of binging or crash dieting, or any quick weight loss schemes are some of the worst things you can do to your fertility.

In fact, whenever weight loss or gain occurs too quickly it can not only throw off your leptin production, it can also directly impact production of hormones necessary for conception. Moreover, from a strictly nutritional standpoint if you do happen to get pregnant while crash dieting, it will dramatically compromise your baby's health and even increase your risk of miscarriage.

At the same time, if you take steps to alter your weight *slowly and sensibly* while keeping good nutrition at the forefront of your plan, your reproductive profile will slowly but surely come back into focus, in a healthful and productive way.

Not only will you be able to get pregnant more quickly and easily, but when you do, your baby will be healthier right from the start.

While I don't advocate any one specific diet to help you achieve your weight loss goals, I would like to offer you the following advice: Six simple steps to healthfully take control of your weight and your fertility, and help you get pregnant fast!

Remember, slow and steady wins the race - so set your goals and go for it in a sane and sensible way!

SIX SIMPLE STEPS FOR ACHIEVING OPTIMAL FERTILITY WEIGHT

1. COUNT CALORIES BY THE WEEK - NOT BY THE DAY!

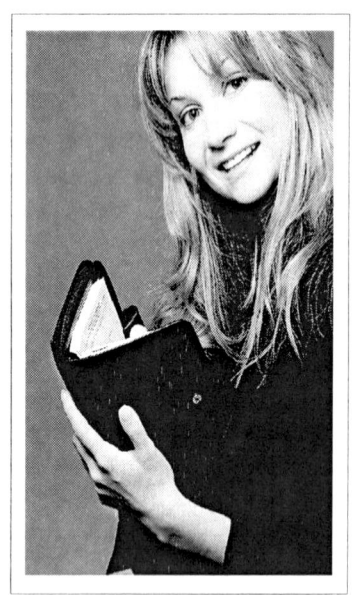

While counting calories is still one of the best ways to control your weight, I have always found that it's much more productive – not to mention easier – to set a weekly caloric goal rather than a daily one. The reason? First off, I've never known a patient to lose or gain weight based on what they ate in a single day! But more importantly, if you happen to eat more on a single day (maybe you're extra hungry or you've been to an event or out to dinner) you won't panic and feel you've "blown" your diet. Sometime within the following two days you simply cut back and eat less and it will all balance out.

By keeping a weekly calorie counting chart – and not a daily one – you'll also have the freedom to eat more of the foods you want when you want them - and worry less about going off your diet.

2. Discover the Magic of Volume Control

I know you've probably heard the term "portion control" before – but this isn't what I mean! I'm talking about the volume of food on your plate relative to its calorie count! Indeed, the one thing I never liked about the concept of "portion control" is that often you can eat a very little bit of food and still come away packing on the pounds. That's because when you eat foods that are calorie dense – such as high fat meals - a very small portion can contain a very big caloric load. So you don't get to eat very much before you have reached your limit.

Conversely, foods such as fruits and vegetables are just the opposite. Their calorie load is so "sparse" that you could fill up three plates and still have relatively few calories. So, you get to eat a lot without consuming a lot of calories.

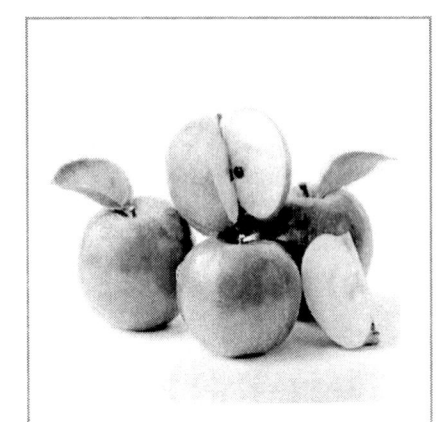

Fruits & Veggies are so low in calories you can eat a ton of them and still not gain weight!

Thus, the secret – or as I like to call it the "magic" - to volume control is to seek out foods that give you the biggest bang for your caloric buck. If you need to lose weight seek out foods that are low in calories – which means you can eat a lot of them, and still lose weight. If you need to gain weight concentrate on calorie-dense foods – meaning you can still eat the amount you are used to, but you'll get those extra pounds you need to get pregnant.

In my book " Eat, Love, Get Pregnant" you'll find over 200 delicious foods that can help you control your weight and increase your fertility at the same time !

3. GET MORE SLEEP

While most folks don't equate weight control with sleep, the truth is, they are intimately entwined! Of course one obvious reason is that when you are sleeping, you can't be eating – so sleeping more at night means less night time snacking! But far more important is the idea that when you are sleep deprived a series of chemical reactions occur that can make it much harder to control your appetite. In fact, I'll bet you've noticed that on the days when you don't get enough sleep you feel hungrier than usual - and usually eat more! By getting adequate sleep, however, you can keep hormone levels on an even keel. And that not only translates into better appetite control, but also better fertility!

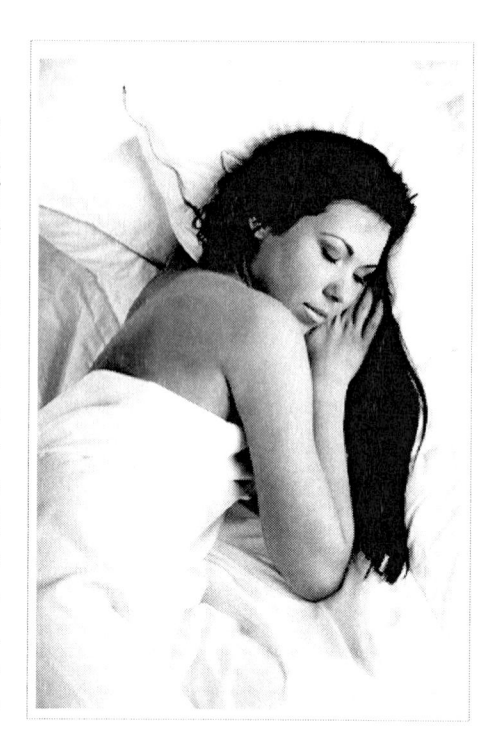

4. EAT MORE WHOLE GRAINS

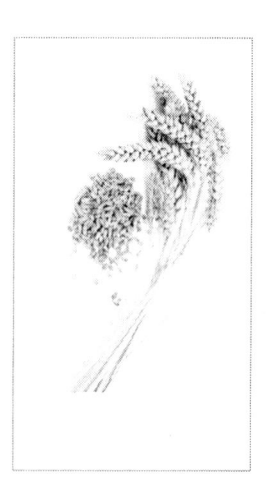

Whole wheat pasta, whole grain muffins, whole grain cereals – any snack or side dish which features a whole grain as the first or second ingredient is not only good for your heart health it's also a great way to control your hunger and feel fuller longer! Whole grains burn slowly – so blood sugar is stabilized. And that means you won't get "pangs" of hunger like you might get an hour or two after eating a piece of cake . Plus - you feel fuller longer!

ENHANCE YOUR FERTILITY WITH WEIGHT CONTROL

5. REDUCE SUGAR INTAKE

Not only will this help with weight control, it will also boost your fertility at the same time. How? First, foods that are high in sugar are loaded with "empty" calories. And by that I mean they may satisfy your appetite for the moment, but soon after you'll feel hungry again – and have an urge to eat even more. So the calories you indulged in are "empty" - because they don't satisfy you for long. But more importantly, there is now evidence to show that eating lots of sugary foods increases your risk of both insulin resistance and type 2 diabetes - two conditions which also interfere with fertility (You'll read more about how and why later in this book). So, by limiting your intake of sweets you'll not only feel better, you'll also have a much easier time controlling your appetite.

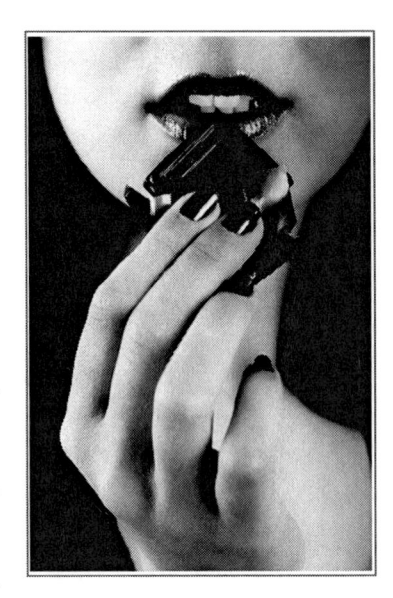

6. REDUCE STRESS

Have you ever noticed that when you're nervous or stressed you eat more? Well that's not just coincidence! Under stress your body churns out a number of hormones, at least some of which influence your appetite. If you were in real physical danger, the extra food would be quickly burned off as you "fight or flee" your stressors. But in the concrete jungle of our modern world, stresses are not a fleeting moment in time, but rather an ongoing state of mind. When this is the case our appetite is always being stimulated – so much so that we often feel hungry all the time, and get little satisfaction from what we do eat. By reducing stress we can keep a lid on some of those stress hormones that would otherwise be wreaking havoc with our appetite.

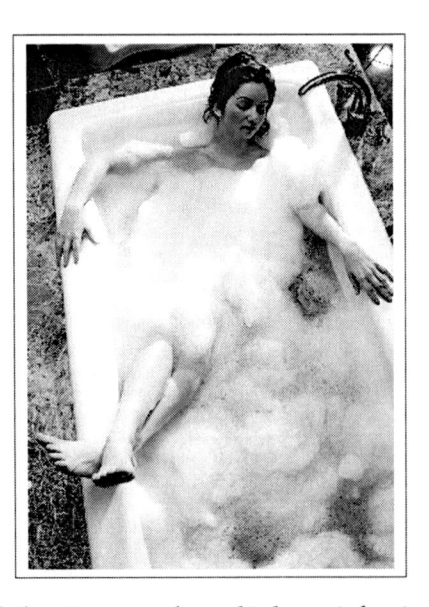

Chapter Five

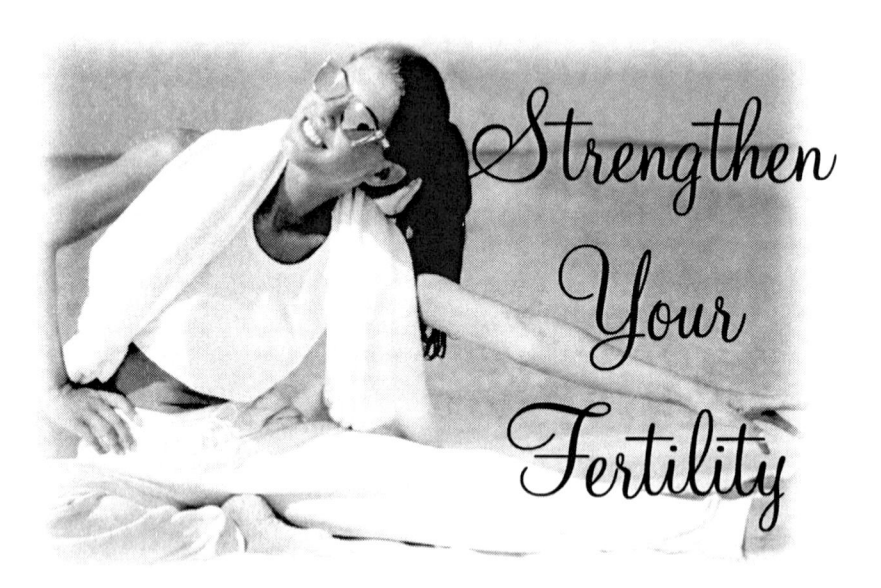

Strengthen Your Fertility

With A Proven Pre Conception Fitness Plan

There is no doubt in my mind that leading an active lifestyle – and getting regular exercise - is the number one way to improve your overall health. Indeed, over the past decade, and particularly within the last five years the amount of research proving the health benefits of regular exercise has been nothing short of astounding.

From prevention of heart disease, high blood pressure, obesity, even cancer – regular exercise is among the best forms of preventive medicine you can find. Andnowhere is this more true than when it comes to enhancing your fertility. In fact, while I have always believed that regular exercise was an important key to getting pregnant fast, I am happy to report that we now have the scientific evidence to show this is true.

At the same time, however, I have sometimes seen fertility problems actually occurring due to exercise. Indeed, when you work out too hard and too long, or when you engage in certain types of physical activity, there is no question that your fertility can suffer. Not only can it make getting pregnant much harder, in some instances it may even keep you from conceiving at all!

That said, you should not use this an excuse not to workout – or become fearful of exercising. The key, of course is to strike a balance – making sure you get enough of the right kind of exercise while cutting down the activities that make getting pregnant harder than it should be. And while I wish there was one general "fertility fitness prescription" I could write for everyone, the truth is that getting pregnant is a highly personalized experience. Your individual body chemistry along with your weight, your diet, your lifestyle, even your age, all figure into your fertility profile – and that means they also influence the kind of specific workouts that will help you get pregnant.

So, rather than try to give you a "one size fits all" fitness solution, I'd like to take a little time to help you understand how fitness affects fertility in general – and the role it can specifically play in your conception plans. I'm hopeful that you will then use what you learn to write your own personal " fertility fitness prescription" - one that will benefit you and your reproductive health the most!

HOW FITNESS AFFECTS FERTILITY: WHAT YOU NEED TO KNOW

As you just read in the previous chapter, body weight, and in particular Body Mass Index or your level of body fat, can have a tremendous influence on your ability to get pregnant. So, in this respect, at least one link between exercise and fertility is obvious: It can help you burn fat so that you can maintain the proper fertility weight.

This is particularly true if you have a tendency to gain weight easily, or perhaps if you are already overweight or even obese. When you exercise you burn calories – and the fewer calories your body has to work with, the more likely it is to burn fat. And, when you burn fat, you lose weight.

But more importantly, at least from a fertility standpoint, when you burn fat, you also help to reduce an estrogen overload in your body. Remember I told you how fat cells are like tiny chemical factories churning out a variety of compounds, including estrogen? As such, when you reduce the number of fat cells in your body, you also reduce the chemical compounds these fat cells produce – including excess hormones, as well as inflammatory chemicals, all of which increase your risk of infertility.

But what if you're already thin – and don't need to burn fat cells? When this is the case it's more about the level of exercise – and the type of activities you do - that counts most. While you may not need to burn fat, your body still requires a certain amount of physical motion every day in order for your reproductive chemistry to function properly.

As you read on you'll discover which activities to engage in – and which ones to avoid- when writing your "fitness prescription". But first, it's important that you learn a little something about your metabolism - the system that links together fitness and fertility.

UNDERSTANDING YOUR METABOLISM : HOW IT AFFECTS YOUR FERTILITY

Most of you are probably already familiar with the term metabolism - the biochemical "engine" governed by your thyroid gland, which, among other things, is responsible for how efficiently you burn calories.

Indeed, through the production of several hormones – including TRH (thyroid releasing hormone which comes from the hypothalamus gland) and TSH(thyroid stimulating hormone from your pituitary gland) - your thyroid gland helps control how quickly and how easily you not only burn calories, but also how efficiently your body uses energy.

When your thyroid gland is working perfectly, calories are burned efficiently and more than enough energy is produced for all your body functions, including reproduction. But all this changes the minute even a slight dip in thyroid function occurs.

Indeed, whether due to illness, diet, or any other number of factors, when the function of your thyroid gland begins to either slow down or speed up , your entire body chemistry – including your fertility – can suffer. What happens?

First, when your thyroid is working under par, you simply stop burning calories as efficiently. This not only causes you to feel sluggish and tired all the time, but it also can cause you to gain weight.

Conversely when your thyroid gland is working overtime, your metabolism runs "fast". This means you *over burn* calories - and that in turn may cause you to have trouble gaining or maintaining weight. Moreover, because you do burn through your calories so quickly, you can feel both jittery and nervous, followed by fatigue and a total lack of energy.

> Your thyroid gland is located in the middle of your neck. When your thyroid gland over produces or under produces hormones, your fertility can be temporarily affected.

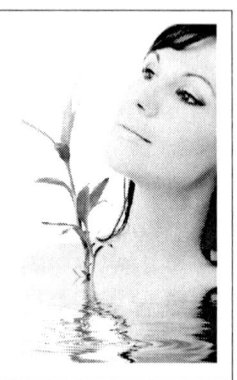

HOW YOUR THYROID AFFECTS YOUR FERTILITY

In addition to controlling your metabolism, your thyroid gland also plays a role in your fertility. And when it's running either too fast or particularly when it is running slow, getting pregnant can be much more difficult. Why?

First, if your thyroid is overactive and your metabolism is running too high, your body simply does not use estrogen as efficiently as it should. This can sometimes result in an insufficient uterine lining – meaning, if you do get pregnant you are at greater risk for miscarriage.

However, when it comes to getting pregnant it has been my experience that a far greater number of problems occur when your metabolism runs too slow – and your thyroid is under active. What happens when this occurs?

As you read earlier, two glands within your brain – the hypothalamus and the pituitary- are responsible for sending the chemical signal to your ovaries to begin producing, and eventually ovulating, eggs. But to do this these two areas of the brain must also interact with your thyroid. Why? It's your thyroid that tells your brain that there is enough energy in your body to support the feeding and nourishing of a baby for nine months.

But what happens when your thyroid is working under par? Your body gets the message that it can't support a pregnancy – so it works against getting pregnant. How?

As your levels of various thyroid hormones decline, it slows the speed at which your body metabolizes all your sex hormones - including estrogen. This interferes with egg production and ovulation on several different levels.

At the same time, your hypothalamus and your pituitary glands sense the decline in thyroid activity, and they respond by trying to jump start your metabolism. This occurs through the release of TRH, which ultimately causes your thyroid gland to release more of the thyroid hormone T4.

While you might think this will normalize your body chemistry and improve your fertility - unfortunately, this isn't the case. Indeed, the production of all this extra TRH prompts your pituitary gland to release prolactin – a chemical that actually suppresses the production of FSH and LH, the chemicals your ovary needs to begin egg production and eventually ovulation.

In fact, while you are breast feeding the production of prolactin is naturally high and acts much like a natural form of birth control. This is one reason that it is much more difficult to become pregnant while you are breast feeding.

However, when you're *trying* to get pregnant, a boost in prolactin production is exactly what you *don't want!* But the good news is – you can do something to keep your thyroid healthy and your fertility functioning normally. As you will discover in just a few minutes, a regular exercise program is often your best "fertility prescription" !

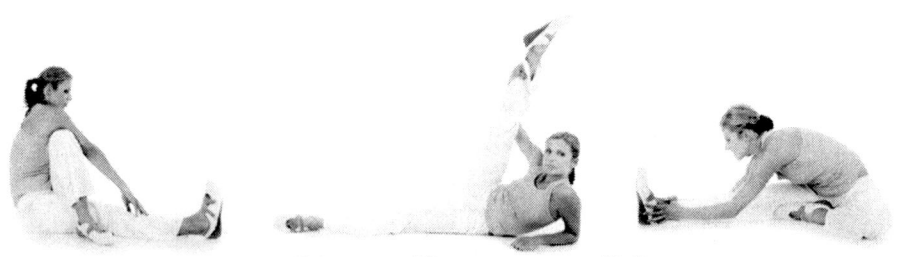

EXERCISE AND YOUR FERTILITY METABOLISM: WHAT ELSE YOU NEED TO KNOW

If you're already an avid exerciser – or even if you just take a run for the bus now and then – you already have some idea of how your body responds to physical activity: Your heart beats faster, blood rushes to your arms and legs, you probably feel a little warm and you may even begin to perspire. All these signs are indications that your body is working harder – with all systems running a little faster than usual.

But physical activity does more than just offer you a passing increase in physiological functions. It also has some lasting effects – including impacting the speed at which your metabolism works.

Indeed, research published in the journal *Neuroendocrinology Letters* in 2005 reports that not only does regular activity increase your metabolic rate, it also effects the level of hormones produced by your thyroid gland. Moreover the more vigorous your activity, the greater the effect on circulating thyroid hormone.

But perhaps even more important, exercise also helps to increase your body's sensitivity to thyroid hormone. And this in turn allows you to better utilize whatever amount of thyroid hormone you are naturally producing. This can be especially important if you are trying to lose weight to increase your fertility.

Indeed, when you diet, your metabolism, and the entire functioning of your thyroid gland slows down to match the lower caloric intake. While eating fewer calories can help you to lose some weight, because your body is now burning fewer calories, the loss won't be as great. This, by the way, is the reason behind weight "plateaus" - times when you continue to diet but your weight loss stops. When this occurs it usually means your metabolism has slowed considerably to match your lower food intake – and so calorie burning slows down as well.

With daily exercise, however, you can keep your metabolism going at a rate closer to how it worked when you were taking in more food . This means fat burning will be much more efficient – and you'll lose weight more easily.

But even more important – at least in regard to your fertility - using exercise to prevent your metabolism from slowing down is a great way to insure a healthy and normal flow of reproductive hormones – from brain chemicals like FSH and LH, to estrogen and progesterone.

The result: When you do reach your ideal weight goal, your body will be primed and ready to get pregnant faster and easier.

Exercise To Optimize Your Fertility

If you're thinking that boosting your metabolism requires lots of vigorous activity for a long period of time, you're in for a surprise! Studies show that just 15 to 20 minutes per day is all you need to keep your thyroid healthy and your metabolism working at optimum levels.

The exercise also doesn't have to be strenuous! As long as the activity raises your heart rate by 30 to 50 beats per minute, then it's likely to have an effect on your thyroid. You can choose walking, swimming, running, dancing, cycling or any type of circuit training. The key is to choose an activity that revs your heart rate – which is a sign that it is also revving your metabolism!

But what happens if you're not on a diet – and your thyroid is running normal – or even high ? Well the interesting thing about these exercises is that they work equally well to normalize a high-normal thyroid, or keep a normal thyroid from going off course.

The key message in all these scenarios is to exercise in moderation! While you don't want to be a couch potato, you also don't want to work out to the point where you will do your body- and your fertility - more harm than good. (Check out the section later in this chapter on what happens to your fertility when you work out too hard!).

EXERCISE AND INFLAMMATION: THE IMPORTANT LINKS

As you read in an earlier chapter, inflammation can be a key factor in not only your overall health, but specifically your fertility. It not only increases problems related to fertility-robbing diseases like endometriosis and PCOS, it can also directly impact fertility by influencing hormone production. This is particularly true if you are overweight, since, as you read previously, fat cells are directly linked to the production of inflammatory compounds. Thus, the more fat cells your body has, the more inflammatory compounds you will have circulating through your system and interfering with hormone production.

So, how can exercise help? Studies show that when you work out on a regular basis, inflammation is reduced body-wide. While links between exercise and weight loss is one way that working out reduces inflammation, it's not the only way. Indeed, some fascinating studies show that exercise can reduce inflammation even when fat burning does not take place.

Indeed, in one study published in the *European Heart Journal*, a group of Finnish researchers found that the level of C-reactive protein or CRP (a marker for inflammation which you read about earlier) actually declines when you are involved in regular forms of exercise. In fact, several studies now support the theory that regular physical activity suppresses the inflammatory process – one reason doctors now believe it helps prevent and treat both cardiovascular disease and type 2 diabetes.

While no one is certain exactly how or why this occurs, one group of Danish researchers published evidence showing exercise helps the body produce anti-inflammatory chemicals, primarily released by bones or muscles during regular physical activity. Of course other researchers have other theories about why it helps, but one thing everyone seems to agree on is that exercise can help reduce inflammation body wide.

I believe these same important anti-inflammatory effects also impact fertility. This is particularly true if you are overweight with an excess fat cells already increasing inflammation. But that said, I also believe it can make a difference if you are of normal weight, or even if you are underweight. How?

In my personal experience, women who suffer from endometriosis – a condition steeped in inflammatory activity – are often "type A" personalities, who are on the thin side, and usually lead a stress-filled life. While these women did not need to exercise to lose weight, certainly I saw that various types of daily workouts of 15 to 20 minutes in duration benefited them greatly. It not only helped in controlling symptoms related to endometriosis – including pelvic pain – it was also helpful in improving their fertility profile overall.

Moreover, sometimes symptoms of this inflammatory disorder can be so subtle you might not even know you are affected until you try to get pregnant - and discover there is a probllem. When this is the case, I have also seen exercise help overcome what seems like "unexplained infertility" - but in reality is really due to mild endometriosis.

But even if you are of normal weight and don't suffer from any inflammatory conditions, you may still benefit from the inflammatory-reducing effects of exercise. First, you will begin reducing your risk of many inflammation-related health conditions, including high blood pressure, heart disease and even some cancers. But moreover, I believe by taking steps to include exercise in your life right now, you will also protect against the "silent" ravages of inflammation that can, over the years, quietly steal your fertility without you even knowing it's occurring.

By comparison, engaging in regular moderate exercise to help reduce inflammation before you see the signs will not only allow you to optimize your fertility now and in the future, but also help protect your overall good health.

WRITING YOUR FERTILITY FITNESS PRESCRIPTION: THE WORKOUTS THAT WORK BEST

As is the case with many factors that influence fertility, when it comes to exercise, moderation is key. And nowhere is this tenet better applied then when it comes to choosing the workouts that work best to encourage fertility.

While it's true that certain types of exercises are definitely more beneficial than others (and you'll learn more about that in a minute), if there is an exercise or a specific type of workout that you really love, then you should continue doing it – as long as you do so in moderation. Indeed, the only fitness regimens that really work, are the ones that you do ! So, above all else, do what you enjoy and enjoy what you do!

That said, as I have mentioned previously, there are certain types of workouts that, for several reasons, appear to offer you not only a beneficial effect when it comes to getting pregnant, but also help you tone, condition and get your body ready for a healthy pregnancy. These include exercises that are generally non-competitive, mildly aerobic (increasing your heart rate by 30 to 50 beats per minutes), and condition the entire body overall without taxing any one particular muscle group. You also want to look for activities that you can do for an extended period of time (up to 40 minutes) without coming away feeling exhausted.

Among the best workouts that accomplish all these things includes:

- Swimming
- Power walking
- Dancing
- Cycling
- Moderate aerobics
- Stretching (which you should perform in conjunction with any workout).
- Tennis (in moderation only, in a non-competitive format)
- Multi activity circuit training (such as what is offered at Curves).

If You Are Overweight ...

If you need to lose weight and want to use exercise to increase calorie burning, these same activities can work for you. However, to turn them from fertility fitness workouts to fat burning activities, you need to do them a little more often and for slightly longer periods of time. If you can do more than one, and alternate them on different days, you may find you will achieve even greater fat burning potential.

What's important to remember, however, is that you don't want to work out to the point where you feel stressed and tired – because neither is good for fertility.

Moreover, if you are overweight and have not exercised for a while, then you need to start slow and build both your endurance and your muscle strength. One of the best ways to do this is by walking. While power walking (a fast paced walk carrying up to two pound weights in each hand) adds some aerobic activity to the regimen that will burn more calories faster, it's also perfectly okay to stroll leisurely, focusing on building your stamina for distance. Indeed, studies show that just the simple activity of continuous walking for up to 20 minutes per day can reduce stress, bring hormones into balance and improve circulation to vital organs, including your ovaries and uterus. There is in fact significant research to show that when blood flow is increased to your reproductive organs, egg production and release occur on a more timely schedule.

If You Are Normal Weight or Underweight ...

If you are underweight or even if your weight is normal, your fertility can still benefit from regular moderate exercise! In fact, I can't stress enough the importance of regular physical activity, no matter your shape or size.

Indeed, it has been my experience that many women who are underweight also suffer from a hormone imbalance that clearly affects fertility. And if this is the case for you – and particularly if your menstrual cycle is somewhat irregular - then certain fitness activities can work to help get your reproductive system back on track. But even if you are of normal weight, with no health problems to interfere with fertility, regular exercise remains important.

What's key in all these circumstances is to select activities that emphasize muscle building and conditioning over fat burning. This includes activities such as walking, weight training, stretching, Tai Chi, or particularly yoga. In fact, as you will read in the section that follows, yoga is one of the universally best workouts for fertility – no matter your weight, shape or size!

> *Hate to exercise? Try "Pilates"! This natural method of stretching and toning the body was developed to help dancers stay in shape without risking injury. A gentle form of exercise it can help you tone muscles, and lose weight without ever getting out of breath!*

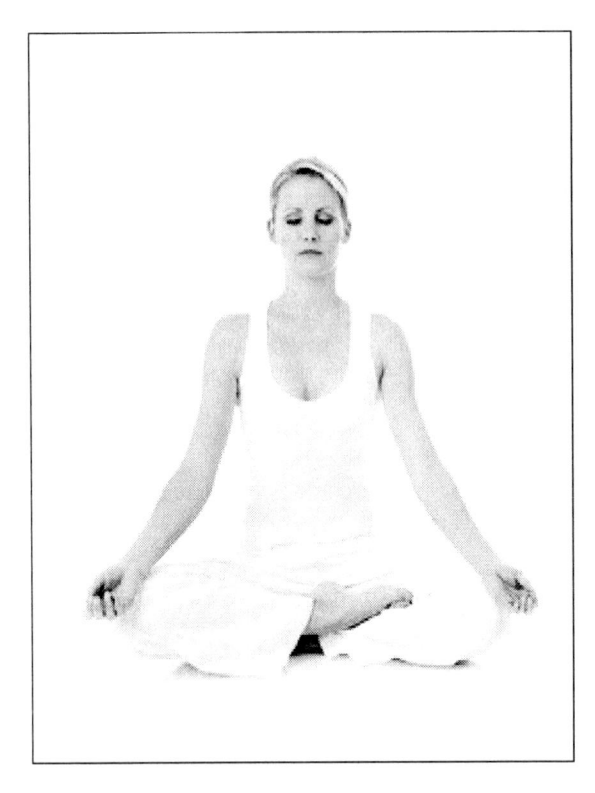

PRACTICE YOGA – GET PREGNANT FASTER !

If I had to choose just one form of exercise that would universally help every woman trying to get pregnant, hands down, my choice would be yoga.

Known as a type of *passive* exercise, yoga helps tone and condition the body via a series of postures (as opposed to movements) designed to strengthen and tone muscles.

It is also one of the only forms of exercise that studies show can have a beneficial effect on both fertility and pregnancy. And how it exerts that positive influence goes right to the heart of what yoga is all about.

Indeed, while most people think of yoga as a form of exercise - and some even regard it as a spiritual belief system - in reality it is actually a proven, scientific way of altering both brain and both chemistry . It accomplishes this through gentle but rigorous exercise, breathing techniques, meditation and ultimately relaxation.

When it comes to fertility, among the most important effects of regular yoga workouts is stress reduction. But it's not just the feeling of being relaxed and more focused that can help you. Indeed, studies show that the stress reduction achieved with yoga has a direct impact on your ability to get pregnant. The pathway is through the hypothalamus – the area of your brain from which all reproductive hormone activity originates. As you will learn in more detail in the next chapter, when stress levels are high your body produces a variety of chemicals and compounds that can dramatically interfere with the functioning of your hypothalamus, and in doing so derail the brain and body chemistry necessary for reproduction.

Yoga works to not only to reduce levels of stress hormones that might otherwise harm your fertility, but in doing so helps all your reproductive hormones work better and more efficiently.

But that's not the only fertility benefit you will receive from this ancient form of exercise. Because studies also show that yoga increases blood flow and circulation, with some of the postures and positions having a direct impact on your pelvis and your reproductive organs. As yoga works to stretch and relax both muscles and connective tissue – particularly in the hips, groin, and lower back – blood flow to the entire pelvic area naturally increases. This not only gives more life-giving oxygen to every cell, but it also helps to remove toxins and other nasty chemicals – some caused by stress – more rapidly from your body. This in turn can lead to more efficient functioning of every organ in your reproductive system – and that in turn can help you get pregnant faster.

Moreover, the practice of yoga also puts a unique kind of emphasis on breathing, helping you to "tune in " to the rhythm of your body. When combined with the stretching movements, studies show this rhythmic breathing helps to release tension, which in turn reduces levels of the stress hormone cortisol – and this is what actually helps increase your chances of getting pregnant. (You'll learn more about stress and its impact on fertility in a later chapter.)

In fact, the principals behind yoga are believed to be so effective in improving pregnancy odds, that today many fertility centers are recommending yoga classes as a way of increasing the success of procedures such as in vitro fertilization.

While many women still require medical interventions to overcome physiologic barriers to pregnancy (such as blocked fallopian tubes or ovarian malfunctions), yoga acts in ways that help the body to work more efficiently and thus better tolerate and better " accept " the fertility treatments.

This in turn increases the chance for a healthy pregnancy – without having to undergo numerous, costly treatments.

For women who don't have medical fertility problems, it works doubly well to support your fertility naturally while encouraging a quicker and easier conception.

NOT ALL FORMS OF YOGA ARE ALIKE

As helpful as yoga can be however, it's important to note there are a number of different forms of this exercise, and not all are beneficial to fertility. For example, Ashtanga Yoga, also known as "power yoga" requires fast paced movements and advanced breathing skills that, for those who are not long practicing devotees may find stressful and difficult to perform.

Likewise, Bikram Yoga, which is practiced in near sauna-like high temperatures also focuses on more complex postures and breathing techniques. If you are not conditioned for this type of activity, Bikram workouts might prove stressful. Plus, should you happen to be pregnant and not know it, the high temperatures associated with this form of exercise might increase your risk of miscarriage.

For most women trying to get pregnant, Hatha Yoga is the most helpful . It also happens to be the most common type of yoga practiced in the US. However, be aware that hatha yoga is also a generic term used to describe the movement and posture segments of all yoga workouts, so not all hatha yoga classes are alike – with some much more complex than others. In fact, some hatha yoga centers actually teach a fourth type of yoga known as "Iyengar". Depending on whom is doing the teaching, this can be a mild and relaxing form of yoga or a bit more strenuous.

The best advice: If you want to use yoga to help you get pregnant faster, I suggest you look into one of the many fertility yoga programs now available around the country . Often referred to as " Conception Yoga" or "Pregnancy Yoga" , these programs are based on the postures and breathing techniques that medical studies have shown are the most likely to benefit women trying to conceive.

If you can't find a "Fertility Yoga" program in your area, then seek out a maternity yoga program – one designed to aid women who are already pregnant. This will not only guarantee it will be a gentle program , but since many of the same postures and techniques that encourage a healthy pregnancy also encourage fertility, it can work to help you get pregnant.

Lastly, remember there are also many books and DVDS featuring yoga for beginners that can put you on the right path to getting pregnant fast!

THE ANTI-FERTILITY WORKOUTS: WHAT TO AVOID

When it comes to your fertility, I would have to say that, overall, doing any type of exercise is more beneficial than doing no exercise at all.

But that said, I would be remiss if I did not remind you that studies do show that certain types of activities, particularly when they are performed excessively – or even obsessively – can work to disrupt hormone activity essential to getting pregnant. In fact, it's not usual for some women to lose their menstrual cycle completely – or to stop ovulating – as a result of doing the wrong types of exercise.

What are the activities that can disrupt your fertility? It's any activity that stresses endurance over toning and conditioning, and causes you to push your body too hard – including marathon running (or any kind of excessive running), training for a triathlon, or any competitive sport training, such as tennis or weight lifting. In fact, even activities I frequently recommend to fertility patients - such as dancing or cycling - can, when taken to extremes, make it harder to get pregnant. In fact, if you are engaged in any type of frequent and vigorous workout program, and you are already experiencing menstrual cycle problems – including irregular cycles, irregular bleeding, or even no cycle at all – then it's a sign you may have to cut back and slow down your fitness activities.

Moreover, I also want to caution you not to use your weight as the barometer of whether working out too hard or too long. Indeed, many of my patients would frequently comment that as long they weren't losing weight they believed they weren't working out too hard or too long. But that can be a deceiving comparison. Why?

When you workout hard you lose fat, but you also build muscle. So, if you weren't overweight to begin with, the muscle may easily replace the fat in terms of the numbers you see on your scale. As such, you might not notice much or even any change in your weight - simply because muscle has replaced fat. But, when it comes to fertility, the number on the scale does not tell the whole story. Regardless of your weight, if you don't have enough body fat, your reproductive chemistry will be compromised. In fact, as you read in the previous chapter, just a small shift below normal is enough to throw your reproductive hormones into a tailspin.

And I can tell you from my personal experience that this is true. Indeed, many of my patients who were female athletes or professional dancers were at or near their correct body weight – and yet they were unable to get pregnant until I explained the importance to gaining back some of the body fat they lost through extensive training.

The good news in all of this: Even if you love to run or engage in other vigorous, endurance sports, you don't have to give them up completely. If you just practice moderation – do less, and do it less often - you can enjoy your favorite activities without posing any risks to your fertility!

FERTILITY & FITNESS: SOME FINAL WORDS OF ADVICE

There is no doubt that we are living in a culture where we tend to spend a lot more time sitting behind a desk than any generation before us. And while I wouldn't go so far as to say our inactivity as a nation is solely responsible for the increase in fertility problems, I do believe exercise can play an important role in helping you get pregnant faster. But that said, not all workouts are equally as beneficial.

To help ensure that your workouts always help and never harm your fertility, I'd like to pass on these few simple guidelines – tenets that have always helped my patients make fitness a healthy and productive part of their fertility plan.

- Whatever activity you choose, always practice moderation. When you are trying to get pregnant never exercise more than three days a week, and always make sure there is at least one day between workouts, necessary for your body to remain strong.
- Don't try to save time by doing all your exercising in one day. Instead, do multiple sessions on different days but keep each session under 40 minutes.
- Don't get compulsive – or competitive – with your fitness routines. While one goal of working out is to build strong muscles and keep your body chemistry humming along, the other goal is to reduce stress. When you toss competition into the equation you defeat some of the purpose.
- Don't be afraid to cut back on – or even cut out - an activity that leaves you feeling drained and strained. If you do feel that way, replace harder workouts with kinder, gentler workouts.
- Finally, use the BMI chart in the previous chapter to monitor your weight loss and make sure that exercise is not causing you to lose too much body fat.

Chapter Six

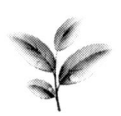

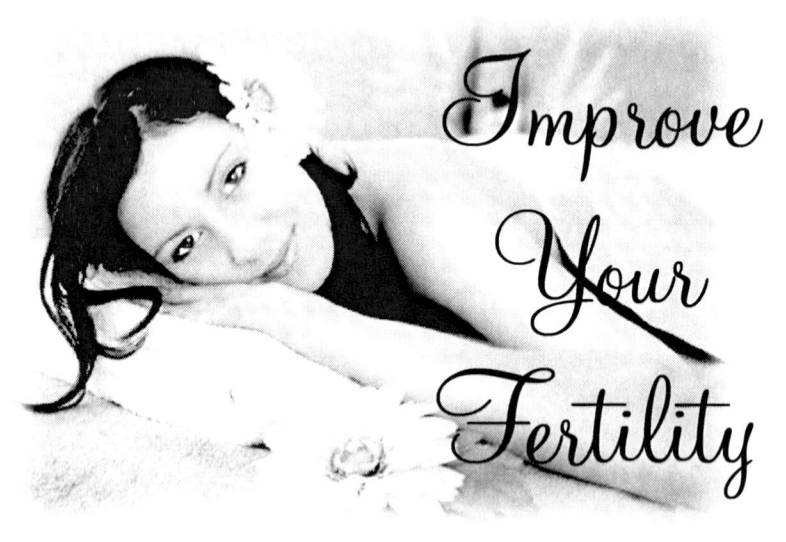

Improve Your Fertility

**With Stress Reduction Strategies
That Really Work!**

A cell phone that is constantly ringing; a screen full of unanswered emails; a boss who just installed a new surveillance camera *right over your desk; and so many* electronic gadgets now stuffed into your handbag or briefcase it takes 15 minutes to find your car keys!

But the minute you do, you dash off to the gym to squeeze in a workout before you race to the market to pick up tonight's dinner, try to remember to get the dry cleaning and return that stack of videos, and still make it home in time to cook the food, get in two loads of laundry and maybe spend a little quality time with your guy! And that's not even counting your social obligations!

If you're like most women this kind of hectic, non-stop activity is a pretty fair rendition of your daily life! In fact, for most of us, living life at break-neck speed has become the new 21st century "norm" - and most of us never realize just how stressed our body and our mind has become in the process.

When you add in recognizable forms of stress - like a demanding boss, a crabby mother-in-law, job insecurities and financial woes - sooner or later you pay the price. For many couples that "price" is infertility - and it's no surprise that the number of even young couples who are affected continues to climb.

Indeed, as our stress levels rise, so too do the difficulties in getting pregnant - affecting everything from egg production and ovulation in women, to sperm count and motility in men, to a reduction in reproductive hormones in both men and women. In fact, studies show that for up to 40% of couples diagnosed with "unexplained infertility", stress is a significant underlying factor, sometimes even blocking the success of assisted reproductive technologies, like IVF.

In one study of IVF patients published recently in the journal *Fertility and Sterility* experts from the University of California at San Diego reported that women who scored highest on a test designed to measure stress ovulated 20% fewer eggs compared to those women who were less stressed. Of those who could produce eggs, the women with the highest levels of stress were 20% less likely to become pregnant.

At the same time, however, we also have studies showing that even if you can't do away with the stressors in your life, learning to better cope with the stresses you do have, can have an enormously positive effect on your fertility.

In the now now-classic study by Harvard's Dr. Alice Domar, women who underwent stress reduction therapy *while* undergoing fertility treatments actually became pregnant quicker and easier than women who simply "suffered in silence" with the anxieties of trying to conceive. This research led to other studies suggesting that every couple could increase their pregnancy rates when they made a conscious effort to counter the effects of stress in their lives. In fact, there is even research that shows stress reduction is an effective way to reduce the risk of miscarriage and premature birth!

In another study published recently in the journal *Human Reproduction*, doctors compared overall pregnancy rates in couples that reported being stressed to those who were not stressed and found that pregnancy was much more likely to occur during months when couples reported feeling happy and relaxed. It was less likely to occur during the months they reported feeling tense or anxious.

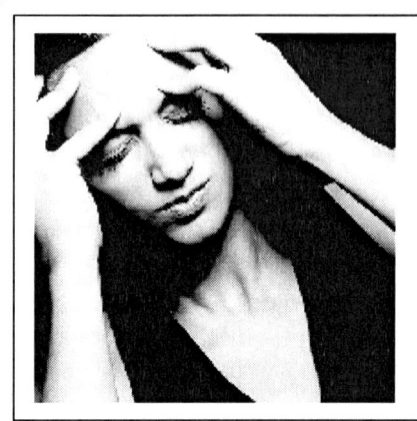

Life can sometimes get so hectic that you end up drowning in a sea of stress without even realizing you're in hot water!

STRESS IN EVERY CORNER OF OUR LIVES

When you stop to think about it, the idea that stress *can* impact fertility isn't really such a far-fetched idea. Indeed, over the past decade and particularly in the last five years we have discovered that many illnesses – including heart disease, high blood pressure, diabetes and even cancer – often have their roots in stress . In fact, today, 60% of all doctor visits are stress-related. Moreover, we also know that reducing stress can reduce your risks of some of these killer diseases.

The problem however, is that many of us don't even realize just how stressed we are! Indeed, while the connections may seem obvious under the scientific microscope, in real life it's not always so easy to recognize or see. In fact, if you are like many of my patients, you and your partner may have become so used to the feeling of being stressed out, that you don't even realize *you are stressed.*

Indeed, as technology came forward with the promise of making our lives easier and less stressful, for many it has had the opposite effect! The quicker you are able to do things, the more determined you became to fill every waking moment with activity – often to the point where any "idle moment" begins to seem like something is wrong!

At the same time, however, I also know that simply telling you to slow down and relax is not going to do much in terms of reducing your overall level of tension. In fact, for many of you, being told that stress is making it harder to get pregnant will actually result in more stress – and an even harder time conceiving!

Instead, what has helped many of my patients - and I what I hope will help you as well - is understanding a bit more about how stress impacts getting pregnant, and in doing so realize how quickly and easily you can take back control of your life - and ultimately your fertility!

Certainly, I don't expect you to give up your cell phone, or turn off your computer any time soon! And in reality there may be nothing you can do about that demanding boss or meddling mother-in-law.

But if you use the information in this chapter wisely, you will not only learn to identify all the ways in which stress is affecting you, but in the process learn how to turn down the volume and change the way your body processes and ultimately responds to that stress. And that is what can help your fertility to blossom!

STRESS AND INFERTILITY:
UNDERSTANDING THE CAUSE AND EFFECT

While the links between stress and fertility are still a relatively new field of study, among most important research to emerge details the impact that every day stressors can have on the brain hormones such as FSH, LH and GnRH - which as you read earlier are all necessary for conception. So how does stress affect this important brain activity?

When you are under chronic stress, a biochemical chain reaction of events causes your brain to secrete a hormone known as CRH - short for corticotrophin releasing hormone. This in turn sends a message to your pituitary to release ACTH (adrenocorticotropic hormone) a powerful peptide hormone which then travels through your bloodstream to your adrenals – two tiny glands that sit just atop your kidneys. When ACTH reaches your adrenals it directs them to release cortisol, the classic "fight or flight" stress hormone that helps prepare your body to " do battle" with your stressor.

On a short term basis, this reaction is actually a good thing. It does, indeed, give your body that extra strength to either flee or fight the stressor. Moreover, once the danger has passed, and the brain perceives that you are again "safe", your body calms down and your hormonal activity all returns to normal.

But what happens when the "danger" doesn't pass – and the stress continues in your life? In simplest terms your body never gets a chance to calm down. Your brain never gets the signal that the danger has passed, so all of the stress hormones I mentioned earlier remain elevated. And that's where the link to infertility really begins.

When stress hormones remain high, your body sends a signal to your brain that all available resources are needed for "combat". To accommodate your body's request for more "fighting energy" your brain responds by shutting down all functions perceived as "unnecessary" to survival. Essentially, anything not involved in helping you fight the stress is "turned off" – and most often, this includes reproduction.

"It is very adaptive to not be wasting resources on reproduction during times of acute stress, [so the body just] shuts down reproduction ....until the stress is gone," says Professor Daniela Kaufer, of the University of California at Berkeley, where she has studied the effects of stress on reproduction.

"These functions go back in evolution a very long time," she says.

Indeed, in an effort to "turn down" your body's activity schedule, your hypothalamus gland suppresses production of GnRH. This in turns down production of FSH and LH - which in turn means that your eggs will not get as powerful a signal to develop, grow or ovulate. And that means your chances of getting pregnant are dramatically diminished.

But there's still more to this complex biochemical picture. In studies conducted by Professor Kaufer and published by the National Academy of Sciences we learned how the stress reaction in the brain not only suppresses the production of hormones necessary to get pregnant, it also boosts activity of a small protein hormone

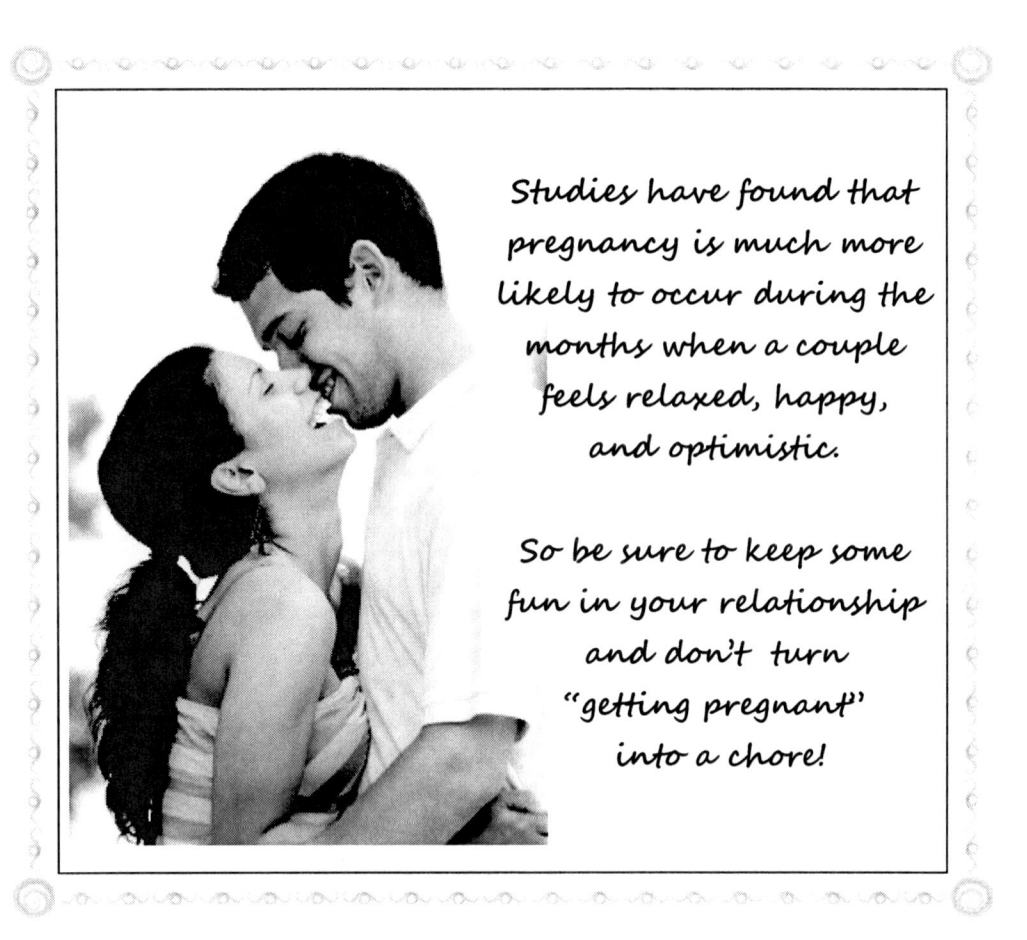

> *Studies have found that pregnancy is much more likely to occur during the months when a couple feels relaxed, happy, and optimistic.*
>
> *So be sure to keep some fun in your relationship and don't turn "getting pregnant" into a chore!*

known as GnIH or gonadatropin inhibitory hormone – a natural biochemical that also works *against fertility*. Indeed, GnIH not only further suppresses production of GnRH, it also works directly to lower production of all sex hormones – putting a kind of 'double whammy' on your fertility !

Moreover, it's not just women who are affected by the process. Indeed, this, and other studies have shown these same stress-induced hormones also impact the production of testosterone, the male hormone necessary for the development of healthy sperm. Without adequate testosterone sperm may not fully develop or mature enough to fertilize an egg – or in the worst case scenario, may not be produced at all.

Chronic Stress Vs Acute Stress: What Affects Fertility The Most

Although studies show that quick, tumultuous bursts of acute stress can have a direct and immediate effect on the production of hormones that inhibit fertility, for the most part, these effects disappear within about 24 hours. So, while having a very bad day at the office, or even experiencing something as dramatic as a car accident or the death of a family member might shut down your reproductive hormones for 24 to 48 hours, studies also show that after this time frame, your body, and your reproductive status returns to normal.

That however, does not seem to be the case when your stress is chronic or ongoing, or if you continue to experience individually stressful experiences in rapid succession. In the UC Berkeley studies on the effects of stress on the hypothalamus, doctors learned that the effects of fertility-inhibiting hormones can linger a lot longer when your stress hangs on, impacting the entire cascade of of hormonal activity necessary for reproduction.

"We know stress effects the top-tier reproductive hormone, GnRH, but we show, in fact, that stress also effects ….GnIH to cause reproductive dysfunction," said lead author Elizabeth Kirby.

In this respect it seems clear that chronic, even low-lying stress can be much worse for your fertility than any single stressful event.

Perhaps the most frustrating aspect of this tenet is that we often don't realize the effect of chronic stress - or even that we are experiencing it. Indeed, in the classic case of "identifying with our captors", our mind begins to view our chronically stressful life as "normal" - so we often don't even realize the impact we are experiencing.

The good news: When you do stop to examine your life and recognize and understand the ways in which stress is affecting you, you can begin to do something about it!

Even better news: While you may not be able to change the factors that are causing you stress, you can definitely change the way your body responds - and in doing so significantly improve your ability to get pregnant!

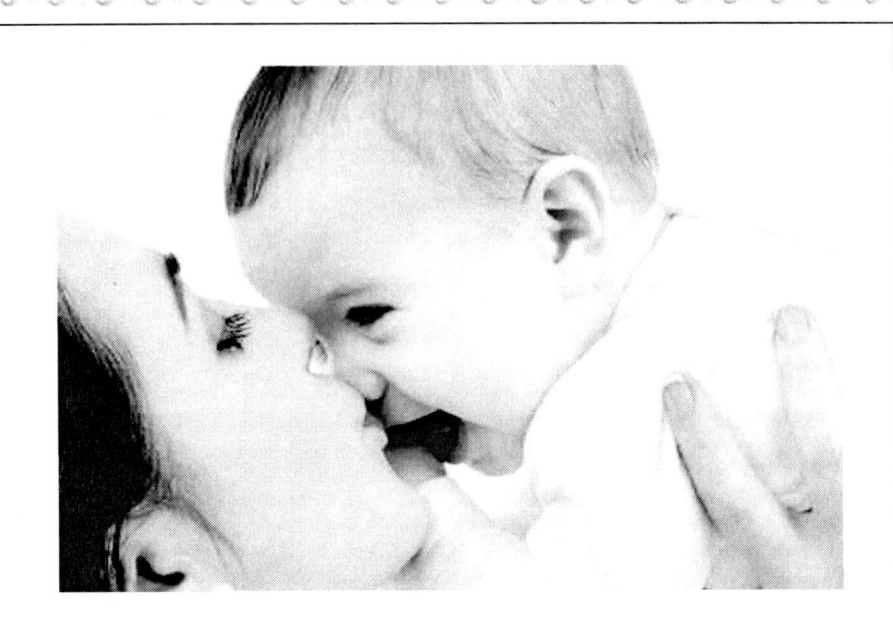

Q: *I've heard that stress can cause a miscarriage. Is this true?*

A: While it's not likely that a single bout of stress can cause you to lose your baby, when stress is ongoing it can reduce proteins within the lining of the uterus that are critical to a successful implantation.

Without these hormones not only will it be difficult for your embryo to attach and begin growing, but the risk of early miscarriage also rises. The best advice is to remain as relaxed as possible during the time you plan to conceive - and to relax as much as possible in the days immediately following attempts at conception. If you do get pregnant then this extra relaxation will help ensure your baby gets the healthiest start in life!

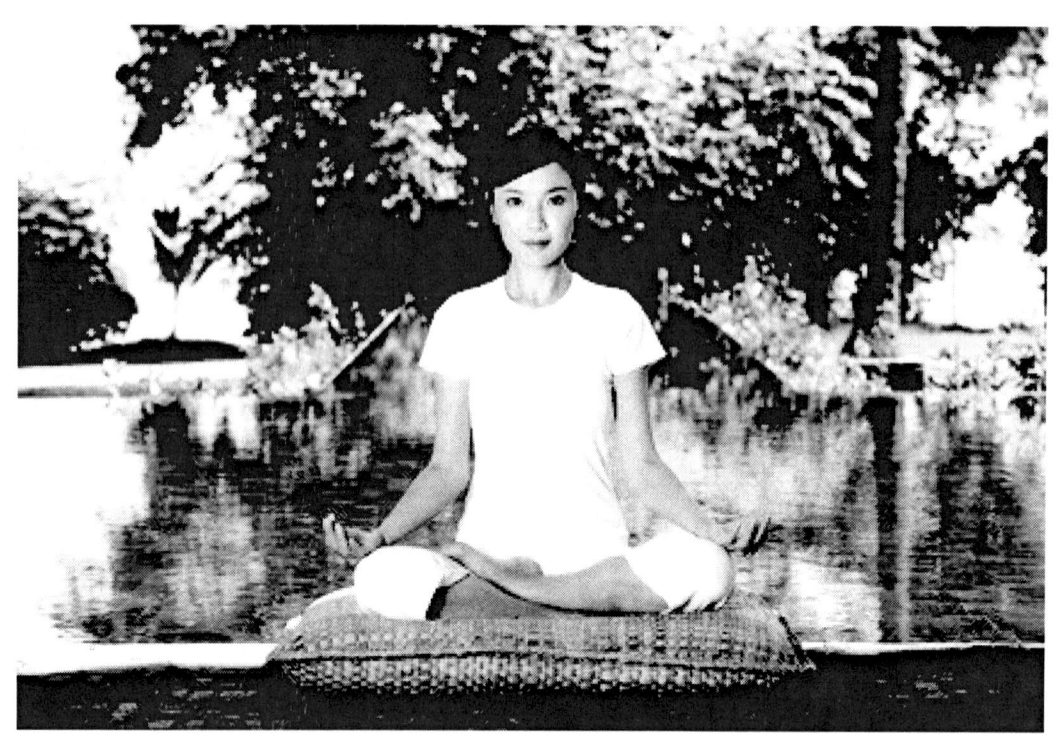

A new study suggests activities like yoga and meditation may help reduce production of chemicals that block conception!

ANCIENT EASTERN ANTI-STRESS FERTILITY BOOSTER CAN CHANGE YOUR LIFE!

For centuries Chinese Medicine doctors have been "prescribing" anti-stress activities like yoga and meditation to increase fertility. And now modern western science has offered proof they might well be the ticket to pregnancy success.

In a major study published in the journal *Fertility and Sterility* researchers from the US National Institutes of Health and the UK's University of Oxford report that women who have a higher level of an enzyme marker for stress have a much more difficult time getting pregnant. And further, that reducing stress levels via such activities as yoga and meditation not only reduces this enzyme, but in the process increases fertility!

The enzyme in question is alpha-amylase, a natural body chemical that rises in response to the production of other natural body chemicals known as catecholamines - hormones which are manufactured as part of the body's "fight or flight" response to stress.

But what does this have to do with pregnancy?

The study followed 274 couples trying to conceive, for a period of 6 months. None of the women had a history of infertility and all used an at-home fertility kit to track their ovulation. On the 6th day of each monthly cycle the women offered a sample of saliva which was tested for the presence of alpha-amylase, as well as the classic stress hormone, cortisol.

What They Found: Women with the highest levels of alpha-amylase were 12% less likely to get pregnant during any given cycle, than women with the lowest levels.

While researchers aren't certain how the enzyme was linked to conception problems, they say early evidence suggests that catecholamines may reduce blood flow to the fallopian tubes, which in turn slows the passage of the fertilized egg to the uterus. By the time the egg does arrive it may simply be "too old" to implant - so a pregnancy does not occur.

As you just read, other theories suggest that high levels of stress hormones interfere with brain chemicals involved in orchestrating egg production and release - so when amylase markers are high it means other stress hormones are also in peak production.

Perhaps most important, the new findings suggest that reducing stress can have an important positive impact on reducing all these potentially harmful chemicals and in the process help you get pregnant faster. Indeed, the researchers on this study suggest that both yoga and meditation may help change the body's chemical responses so that even if you are under stress, your fertility won't be as easily affected. Indeed, for centuries Chinese Medicine doctors have been saying the same thing - and now western doctors seem to have the evidence they were right!

More Coping Mechanisms That Boost Fertility

While yoga and meditation are certainly two important ways to decrease stress and improve fertility, they are certainly not the only path to getting pregnant! Indeed, when it comes to stress reduction I have always believed that whatever activities make *you* feel happy and relaxed are the activities that will also promote *your fertility*. So, whether it's reading, gardening, going for a walk or a run, doing crafts, knitting, or going out dancing - if it helps you feel better than it's going to have stress reduction effects - and positive effects on your fertility.

Of course if you're like many of my patients, you know what to do to relax – you can just never find the time to do it!

Because so many of my patients remain leading women in the fields of entertainment, music, fashion and the arts, telling them to relax is a little like telling a clock to stop ticking – they could never do it! Indeed, the sad reality is that for all us, sooner or later everything harkens back to our hectic life and our busy lifestyles.

So, in this respect I fully understand that trying to "schedule" in time for relaxation can sometimes add to our stress. But the good news is you can still take advantage of all that relaxation has to offer – and do it in with minimal time and effort!

To help you do just that, I've combed the research to come up ten quick and easy things you can do beginning right now, to start reducing your level of stress and encourage your fertility - even with the busiest, most hectic schedule. It's my hope that at least some of them will intrigue and interest you - and eventually become part of your daily living.

And remember, since stress affects not just your fertility but also your partner's, (and you can read more about that in the chapter on male fertility), be sure to share these activities with him – or maybe even find time to do them together!

Of course it's also important to remain cognizant of the situations in your life that cause you the most stress - and when you can, avoid them. This is particularly important during the months you are actively trying to conceive.

But when you can't, be doubly sure to put the following ten tips into motion, so you can begin to counter the effects of your stress in a positive and healthful way.

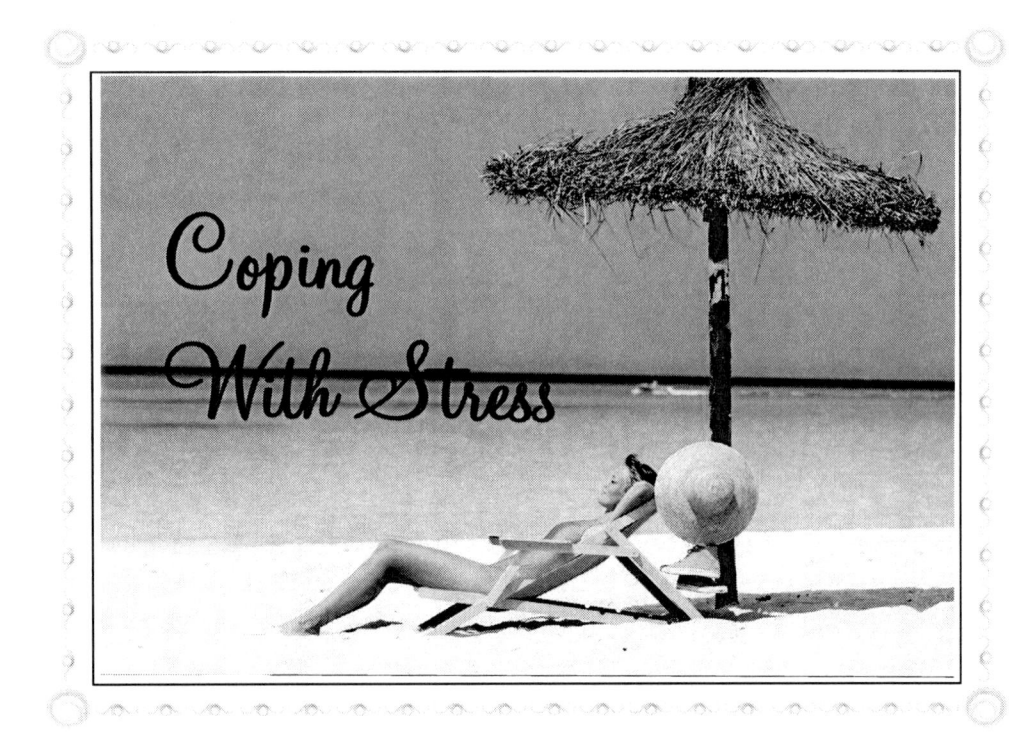

10 Things You Can Do Right Now To Improve Your Fertility

Stress Buster # 1: Breathe ... and Conceive!

The concept seems almost magical: Take deep breaths and get pregnant faster. But in truth, it really works - and there's no magic involved! Indeed, scores of studies have demonstrated the power of controlled, deep breathing to not only induce a state of relaxation, but also have a direct impact on the ebb and flow of hormones, including those linked to stress. As such, it's not hard to see how deep breathing can ultimately work to promote fertility.

And in fact, this is exactly what Harvard's Dr. Alice Domar found in one of her now classic case studies on infertility. Here, 132 women all of whom were having problems conceiving, were enrolled in a stress reduction program that focused on deep breathing exercises along with several other mind-body relaxation techniques. The result: Within six months of beginning the study, 42% of the women were able to get pregnant – compared with just 20% who did not participate in the stress reduction program.

Five For Five Deep Breathing Fertility Exercise

If you want to give deep breathing a try, here's a quick easy way to get started: With your hands placed gently over your tummy, inhale, count to five, then exhale.

Do this five times – which should take about 5 minutes. Repeat the exercise 5 times during the day for a total of 25 minutes of deep breathing. You should see a noticeable difference in your level of daily tension within 5 days or less!

In addition to this deep breathing exercise you should also consider getting involved in a yoga program.

As you read in the previous chapter, yoga postures can have a positive effect body-wide and can actually increase fertility. In addition, however, the breathing exercises that accompany yoga movements are another great way to help you relax and encourage your fertility

STRESS BUSTER # 2: TALK SOFTLY!

Have you ever noticed that when you are nervous or tense your voice can become louder and the pitch higher than normal? This is because tension causes a tightening of all your muscles, including those that control your vocal cords. The tightening motion then feeds back to the brain that you are really tense, which encourages the production of more stress hormones and more muscle constriction.

But according to studies in the *Journal of Behavioral Medicine*, you can break the feedback loop and "trick" your body into relaxing by making a conscious effort to soften and lower your voice. This slows down your heart rate which ultimately sends a signal to your brain that the stress crisis is over - which in turn helps dampen down the production of those stress hormones. The fewer stress hormones your body produces, the easier it is for your reproductive hormones to function optimally.

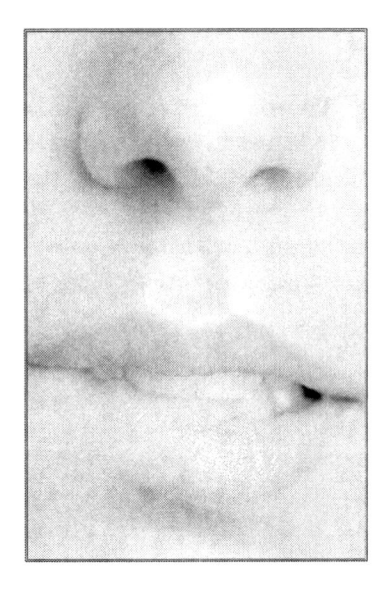

Soft Talk Fertility Exercise

While it's not always easy to stop a tension tailspin in motion, here's a practice method that can eventually become a stress coping tool. Each time a small stress occurs – you are stuck in traffic, your boss chews you out for something that's not your fault, dinner burns or the washing machine floods, stop, take a breath, close your eyes, and as calmly as you can *whisper* the following phrase: " I am in complete control and I am able to handle everything that comes my way today." Softly repeat the phrase four or five times – and you should begin to feel a sense of warm relaxation spreading throughout your body as your muscles begin to relax.

Be it your spouse, your mom, your best friend or your puppy or kitten, giving a hug is a major stress reducer. If you get one back, even better! How does it work?

In research conducted at the University of North Carolina, doctors discovered that when we hug – or when we are hugged – our body produces more of a hormone known as "oxytocin", which in turn helps reduce the production of stress hormones.

In fact, one reason why many women report feeling so serene when they breast feed is because oxytocin is produced in larger amounts during this activity.

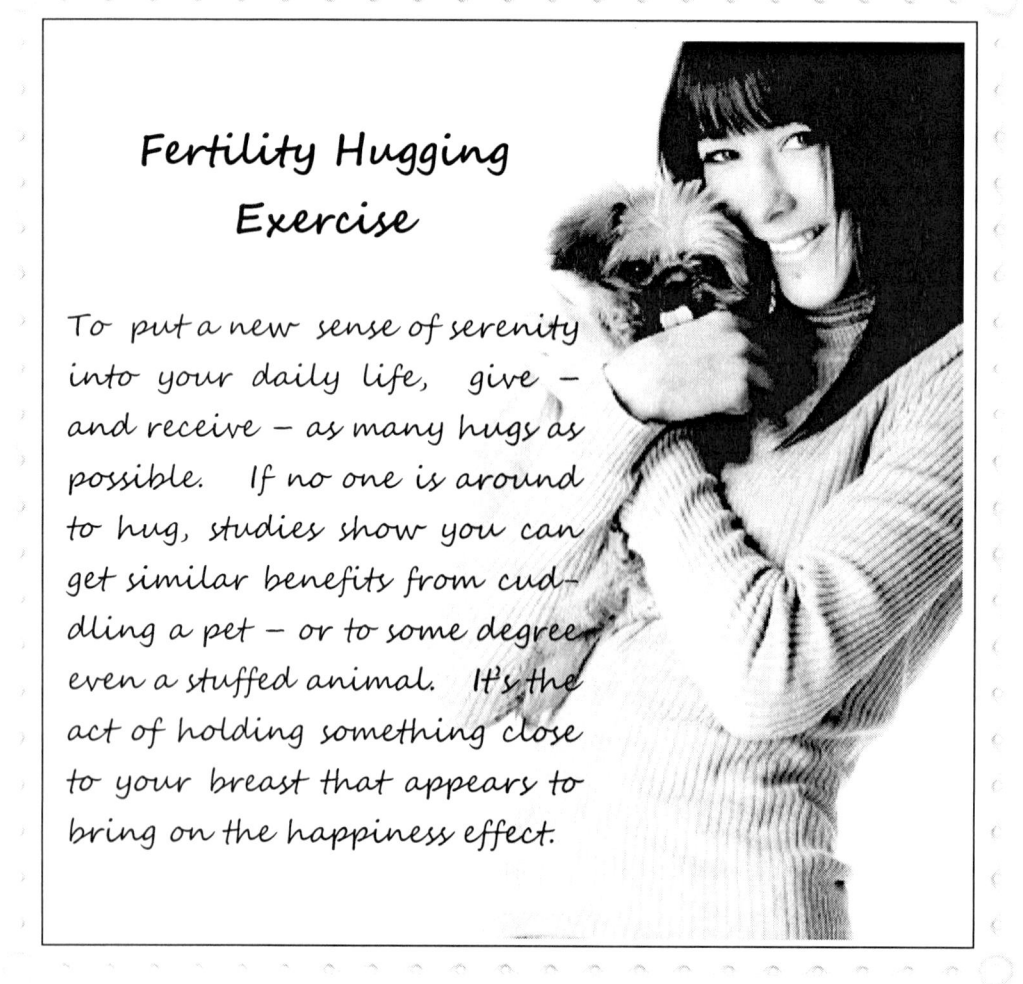

Fertility Hugging Exercise

To put a new sense of serenity into your daily life, give – and receive – as many hugs as possible. If no one is around to hug, studies show you can get similar benefits from cuddling a pet – or to some degree, even a stuffed animal. It's the act of holding something close to your breast that appears to bring on the happiness effect.

> *Concentrating on the sights and sounds around you is one way to reduce stress and allow your body to relax. Next time you're taking a bath clear your mind and just think about the feel of the water on your skin!*

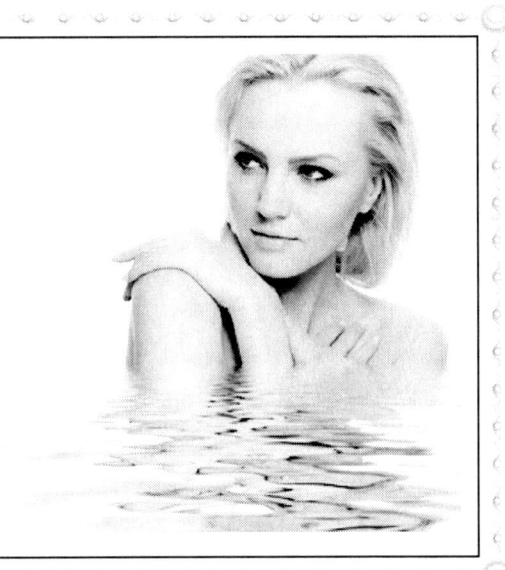

STRESS BUSTER # 4: MINDFUL MEDITATION

Studies have long shown that meditating – the act of quieting the mind and focusing on, well, *nothing* is one way to relieve stress that's locked inside your thought process. Indeed, the more you concentrate on your problems- and think about them in a non-productive way – the more stressed you will become. When the thought you're *most stressed* about is your fertility, then the effect puts a double whammy on hormones linked to getting pregnant.

Meditating works by putting your thought process on a virtual "vacation" – temporarily removing the stress and giving your mind, and consequently your body, a break. Not only is this good for your cardiovascular health – and your immune system – studies show it's also good for your fertility.

In one study of women under going IVF treatments at a fertility clinic in Barcelona, Spain, doctors found that those who participated in relaxation therapies such as meditation had a much higher rate of successful embryo implantation than those who did not utilize this great form of stress reduction.

Writing in the *Journal of Human Reproduction* they suggest that in addition to improving quality of life, relaxation therapies have a direct impact on the rate of pregnancy.

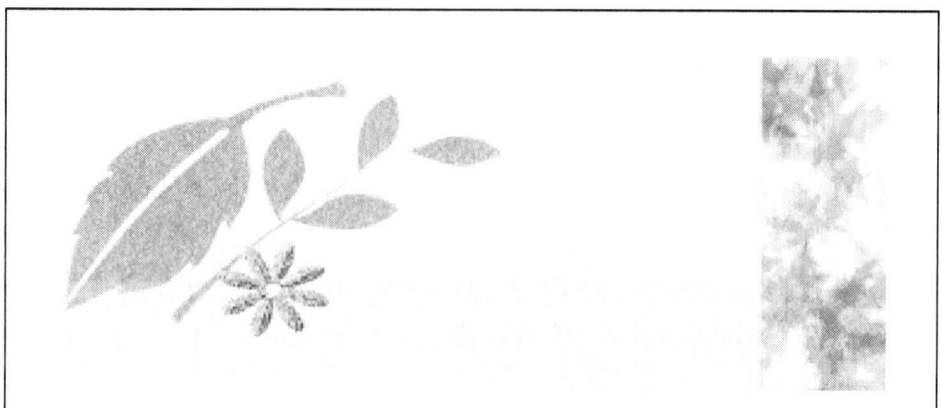

Mindful Meditation Exercise For Fertility:

If you've always wanted to try meditation but didn't know where or how to start, then a relatively simple method known "mindful mediation" might be right for you.

Here, you simply sit down in a comfortable chair and with your eyes closed, concentrate on nothing but the sound of your breathing. Breathe normally, but simply pay attention to your inhales and exhales. If your mind wanders, don't stress about it, just keep bringing it back to concentrating on breathing.

If this seems too boring – and you find your mind being continually distracted – add a word or phrase to the rhythm of your breathing, and say it, either out loud or to yourself, as you breathe in and out. For a doubly good effect, choose a short positive phrase that has to do with fertility – such as " Pregnancy Now " or "Happy Conception" or "Motherhood is coming". Say the phrase once while inhaling and once while exhaling – and try not to think about anything but the phrase and your breathing. Do this for up to 20 minutes once daily for optimum results.

STRESS BUSTER # 5 : CHANTING

Sound a little too "Age of Aquarius" for you? That's what many of my patients have said! But once they give it a try, chanting often becomes their favorite way to relax.

How does it work? Repetition is the key!

Indeed, studies show that repetition of any activity induces a meditative state of relaxation that can actually change brain wave activity.

Theoretically any repetitive activity can do the same thing (it's one reason why so many pregnant women take up knitting - it's the repetitive action that is both calming and a bit addictive).

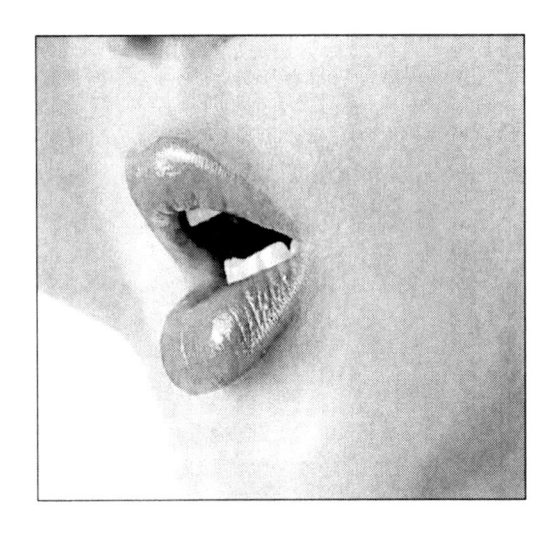

But when you combine repetition with the audible sound of chanting you get double the effect!

Indeed, studies show that sounds produced while in a relaxed, meditative state can actually penetrate muscles, bones and organs causing cells to change in response to certain frequencies.

Sound can also help stimulate the secretion of stress-reducing hormones and may even modify brain waves involved in the production of reproductive hormones.

So as long as you are chanting something positive - a phrase that doesn't stress you out or bring sadness to your heart - then the overall effects should be good for your health and helpful to your fertility.

Fertility Chanting Exercise

Find a comfy position – in your favorite chair, on the floor with a stack of pillows, even in bed !

Make sure you're wearing unrestrictive clothing – or at least something that doesn't tug, bind, pull or pinch your skin , which can be distracting.

Now choose a phrase that feels comfortable for you to say.

It can be a line from a favorite song or poem, or any positive affirmation about fertility – such as "I am fertile, I will be a great mother" or " Pregnancy is mine, pregnancy will happen" etc. Just make sure the line has a positive life force *and* that the string of sounds you utter when you say them feels comfortable and easy.

Once you have that in place, close your eyes and simply begin repeating the phrase, aiming for a rhythmic cyclical repetition.

You can start slow and gradually speed up or keep your tempo even, whatever feels best to you.

You can also say the phrase as loudly, or as softly as is necessary (don't want to scare the neighbors!) as long as it's audible to you. Try to feel the motion or the rhythm of the phrase and if feels good, let your body move or sway to the rhythm you create.

Ten to fifteen minutes of chanting once a day – or every other day – is all you need to reduce stress and get your fertility hormones humming along!

Stress Buster # 6: Sensory Perception Relaxation

If you're a busy woman with a packed schedule, then sensory perception relaxation is for you - simply because it allows you to do what you do normally, but in a way that promotes relaxation.

In this technique, you simply heighten your sensory awareness during whatever activity you are already performing – paying attention to the smells, sounds and tactile feel of things that you normally don't even notice.

This works as a diversion to draw your brain's attention away from whatever is stressing you – either at the moment, or any long term worries on your mind. This in turn disrupts the stress response, reduces the flow of harmful brain chemicals and helps protect fertility.

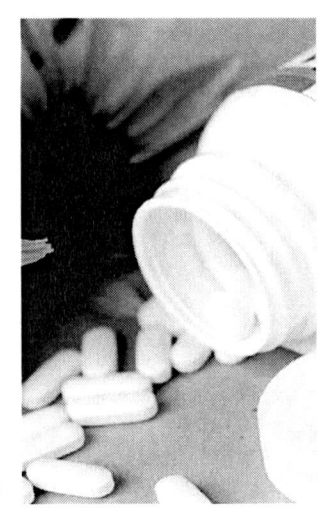

Q: *I've heard that using tranquilizers to reduce stress can harm my fertility - is this true?*

A: When used on a short term basis most tranquillizers won't harm fertility. But that said, long term use of some types has been known to disrupt the menstrual cycle and could make getting pregnant more difficult.

If possible, try all natural stress reduction such as yoga, meditation and getting enough rest! These things will not only reduce your stress but also increase your fertility!

If you have trouble sleeping try a gentle herbal remedy such as Valerian root - or even a cup of warm milk before bedtime. Both have been shown to bring on natural, relaxing sleepiness!

Sensory Perception Fertility Exercise:

The next time you are washing the dishes – or perhaps doing hand laundry – concentrate on every sensory stimulation around you. Think about how the warm water feels on your hands or the smooth feel of the slippery soap suds. Put your attentions on the smoothness of each plate or the squeaky clean feel of each glass – or if you are doing laundry, the silkiness of the fabric or the weight of it in your hand after it is wet.

If you are using aromatic soaps, inhale deeply and concentrate on the pleasant smells and let your mind drift into the fragrance. You can also concentrate on any sound in your immediate vicinity – the water running, or the sound it makes as it splashes into the sink, the clinking of the glassware, the gentle swish of the fabric.

Concentrate on all of the "sensory" perceptions involved in whatever you are doing and for the moment think only about those things.

And what if you're on a crowded bus or stuck in traffic – and there is nothing pleasant around you?

Then turn your thoughts inward to the feel of that soft scarf around your neck, how your gloves feel on your hands, or even the silky smoothness of your hair. The key is to engage your senses and your stress will melt away.

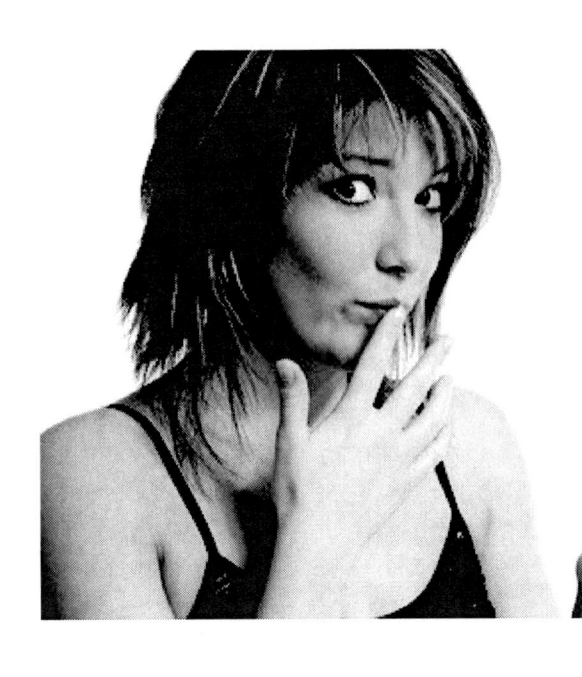

Stress Buster # 7: Anti Stress Foods

For many women – as well as men – food is a source of stress-relieving comfort

The problem is, however, that for most of us our "stress food " choices rarely lead to long term *stress control.*

While that five pound box of chocolates, quart of ice cream or giant bowl of Mac & Cheese may temporarily make you feel better, the "after effects" , which include drops in blood sugar and increases in inflammation – can actually become a source of more stress.

What's more if you are trying to lose weight to increase your fertility, then turning to food to manage your stress can have other complications as well, both emotional and physical.

At the same time, there are foods which, for a variety of reasons, have properties that work to *relieve* and even *reduce* stress - mostly by reducing the production of stress hormones. Or, in some instances, countering their effects. Filling up on these foods is a plus- during times of stress.

So if you're a stress-eater, no need to quit! Just turn the page and you can learn how to select foods that offer comfort - and reduce stress at the same time!

THE ANTI-STRESS FOODS TO INCLUDE IN YOUR DIET :

GREEN TEA – Japanese research confirms that drinking just three cups a day can decrease stress hormones up to 30%!

WHOLE WHEAT MUFFINS, PASTA OR PIZZA – Anything made with whole grains are loaded with fiber – and that can help modulate blood sugar levels which in turn keeps you from feeling jittery and stressing out. It can also help you feel fuller longer – and that can also lead to feelings of satisfaction and less stress.

YOGURT, ICE CREAM OR MILK - The key here is the calcium content which has a calming effect on the body. According to a 2005 study from the *Archives of Internal Medicine,* calcium is an effective way to beat some of the symptoms of PMS. It works by reducing brain activity linked to a hormone imbalance. Since some of these same hormones are also involved in fertility, it seems reasonable to suggest that increasing your intake of foods high in calcium will yield similar beneficial results. Remember though, some of these foods can be high in calories – and you only need a little to get results.

NUTS – PARTICULARLY ALMONDS, PISTACHIOS AND WALNUTS - Almonds are loaded with B vitamins which can counter some of the effects of stress hormones - so they're always a great choice! Also try eating almond butter on days when you feel particularly stressed – many people report it has a calming effect. Moreover both pistachios and walnuts can calm a racing heart, thereby helping to reduce the production of stress hormones.

In a 2007 Penn State University study doctors found that a handful of pistachio nuts a day lowers blood pressure which in turn helps temper the body's stress reactions. Walnuts have also been found to impact blood pressure, helping levels to drop even while you are under stress.

STRESS BUSTER # 8: THE SCENT OF RELAXATION

If you're always on the go you can carry some instant relaxation in your pocket – *literally*.

The key is aromatherapy – the use of certain scents to help blunt your body's stress response, reduce the production of harmful stress chemicals and in some instances even give your fertility a boost!

Indeed, studies show that our sense of smell is a direct pathway to the brain, helping to influence the production of feel-good chemicals like dopamine and serotonin, which can play a huge role in keeping stress responses low. Smell the "right" scents and your brain reacts in a calming way!

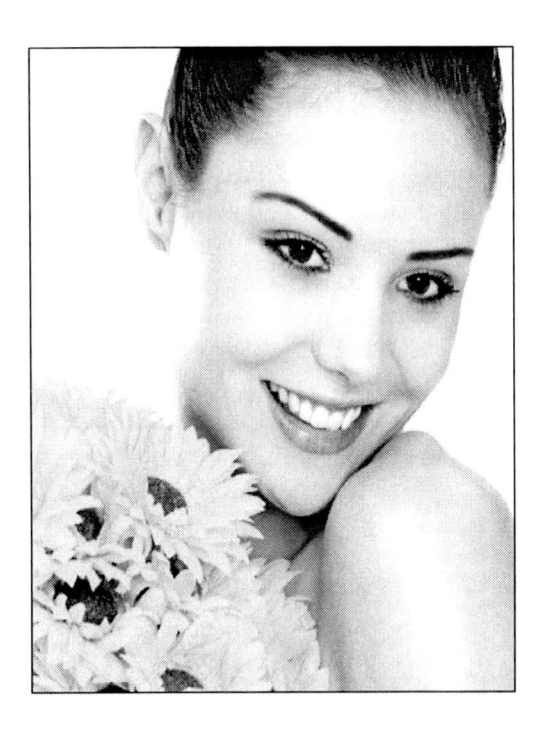

Moreover, new research published in the journal of *Agricultural and Food Chemistry* found that an aromatic compound known as linalool – found in many fruits and vegetables – causes a measurable reduction in cortisol, the key stress hormone found to influence infertility. The same scent also helps calm down over 100 genes involved in the stress response!

So the next time tensions begin to mount up, take a quick trip to your local grocery store and spend 15 or 20 minutes "inhaling" in the fresh fruit and produce section! Not only will the collective scents help calm you down, they may also inspire you to eat more healthfully too!

Your Fertility Scent Prescription:

You can keep a hankie or some cotton balls soaked in these scents in your purse and take a whiff anytime you need an instant stress reducer!

- **CITRUS FRUITS** - Oranges, lemons and limes, plus apples, pears, broccoli and cabbage contain lots of linalool. Keep bowls of them around the house and inhale the scent particularly when feeling stressed.

- **COFFEE BEANS** - While coffee itself may not be so great for your fertility (see my chapter on food and fertility), the scent of coffee beans can have a positive effect on stress. According to studies at Vanderbilt University inhaling the scent of coffee activates anti-anxiety genes, which in turn help increase production of stress-fighting antioxidants.

- **LILLY OF THE VALLEY** - If you're feeling tense try a spritz of any fragrance containing notes of the flower Lilly of the Valley. In studies conducted at the University of Cincinnati, Lilly of the Valley was shown to reduce stress by up to 25%, mostly by influencing the production of Alpha waves in the brain. They help promote feelings of tranquility and calmness without making you feel groggy or tired.

- **LAVENDER** - In hospitals in Oxford, England essential oil of lavender, along with the scents of marjoram, geranium, mandarin and cardamom have all but replaced chemical sedatives in helping patients to calm down and relax. Plus, all have been shown to lower blood pressure as they reduce stress.

- **VANILLA** - Long known for it's calming properties, vanilla oil can be an instant stress reducer, helping you feel immediately calmer in almost any stressful situation. It can also work long term to help keep stress hormones from raging out of control.

STRESS BUSTER # 9 : MASSAGE THERAPY

Not only is there some great evidence showing that massage therapy reduces stress, there are also a number of fertility doctors who report that it increases the success rate of an embryo implantation, and may also increase pregnancy rates.

How does it work?

By combining the therapeutic benefits of human touch (which much like hugging helps reduce stress levels) with an increase in blood flow and circulation, a reduction in muscle tension, and the therapeutic effects of sensory perception, massage works on many different pathways to mediate the production of stress hormones as well as increase healthy blood flow to all the vital organs – including those in the reproductive system.

MASSAGE THERAPY TIPS:

- If you can, spring for a professional massage whenever you feel particularly stressed, or when stress becomes chronic and ongoing.

- If you can't afford a professional massage, rent or buy a massage video so that you and your partner can learn how to reduce each other's stress. Schedule your massages on alternating nights so each of you can gain the full benefits of the relaxation.

- Try self massage! If there is simply no one around when you're feeling the most stressed, don't overlook the power of a self- massage. Especially effective is a self-foot massage, but you can also gently massage your own legs, arms and especially your hands and gain some important therapeutic, stress reducing benefits.

- To increase your chances of getting pregnant, have your partner give you a foot massage just prior to making love. Preliminary study evidence and some anecdotal reports indicate that a lower body massage, particularly foot massage, given just before an insemination or an embryo transfer increases the rate of pregnancy. Doing the same thing before trying for a natural conception could have similar effects.

STRESS BUSTER # 10: PUT ON YOUR DANCIN' SHOES!

As anyone who's ever spent an evening watching Dancing With The Stars can tell you, dancing is a wonderful and fun activity. But did you know it's also a potent stress reliever that could help you get pregnant? It's true!

Studies in both Germany and at the University of New England found that dance lowers levels of stress hormones that otherwise interfere with conception. Among the most stress-relieving of all dances is the tango - which studies show can dramatically lower levels of cortisol. Experts say it also evokes a state of "mindful mediation" that is similar to Yoga! Plus, the socializing aspect of dancing is also stress relieving. So put on your dancin' shoes!

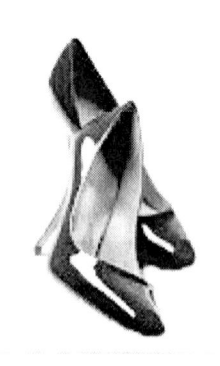

Your Dance Prescription:

Because dancing with a partner to music appears to have the most positive effects on stress reduction, do try to get your partner up on his feet along with you! But if that just isn't going to happen, plug in your Ipod and dance to your own beat! Studies show there are still many positive stress reducing effects from dancing alone.

Moreover, other studies have shown that listening to music can actually alter your brain waves and change the way your entire body chemistry works - particularly the area of the brain where mood enhancing bio-chemicals are made. Since this is the same area of the brain where fertility signals also originate, it would not be surprising to discover that music may also enhance fertility!

Some Final Words:

Relax, Smile and Get Pregnant !

As hard as it may be to believe that simple things such as deep breathing , talking softly or dancing can help you get pregnant faster, I can promise you the effects of all 10 stress reduction tips can and will yield a positive result. But even more important than taking steps to reduce your stress is making a conscious effort to cultivate positive emotions about getting pregnant.

Of course I know you are looking forward to being a mother – and that happiness abounds when you even think about having a baby. But what I mean is to take those positive emotions and carry them over to how you feel about *getting pregnant* . This is important whether you are just starting on your road to conception, or particularly if you have been trying for a while and can't seem to make it happen.

Why does your attitude matter? In much the way that stress can impact the production of reproductive hormones, so can a negative state of mind. When you have negative thoughts, when you dwell on all the things that aren't going right in your life, when you focus on what you might not accomplish or what you don't have, you affect your brain chemistry in a negative way. While the effects on your reproductive hormones aren't quite as profound as when you are under extreme stress, still, I believe that over time it does make an important difference.

As you go through the remainder of this book, you will find that at least some of the suggestions I make may involve changes in your life and your lifestyle . In some instances you may find yourself giving up life long habits or changing your diet in a way that may exclude or reduce your intake of some of your favorite foods. Whatever the case is, make sure that whatever changes you do make to increase your fertility are viewed in a positive light. If you feel a sense of deprivation or resentment about the changes you make, the enhancements won't have quite the same level of positive effect. They can still help, of course, but the results might not be as quick or as fruitful.

The point I really want to emphasize is that it's not just stressful emotions that can disrupt your fertility, but also, that thinking happy, positive thoughts about getting pregnant can enhance your chances of a faster, easier, and perhaps even a healthier pregnancy.

So even during your most stressful moments, whether they are caused by situations under your control or not, it's important that you put a barrier between your negative thoughts and your goal of getting pregnant. When it comes to conception remain as positive as you can – and that goes for the way you relate to your partner as well. Too many times I have seen couples turn on each other – rather than *to each other* – as soon as conception problems arise. They start out blaming themselves, but then quickly progress to blaming each other – and the stress that this can cause only takes them farther from their parenting dreams.

So my advice to you is to not just relax more and try to control your stress, but also to let the loving feelings you and your partner have for each other prevail – both in the bedroom and out of the bedroom! Be kind to each other and make this goal of having a baby a loving adventure that brings smiles to your lips and a warm glow to your hearts– no matter what the circumstances may be.

By remaining positive about your decision to start or continue your family, and remaining joyously hopeful about your ability to do so will, I promise you, boost your fertility and bring you both that much closer to realizing your parenting dreams.

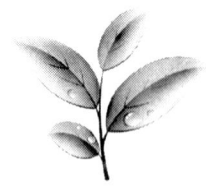

Chapter Seven

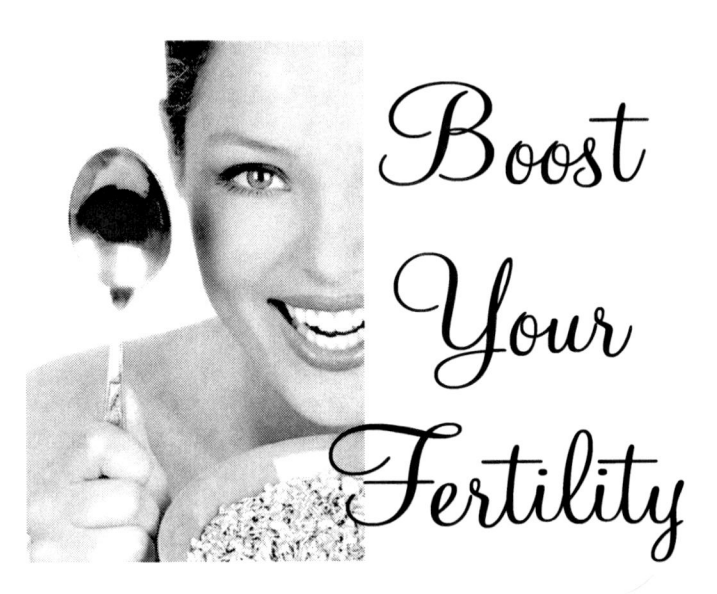

Boost Your Fertility
With Foods That Make A Difference!

It's hard to open a magazine or go online and not see a story about diet! Indeed, everywhere we look food seems to play an increasingly important role in our health – and I'm not just talking about weight control.

In fact, it seems like that coy old adage "You are what you eat" is coming true in more ways than one.

Over the past decade, and particularly in the last several years researchers have discovered a multitude of ways in which what you eat – and sometimes what you don't put on your dinner plate – can play an enormous role in everything from preventing heart disease and diabetes, to reducing blood pressure, sometimes even protecting you from cancer. Research shows there may even be links between diet and the prevention of certain auto immune diseases most likely to impact women, including multiple sclerosis, Lupus and fibromyalgia.

And now I am happy to tell you that in the last several years science has also added boosting fertility to that list of "food miracles". Today we have the medical studies to prove what I, and many of my colleagues all around the globe have believed for decades: What you eat – and what you avoid eating – can make a huge difference in how quickly and easily you get pregnant. For some of you reading this book, your diet – and the nutrients you consume every day – may even be the deciding factor that ultimately makes your dreams of motherhood come true!

Having grown up and received my medical training in Denmark and other European countries - where natural treatments have always prevailed - I have seen firsthand the powerful difference that diet can make in the health of my patients and their families. In fact I have long believed that counseling my fertility and obstetrical patients on the importance of eating healthy is one of the most beneficial pieces of "medical" advice I can offer them.

But there's even more to this concept than just eating healthy. Throughout years of experience working with infertility patients I also came to see that certain types of diets, and even more specifically, certain types of foods, appear to have a *direct impact on getting pregnant* – in not only women, but also men. Remember, while your baby will be conceived, nourished and grow inside your body, one half of the success of your pregnancy is still linked to your partner, and in particular the health of his sperm.

So it's important to realize that it's not just your pre-conception diet that matters, but *his* as well. And later in this book you'll learn about some important things your partner can do – and the foods he should eat – to encourage the healthiest sperm possible.

But what's also important to remember is that it's not just what you and your partner eat that matters, it's also what you avoid eating that makes a difference as well. Indeed, the foods that you leave off your pantry shelves can be as important as the foods you include. While the research in this area has been a little less publicized, I can tell you without hesitation that there are certain common and popular foods that can quickly and easily derail your fertility – and make it much harder for you to get pregnant, even when your reproductive system is healthy and free of problems.

The bottom line: Food can be your fertility's best ally – or its worst enemy - but most important, you have the power to choose!

But how do you start to make these choices? It begins with understanding a little something about the three main food groups – carbohydrates, proteins and fats – and how they act and interact with your reproductive system and with each other, to help encourage a quick and easy pregnancy.

COMFORT "CARBS" AND GETTING PREGNANT

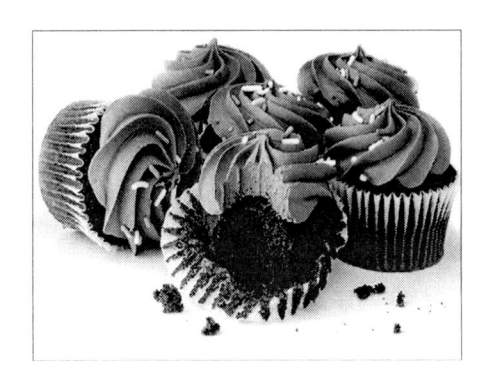

If you're like most of my patients, it's highly likely that in the days just prior to your menstrual cycle food takes on a much more important meaning! I'm talking about food cravings – and for many women goodies like chocolate, pasta and bags of chips rank high on that must-have pre-menstrual list.

Well the fact that you do crave them is no accident. The reason? Most pre-menstrual snack cravings fall into just a single food-group known as carbohydrates. And, in fact, the carb cravings you have during your "time of the month" – when reproductive hormones are raging - is the first clue that they may somehow be tied in to getting pregnant. And in fact they are.

But if you're thinking that all you need do is load up on carbs to help you get pregnant, it's time to put down that fork and listen up: While some carbohydrates can definitely encourage your chances of conceiving, others can hamper or even block conception efforts. Discovering which carbs fall on which side of the fertility fence is the first step in creating a food plan that will enhance your chances of getting pregnant.

CARBOHYDRATES AND CONCEPTION: WHAT YOU MUST KNOW

When most of you hear the word "carbohydrates" I'd bet that that the foods which come to mind are the yummy items in this category - "comfort" carbs like bread, pasta, cake, cookies and chips, as well as sugary foods such as chocolate bars and other types of candy or soft drinks.

As a whole, these types of "comfort foods" fall under the heading of "simple carbs" – called so because once ingested they quickly breakdown into sugars which are then rapidly released into your bloodstream. You may have also heard these types of carbohydrates referred to as foods with a 'high glycemic load". In simple terms this means they have the capacity to release lots of sugar into the bloodstream at a fairly rapid rate.

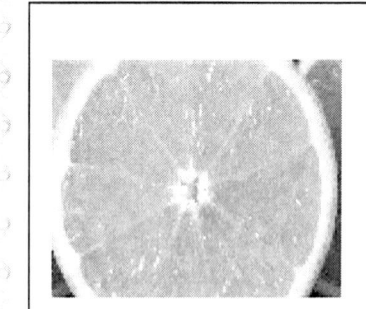

> *Fresh fruits and vegetables along with whole grains such as wheat, oats and rye are all complex carbohydrates – one food group that is especially important for boosting fertility!*

But while these carbohydrates may be the ones you are most familiar with, it's important to remember they make up only one-half of the carbohydrate story. Because this food group also includes fruits, vegetables, and whole grains such as wheat, oats and rye. Together these foods are known as "complex carbohydrates" – so named because digestion takes longer *and* because the end result is a slow release of sugar into the bloodstream. Because that release is slow these foods are known to have a "low glycemic load" - or more simply put, they digest much more slowly, therefore they do not release a lot of sugar at once. And that in turn helps you maintain a steady sugar level.

So what does all this have to do with getting pregnant? Many believe that the way in which your body metabolizes the "sugar load" related to simple carbohydrate consumption can impact at least some of the hormonal activity necessary for getting pregnant. How does this occur?

It all begins with a hormone known as "insulin". Secreted after every meal by your pancreas (an organ that sits smack in the middle of your abdomen), insulin is a hormone that helps clear sugar from your blood and hustle it into your cells where it is converted into energy.

In fact, insulin acts like a sort of "door knocker" that tells cells to "open up" and let the sugars in. Because "simple" or "quick burning" carbohydrates - like white bread, cake or cookies - are quickly converted into sugars, your body must quickly produce a significant amount of insulin in order to begin that "door knocking" process and get the sugar out of your blood and into your cells. When your intake of these foods is small – or you eat them only occasionally –these quick releases of insulin don't have any lasting negative effects.

Over time, however, eating a diet high in these "quick burning " or "simple" carbohydrates can begin to change the entire insulin clearing process. Indeed the more often your cells are bombarded with insulin's "knock", the less responsive they get. And the less responsive they get, the more insulin that is required to get those cells to "open up" so that the sugar can be cleared from the blood. This condition is known as "insulin resistance" - and it is here where the impact on your fertility really begins.

More specifically, because insulin is a hormone, its production and release is part of a network of finely tuned and balanced hormonal activity, at least some of which is involved in egg production and release. So, when your body is continually forced to produce a lot of insulin - as is the case when your diet is high in simple carbohydrates - other hormones affected by insulin levels also go out of balance.

Over time, the entire hormonal network necessary for conception can become disrupted – and it occurs in a number of key ways. Among the most important, however - at least in terms of your fertility - is an increase in the production of androgens - male hormones such as testosterone.

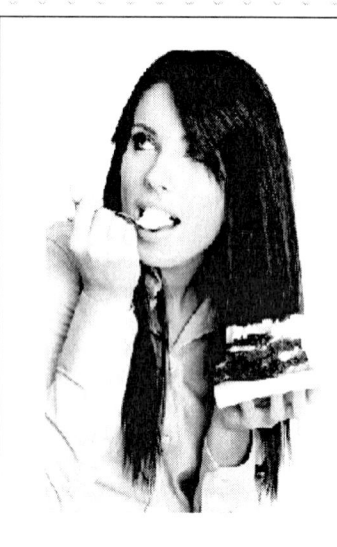

> *In one Harvard University study doctors found that women who consumed a diet high in "simple" carbohydrates – like cake, cookies and white bread – were 92% more likely to have fertility problems – and a harder time getting pregnant!*

Normally, testosterone is produced by your ovaries, but in a very tiny amount. It's both advantageous and necessary – *in this small amount.* However, when insulin levels are consistently high, it sends a message to the ovaries to step up testosterone production – and in turn slow down or even stoop producing estrogen. Once this happens, it dramatically affects both your ability to make a healthy egg, or to release - or ovulate - any eggs you do make.

Eventually, if left to continue long enough – some women may stop ovulating completely. This is often the case for those who develop an insulin-related fertility-robbing condition known as PCOS or Poly Cystic Ovarian Syndrome, a problem you'll learn more about later in this book.

But even if you don't have PCOS, eating a diet high in simple carbohydrates can still cause enough of an impact on your body so that eventually your fertility is affected. Not only will it be harder to get pregnant, but if left to go on long enough, without treatment it can become impossible.

And in fact, this is exactly what a group of Harvard researchers recently discovered when they analyzed data from the massive, nationwide Nurses Study – a research project involving over 18,000 women.

What the Harvard group found: Women who consume a diet high in quick-burning "simple" carbohydrates, are a whopping 92 percent more likely to experience ovulatory – related infertility problems then women who eat less of these foods! Indeed, in many instances, continually snacking on products made from white flour - including bread, cake, and cookies, or eating a lot of white potatoes and white rice actually blocked fertility and kept these women from getting pregnant. And this finding held true even after they factored in the effects of age, smoking and consumption of animal fat – another food type related to fertility that we'll discuss in a few moments.

THE CARBOHYDRATES THAT CAN HELP YOU GET PREGNANT

So, by now you might be thinking that the way to get pregnant fast is to simply *stop* eating all carbohydrates - no matter your food cravings. But that would be wrong! Because what researchers also discovered is that some carbohydrates are definitely necessary to promote fertility – and some can even help you get pregnant faster!

Remember you read earlier that not all carbohydrates are alike? Indeed, the Nurses' Health Study also found that women who ate diets high in "complex carbohydrates" – including fruits, vegetables, and whole grains - were actually able to *decrease* their risk of ovulatory-related problems and get pregnant faster and easier.

This finding dovetails perfectly with previous research showing that most slow burning carbohydrates are also high in fiber - an important non-nutritive compound that not only helps keep blood sugar balanced, but also works to pull heart-harming cholesterol from your blood. Indeed, the American Dietetic Association has confirmed that fiber is an essential element for controlling blood sugar as well as helping to control weight – two factors that also play an important role in getting pregnant.

So, while it's clear that your body – and your fertility - need carbohydrates in order to function properly, by reducing your intake of simple carbohydrates (like white rice, potatoes, and anything made from white flour or sugar) and loading up on complex carbohydrates (like whole grain cereals, and plenty of fruits and vegetables) you can optimize your fertility and increase your chances of getting pregnant quicker and easier. Not coincidentally, the same foods that are good for fertility are also good for your heart – and may help you to live a longer and healthier life!

Your Fertility Prescription: The Carbohydrates That Can Help You Get Pregnant

So what carbs should you eat to boost your fertility – and which ones should you avoid? Here's a quick summary guide to help you make your choices!

The Good Carbs To Eat:
Whole grain bread; whole grain pasta; spelt (a grain) ; oatmeal; buckwheat; barley; brown rice; whole grain cereals like Cheerios, Special K, Complete or Total; apples, apricots, blueberries; cantaloupe; grapefruit; strawberries; cabbage, broccoli; cauliflower; yams; pumpkin; soy beans; lupin; tomatoes.

The Carbs To Reduce or Avoid:
Cake; candy; soda; anything sweetened with high fructose corn syrup; cupcakes; French fries; donuts; white bread; white rice; mashed, boiled or baked white potatoes (cold potato salad is okay in moderation); fruit juices; sweetened cereals; rolls; pies; potato chips; pretzels.

For a more complete list of both good carbs and bad ones, plus other dietary factors to consider in each of these foods, please see my book Eat, Love, Get Pregnant! which is loaded with over 200 foods that can increase your fertility and help you get pregnant.

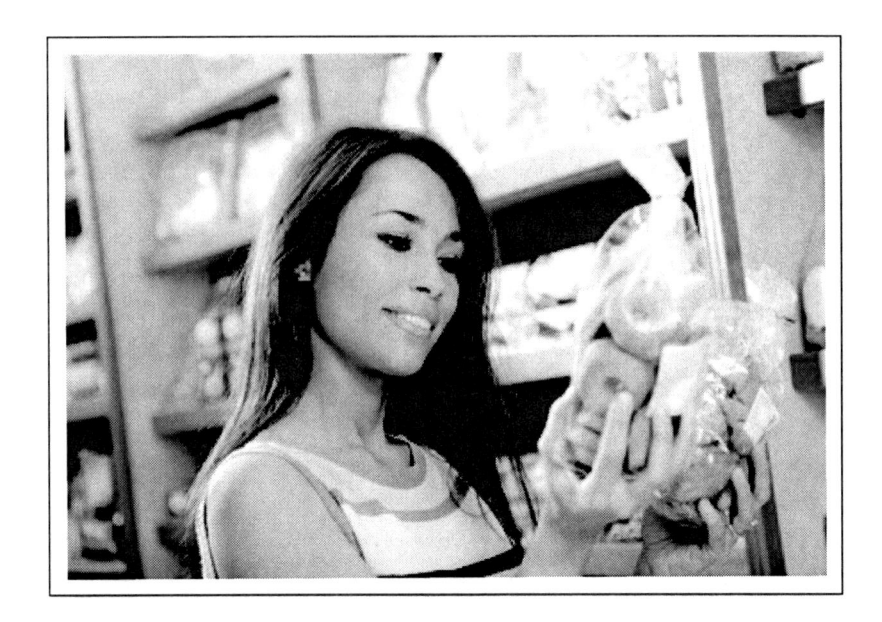

THE HIDDEN FOOD ALLERGY
THAT CAUSES INFERTILITY

If you and your partner are one of millions of couples worldwide grappling with a diagnosis of "unexplained Infertility" then you already know how frustrating this condition can be. While doctors are quick to pinpoint that "something " is wrong - they seldom can tell you what, or what can specifically help you to get pregnant.

Now, however, a growing body of evidence has begun to shed light on a new diagnosis of unexplained infertility - and one that just might put you on the fast track to conception.

The problem is celiac disease - sometimes referred to as a "gluten allergy". While once thought to be a rare, inherited genetic condition, it is now been believed to affect over 2 million people in the United State alone - and many more may be undiagnosed.

"Approximately 3 million suffer needlessly, undiagnosed with this condition - most never realizing that a change in diet could change their life ", said Alice Bast, Executive Director of the National Foundation for Celiac Awareness in a recent interview.

Of those couples affected by unexplained infertility, *we now know that for almost half,* gluten allergy may be the cause or a significant contributing factor.

And while for some of you the symptoms are easy to recognize - including a history of gastrointestinal upsets, diarrhea, gas and bloating), for many others signs are much more vague, making the condition much harder to recognize. Indeed, problems can be as diverse as headaches, joint pain, "brain fog", fatigue, loss of energy, irregular menstrual cycles, anemia, and in many instances, unexplained infertility.

According to the National Foundation for Celiac Awareness, on average it can take 10 years - or sometimes more - for people to get the correct diagnosis.

Understanding The Links Between Diet, Celiac disease & Infertility

In order to absorb nutrients from food, your intestines come equipped with tiny hair-like projections called villi. Think of these as tiny pond-fronds moving back and forth, helping to pull the nutrients from foods and send them into your blood stream.

In those who have celiac disease, eating products rich in gluten (a type of protein commonly found in rye, wheat and barley) ignites an immunologic firestorm that causes the body to produce toxins. It is these toxins that damage the villi, causing them to lie flat. When this happens nutrients are not properly absorbed - including those from proteins, carbohydrates, and fats, as well as vitamins and minerals and in some cases even water and bile salts.

But that's not the only problem that occurs. Increasingly research suggests these same toxins create body-wide inflammation capable of affecting your health from head to toe - **including your fertility.**

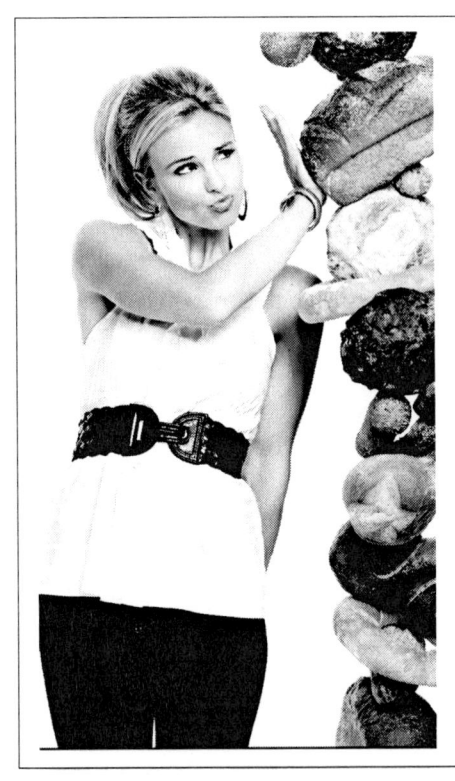

> "THE VIEW" co-host Elisabeth Hasselbeck is one of millions of women diagnosed with celiac disease. Hasselbeck discovered her problem when she was unable to get pregnant! Once she went on a gluten-free diet, not only did her symptoms clear, but she was able to quickly and easily conceive!
> Read more about her story in her book, "The G Free Diet".

- Researchers at Molinette Hospital in Turin Italy report that early findings of a study of women with celiac disease indicate the rate of "unexplained infertility could be as much as 3.5% higher than in the general population. They also suggest celiac disease increases the risk of miscarriage and low birth weight babies.
- Doctors from Tampere University Hospital and Medical School at the University of Tampere, in Finland found that the rate of celiac disease among women reporting infertility was 4.1%.
- In a study conducted by physicians at Thomas Jefferson University Hospital in Philadelphia doctors found that the rate of recurring pregnancy loss is four times higher in women with celiac disease.
- In a meta-analysis study conducted jointly by doctors at the Technion School of Medicine in Haifa, Israel and St. Luke's Roosevelt Medical Center in New York City, doctors concluded that not only is there a strong association between celiac disease and infertility, it also remains a condition continually overlooked by many obstetricians and even fertility doctors.

Indeed, while it may be easy to see how this condition can impact your stomach health, the links to fertility as well as miscarriage are a bit less obvious.

Still, many doctors believe the immune responses linked to Celiac disease, including the production of toxins, have a detrimental affect on the menstrual cycle and disrupt ovulation. How does this occur?

Celiac expert Dr. Alex Shikhman believes it may be through the increased production of a hormone known as prolactin.

" Studies show that when women sensitive to gluten eat this protein, it typically causes an upswing in the production of prolactin," says Shikhman, director of the Institute for Specialized Medicine in Del Mar, California.

Produced by the pituitary gland, and secreted in small amounts in both men and women, prolactin is the hormone that naturally increases during pregnancy in order to help prepare your body for breastfeeding. But it also does something else: In high amounts prolactin can turn off production of brain chemicals linked to both egg production and release. These include FSH, which stimulates eggs to grow, and LH, which prompts ovulation. In fact, one of the reasons most women don't get pregnant while they are breastfeeding is because high levels of prolactin keep them ovulating.

At the same time, however, if you want to get pregnant, the production of FSH and LH is critical. So it's easy to see how high prolactin levels can keep you from conceiving.

But I believe it's not just high prolactin levels, which contribute to gluten-related infertility. Since the very nature of a gluten allergy means that you are absorbing far less nutrients from your foods and even your vitamin supplements, I also believe this condition can lead to a deficiency of factors that I know are essential to getting pregnant - particularly the B vitamins, plus vitamins C, D and A, as well as minerals like calcium and iron.

In fact, as you will discover over the next few chapters, whenever any of these nutrients are in short supply getting pregnant can be much more difficult. As such,

> ## Male Fertility Affected By Gluten Foods Too!
>
> It's important to note that it's not just female fertility that's affected by a reaction to gluten. Studies show it can also affect men increasing the production of defective sperm making it much more difficult to conceive.

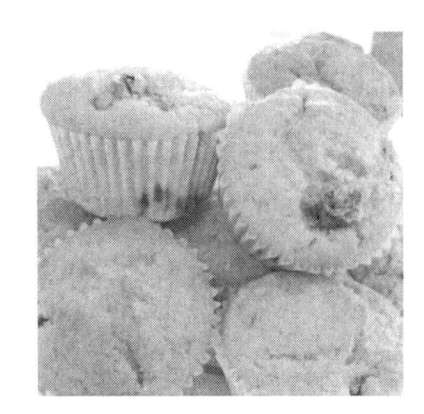

any problems that cause a decrease in nutrients, including irritable bowel syndrome or a poor diet, can be a factor in unexplained infertility - but certainly a gluten intolerance is one major cause of these problems.

Moreover, Dr. Shikhman has been gathering data suggesting there may be a link between gluten allergy and endometriosis, the menstrual related disorder that is also a leading cause of infertility in young women. (See Chapter 16). According to his preliminary research, when caught in its earliest stages, mild endometriosis responds to a gluten-free diet - meaning that not only does the endometriosis clear, but so do the related fertility problems.

Additionally, it's important to point out that it's not just women who can be affected by a gluten allergy or sensitivity. Indeed, some studies show that men who are sensitive to gluten also experience problems with sperm production - including producing sperm that are misshapen or in other ways defective. And this too can often contribute to a couple's diagnosis of unexplained infertility.

Diet And Recurring Miscarriage

In addition to making it harder to get pregnant, if you do happen to conceive, celiac disease can also increase your risk of recurring or chronic miscarriage. How does this occur?

One theory links the problem to a blood protein known as antiphospholipid antibodies. Normally, the membranes of all your cells contain molecules called phospholipids. Some of these molecules contain a glue-like substance that actually helps the cells of your placenta (the sac that surrounds and nourishes your baby in the womb) to fuse together and grow. When the body produces antibodies to phospholipids, it causes tiny blood clots to form within the placenta, thus blocking nutrients from reaching your baby. When your baby can't be nourished, growth and development can become so restricted, a miscarriage results.

In women who have Celiac disease, Dr. Shikhman says the production of these antibodies can soar - along with the risk of miscarriage.

"There is a very strong link between antiphospholipid antibody syndrome and gluten intolerance - and consequently, an increased risk of miscarriage," he says.

Moreover, when a mother has poor nutrition, before and right after conception, studies show that the risk of miscarriage increases. As such, it stands to reason that if you are not absorbing the proper amounts of nutrients from your foods or your prenatal vitamins, then your baby will not be receiving the proper nourishment necessary to survive and thrive. So even without the antiphospholipid antibody syndrome, still, your risk of miscarriage would naturally increase.

What Causes A Celiac Disease?

While the exact cause of celiac disease is not known, it is considered an autoimmune disease, a condition wherein your body's immune system attacks it own tissue. And, it can also be hereditary. About 1 in 133 Americans have the condition, but that number rises to 1 in 22 for if you have a family member who is also affected. But just having the gene isn't enough to cause you to develop the problem. Indeed, it is only when factors in your life and your lifestyle come together with your genetic history that the condition takes hold.

For reasons we don't yet understand, problems can arise after a health trauma, such as an infection or injury, or sometimes, after pregnancy, or after a surgery. That said, the disease would not appear until gluten is consumed.

For many men and women the signs and symptoms of celiac disease are easy to spot: You simply don't feel well after eating foods that contain wheat, rye, or barley - such as breads , cereal, or pasta. Problems can include bloating, gas, diarrhea, and other gastrointestinal upsets that are had to miss.

Unfortunately , however, too many doctors still misdiagnose this condition, instead labeling these patients as having irritable bowel syndrome (IBS), an entirely different condition requiring altogether different treatment.

But this condition is also misdiagnosed for another reason: Sometimes the telltale gastrointestinal symptoms can be minor or even non-existent. Instead, other symptoms move to the forefront, some of them quite diverse. These can include: unexplained weight loss or gain; unexplained iron deficiency or anemia ; vitamin K deficiency ; bone or joint pain ; depression or anxiety; fatigue, weakness, or loss of energy; irregular menstrual cycles.; canker sores in the mouth; blistery, itchy skin rashes; tooth discoloration or loss of enamel; unexplained infertility; chronic miscarriage.

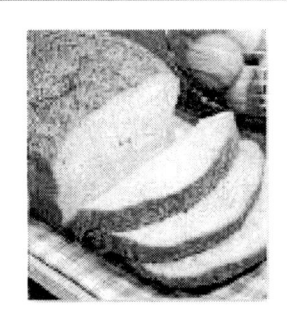

> **Q:** *Is there a difference between celiac disease, wheat allergy & gluten intolerance - or are they all the same thing?*
>
> **A:** Though the terms are often used interchangeably, they are different conditions. Celiac disease is an autoimmune disorder wherein the body's immune system attacks normal intestinal tissue, in response to eating gluten. Because of this, people with celiac disease are at risk for mal absorption of food in the GI tract, causing the nutritional deficiencies & other snafus related to infertility. A wheat allergy or a gluten intolerance are not auto immune diseases, and as such do not put you in the same risk category for infertility.

Do You Have A Gluten Problem : How To Tell

If, in fact, you do have any of the symptoms just mentioned, and particularly if you have more than one, then I recommend that you speak to your doctor about the following blood tests used to diagnose celiac disease:

* Total IgA
* IgA anti-tissue transglutaminase (tTG)
* IgA antiendomysial antibody immunofluorescence (EMA)

If IgA is deficient, the tTG test should also be ordered. At the discretion of the doctor, antigliaden IgG may also help nail down the problem.

Depending on the results of these tests your doctor may also order a biopsy of your stomach lining to know for certain if gluten sensitivity is your problem.

IMPORTANT TO NOTE: You must be eating gluten foods at the time of your testing in order to get the proper diagnosis. So, if you believe you may have issues with gluten and want to be tested, don't change your diet until after the tests are done.

The longer you have been living with celiac disease, and the degree to which you are affected, can make a huge difference in terms of how long it may take to heal your intestines, get your villi "back on their feet" and your nutrient absorption profile back to normal. For some it may be only a matter of months, for others it could take several years before a complete healing occurs.

THE GOOD NEWS: If it turns out you are gluten -sensitive, as soon as you eliminate these foods from your diet, the healing process begins almost immediately. And this means that every day you stay away from these foods you are one step closer to getting pregnant! In fact, studies show that for many women there can be a remarkable turn around in just a few months time.

Indeed, with an increased ability to absorb nutrients, and the reduction of inflammation caused by the toxic reaction to gluten, experts say that for many couples, unexplained infertility all but disappears! For women who are having repeated miscarriages, a healthy pregnancy is often eminent once these gluten-rich foods are eliminated.

What's key to remember, however, is that diet IS the only cure for celiac disease. Moreover, there is no such thing as "cutting down" or eating " just a little". Indeed, when this condition exists, even the smallest amount of gluten is enough to kick start the inflammatory process and begin the production of toxins that not only harm your health, but also your fertility.

Once diagnosed, there are many books that can help you plan your diet. If you visit GreenFertility.com we'll help you find the best places to buy gluten-free foods - even online! While eating out can be more of a challenge, it can be easy if you stick to natural whole foods like fresh meats, fruits and vegetables.

FIND THE HIDDEN SOURCES OF GLUTEN IN YOUR DIET !

To help you get started in hunting down some of the "hidden" sources of gluten in your diet, what follows is a partial list of where to look. Remember, even in small amounts gluten can be harmful, so if you are diagnosed with this condition, you must read all food labels!

* Breads, crackers, cookies, cakes, pie crust and pizza crust, cereal, pasta or macaroni made from wheat, rye or barley.
* Prepared foods such as frozen dinners, French fries, rice mixes
* Lunch meats, frankfurters, sausages, egg substitutes.)
* Canned soups, broths and soup mixes
* Vegetables in sauce, creamed vegetables, breaded vegetables, some baked beans and some prepared vegetables and salads.
* Malted milk, cocoa mixes, some chocolate milk, nondairy creamers, some flavored coffee and some herbal tea.
* Some alcoholic drinks such as ale, beer, gin and whiskey
* Some flavored yogurts, frozen yogurts and ice creams
* Some processed cheeses such as bleu, stilton, Roquefort and gorgonzola
* Fats found in some commercial salad dressings, wheat germ oil and many commercial gravies and sauces
* Candy bars or candies which are dusted with wheat flour; butterscotch chips, licorice and flavored syrups
* Dried fruits dusted with wheat flour, some prepared fruits and pie fillings
* Flavorings such as curry powder, meat sauces, ketchup, mustard, horseradish, chip dips, most soy sauce, some distilled white vinegar, some cinnamon, some salad dressings, flavoring extracts, seasoning mixes, and bouillon .

It is also important to note than gluten is found in the communion wafers used during certain religious services.

Additionally, some vitamin pills and herbal supplements also use gluten as a binding agent, and you may even find it in some lipsticks, postage stamps and adhesive used on envelopes.

Ingredients which are actually "gluten" in disguise include: Bulgur, Bran, Brown rice syrup, Durum, Farina, Graham, hydrolyzed vegetable protein, Kaska, Kamut, Kasha, Malt extract or flavorings, Malt vinegar, Matzo meal, Oat gum, Semolina, Spelt, Teff, Triticale.

Additionally, some people with gluten intolerance also cannot tolerate oats, while others have no reaction to this grain . Currently research is underway to determine how oats are likely to affect individuals with gluten intolerance. Until more conclusive information is available, experts at the National Institutes of Health suggest folks with gluten allergies should also avoid eating oats and products made from oats unless their physician has instructed them otherwise.

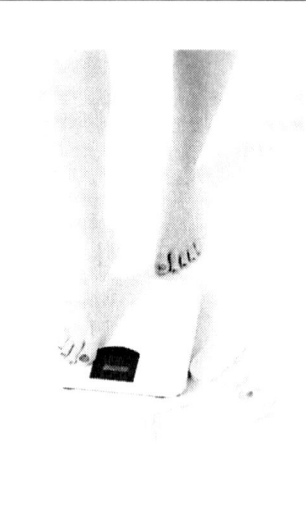

Weight Loss Bonus!

In addition to being a factor in infertility, for many women with undiagnosed celiac disease losing weight can be very difficult. The good news: Once you start your gluten-free diet you may lose weight quicker and easier - & that can boost your fertility!

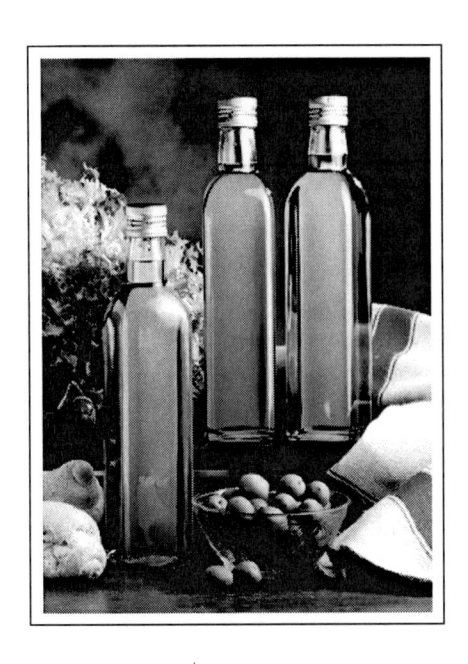

The Secret Is Out: Fats Help Fertility!

Once upon a time – in the *not too distant past* – fat was the enemy! And I'm not just talking about body fat, but *dietary fat* – all those juicy burgers and plates of French fries, each loaded with not only lots of fat grams, but also lots of calories!

Indeed, over the past decade we have come to see that foods high in fat are intimately linked to a variety of illnesses, including high blood pressure, an increased risk of stroke and an increased risk of heart disease, and possibly some cancers.

And certainly we know that fatty foods have a reputation for making us put on the pounds quickly – another link to all these diseases.

But one of the most important facts that has come to light over recent years is that much like carbohydrates, not all fats are alike! While some are clearly bad for your health – and super bad for your fertility - others can improve your overall health, decrease your risk of disease, even help you get pregnant. And these are the "good fats" I want to tell you a little something about right now!

The Good Fats That Help You Get Pregnant Faster!

While not all fats all created equal, when it comes to the "good" fertility fats, those at the very top of the list are known as MUFAs – short for mono-unsaturated fats. Derived from sources such as olives, nuts and fruits like avocados, these fats help the body to function more healthfully, including decreasing some of the effects of "bad fats", such as high cholesterol. In addition, when paired with a number of fertility nutrients – which you'll learn about in the next chapter – these "healthy fats" work even better to stabilize blood sugar levels and in the process normalize the hormone functions necessary for optimum fertility.

Moreover, there is good evidence to show that replacing saturated fats – like the kind found in red meat, for example - with mono-unsaturated fats from vegetables - will not only help you to lose weight, but from a fertility standpoint, will also help you get pregnant.

How? The "good fats" work primarily by decreasing the power of inflammatory compounds that would otherwise harm your fertility. Not only do they reduce their risks, but on their own these anti-inflammatory "good fats" work to protect you against a host of inflammatory conditions that work to harm fertility, such as endometriosis. Examples of the MUFA "good fats" that can help you get pregnant include: Olive oil; grape seed oil; canola oil; walnut oil and mayonnaise made with any of these oils.

> Omega -3 fatty acids are among the most important fertility nutrients you can eat! Find them in foods like salmon and tuna, walnuts, flax seeds, or foods fortified with DHA.

But MUFAs are not alone on the healthy pantry shelf. Right alongside them are another group of healthy fats known as PUFAs – short for polyunsaturated fats. Among this group are what are known as "essential fatty acids" or EFAs - key factors necessary to maintain healthy cells throughout your body. In fact, EFAs play an even more vital role in your overall good health and your fertility by directly impacting the production of hormone-like compounds that help to regulate blood pressure, blood clotting, and blood fats, as well as insulin production.

Most important – at least in terms of your fertility – are two particular EFAs known as Omega-3 and Omega-6. What's particularly important about these two compounds is that while they are essential to your health, they are the only two essential fatty acids that your body *cannot manufacture on its own* - you need to get them from foods or supplements. And, you need them to get pregnant!

OMEGA - 3 : THE SUPER SONIC ANTI-INFLAMMATORY FERTILITY BOOSTER

While both Omega-3 and Omega-6 are important, when it comes to boosting fertility, it is Omega-3 fatty acids that hold the most significance. In particular it is two specific Omega-3 fatty acids - compounds known as eicosapentaenoic acid (EPA) and docosahexaenoic acid (DHA) – that can make the biggest dietary difference in how quickly you get pregnant.

Found in foods such as cold water fish, flax seeds and walnuts, these compounds appear to have a direct impact on ovulation, as well as working hard to protect you from the fertility robbing effects of a high carbohydrate diet and in particular, insulin resistance.

While this is significant for all women, it is vitally important if you have been diagnosed with PCOS. Indeed, in one study published in the *Journal of Clinical Endocrinology and Metabolism* in 2004 researchers found that simply adding more Omega-3 to the daily diet had enough of an impact on hormonal production to kick start ovulation in women with PCOS who were not ovulating at all! Other research has shown these essential fatty acids can have powerful anti-inflammatory effects on endometriosis – and in the process help reverse many of its fertility-robbing effects.

But it's not just women with these specific conditions who can benefit from these powerful natural compounds. Indeed, studies have shown that Omega-3 fatty acids can encourage conception in every woman, primarily by reducing the inflammation that frequently leads to fertility-disrupting hormone imbalances.

Once you are pregnant, Omega-3 fatty acids kick in immediately, helping to promote your baby's growth and development by increasing blood flow to the placenta - the sac that protects and nourishes the embryo in your womb.

Moreover, a diet rich in Omega-3 fatty acids both before and after you get pregnant can help reduce your risk of premature birth, and may help you avoid pre eclampsia (a dangerous rise in blood pressure that can occur during pregnancy) as well as post partum depression. According to research published in the *Journal of the American Dietetic Association*, eating foods rich in Omega-3 during pregnancy can also reduce the risk of gestational diabetes. And if that were not enough to convince you to add these healthful foods to your diet, studies also show moms who consume lots of heart-healthy Omega-3 foods before and during pregnancy may give birth to a smarter baby - with all indications that this compound contributes to brain development in the womb and encourages a higher level of intelligence later in life!

KEEP THE BALANCE AND GET PREGNANT FASTER!

As important as Omega-3 is to your health and your fertility, you'll derive the most benefits when you combine the nutrient in this group in the proper balance with foods containing Omega-6. Why does this matter?

First, Omega-6 fatty acids also possess powerful anti-inflammatory factors – compounds that also play an important role in getting pregnant. But the caveat here is that they only act as an anti-inflammatory when consumed in balance with Omega-3 fatty acids. Indeed, when the balance is off and your intake of Omega-3 is in short supply, then Omega-6 fatty acids actually become a *source* of inflammation in your body, interfering with both fertility and pregnancy, as well as increasing your risk of diabetes and heart disease.

Moreover, when your intake of Omega-6 rises too high – with no balance from Omega-3 - it promotes the formation of blood clots. This not only increases your risk of heart attack and stroke, but also your risk of early miscarriage. In fact I have seen a number of patients who, while believing they could not get pregnant, were actually conceiving, but losing their pregnancy very early on. For many, simply balancing their intake of Omega-3 and Omega-6 fatty acids helped them overcome early pregnancy loss and go on to deliver healthy babies.

In fact, the very latest research shows that the most promising health effects of essential fatty acids overall are achieved through a proper balance of Omega-3 and Omega-6. The ratio to shoot for is roughly four parts Omega-3 to one part Omega-6. While this may sound like it involves some complicated mathematics, it's really just a matter of eating a balanced, healthy diet! In my book *"Eat, Love, Get Pregnant"*, you will find a complete chart of over 100 of the most common foods scientifically proven to increase fertility, along with data on how each food stacks up in terms of Omega-3 and Omega-6 protection.

ONE FINAL CAUTION: KNOW YOUR OMEGA -3

While loading up your diet with foods rich in Omega-3 fatty acids in one way to help insure your fertility, finding the right sources is also important.

While fish remains the most potent and complete source, there are many foods which contain Omega-3 acids, as well, including walnuts, flax seed oil, and some mayonnaise brands. But nutritionist and dietitian Elizabeth Somer, RD says if you rely only on these forms of Omega-3, you might not be getting the benefits you need.

"What you get in foods like walnuts and flax seed oil is an Omega-3 acid known as ALA -- alpha-linoleic acid," says Somer. While it's good for your health, she says, to gain the full benefits of Omega-3 it requires the body to convert ALA to DHA – the kind of Omega-3 found helpful to fertility.

> *It's important to realize that not all Omega-3 sources are alike ...so choose wisely to get the best fertility result!*

The problem with the conversion, says Somer, is a variety of individual health factors, including our overall nutritional status, can sometimes hamper that process. So you might end up with less protection than you think you're getting - and maybe even more of an imbalance between Omega-3 and Omega-6 than you realize.

The good news: There is a variety of foods now available that are fortified with DHA so no conversion process is necessary! These include certain brands of eggs, egg whites, soy milk, whole wheat bread and cereal. To make sure you're getting a product fortified with not just Omega-3 but specifically DHA, read the label!

Also remember, you can take Omega-3 supplements, alone, or in conjunction with Omega-3 rich foods to ensure you are getting the right amount. A little later in this book you'll learn more about Omega-3 supplements –and how to use them to balance your intake of Omega-6 even if your diet is less than perfect!

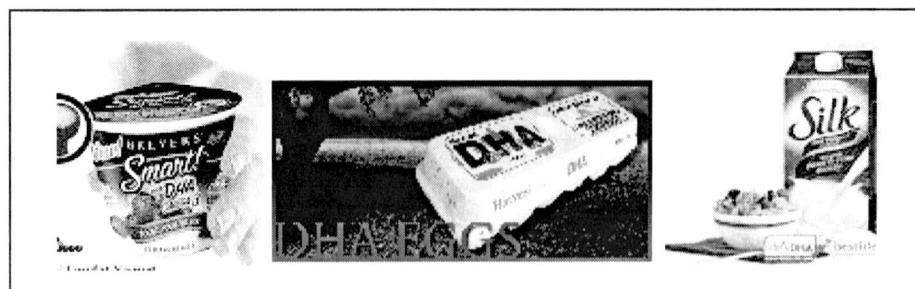

Today many products including some yogurts, eggs, soy milk, and mayonnaise are fortified with DHA – which means they can add to your daily requirement of essential fatty acids!

THE FATS THAT CAN HARM YOUR FERTILITY: WHAT YOU NEED TO KNOW

As you just read, there are certainly types of dietary fat that can make a huge difference in helping you get pregnant fast. But at the same time we discovered the power of "good fats" to enhance your fertility, we have also learned more about the fertility robbing effects of the "bad fats" - foods that are still considered to be the enemy when it comes to getting pregnant.

Among the most troubling of these enemy fats are known as *trans fats*. These are man-made compounds that occur during the conversion of a liquid oil into a solid shortening – the type used in many commercial baked goods and fast foods to extend their shelf life. The problem is that while these hybrid shortenings may extend the life of the foods on supermarket shelves, the trans fats that result do the opposite for those of us who consume these foods. In short, trans fats are now believed to be a direct link to heart disease, insulin resistance, type 2 diabetes – and now, infertility.

Indeed, in one study recently published in a leading nutrition journal researchers found that women whose diet included just four grams of trans fats per day had a whopping 93% increase in fertility-related ovulation problems.

How do trans fats harm your chances of getting pregnant? While no one knows for certain, many believe they incite inflammatory reactions within the body – a situation which not only impacts ovulation, but may even affect the health of your fallopian tubes. Trans fats also impact the way sugar is metabolized so, like quick-burning carbohydrates, they may play a role in exacerbating insulin sensitivity. As you read earlier this can impact ovarian function, and particularly egg production and release.

Moreover, my personal research and experience has shown that trans fats may also be a major contributing factor to the menstrual related disorder endometriosis – which, not coincidentally is also a leading cause of infertility, particularly among younger women. You'll learn more about this disorder – and the food and lifestyle factors that affect it - later in this book.

The good news: Whether you have endometriosis or not, by simply reducing your consumption of foods high in trans fat you can improve not just your fertility but your overall health - and get pregnant faster!

But the news gets even better: Today cutting trans fats from your diet is actually easier than ever thanks to some major changes within the food industry itself. Indeed, many companies are now making a real effort to cut the use of trans fats in food preparation, and many restaurants are cutting down or cutting out recipes that use ingredients containing trans fats.

In Denmark, where I grew up, the impact of dietary fat has always been a major concern – which is why I wasn't at all surprised to learn that in 2003 my home country became the first nation to ban completely the use of trans fats in any commercial food products.

Today, many countries and major cities, including New York City, which I have called home for over 40 years, have followed suit, instilling a similar ban on trans fats served in restaurant food. What's more, fast food chains like KFC, Taco Bell, Wendy's, Chili's and Starbucks have all announced efforts to eliminate or dramatically reduce trans fats in their products.

AVOIDING TRANS FATS: WHAT YOU CAN DO

Thanks in part to new FDA guidelines requiring food companies to list the amount of trans fat in every processed and packaged food, it's a lot easier to make healthy food choices. The new guidelines that quickly ratted out the "bad guys" now means there are fewer foods that are high in trans fat lurking on supermarket shelves. I predict that in years to come there will be fewer still – so making healthy choices will become even easier.

For right now, however, the best way to reduce your intake of trans fats is to simply read the labels of every packaged food you purchase and specifically look for the amount of trans fat listed, paying close attention to the correlation between the levels and the serving size.

Also important to remember: While many snacks and fast foods now boast they contain " NO TRANS FAT", legally this means they can still contain up to .5 or one-half gram of trans fats per serving. Since we all know that serving sizes are deceiving (studies show most of us automatically double the serving size, particularly when eating prepared foods), it's easy to see how you can easily consume four grams or more of trans fat a day, even if you think you aren't getting any! Add to this the foods that you know contain significant trans fats and you eat them anyway – such as French fries or a doughnut – and it's even easier to hit or even surpass that fertility-robbing four grams of trans fat a day and still believe you are eating healthy.

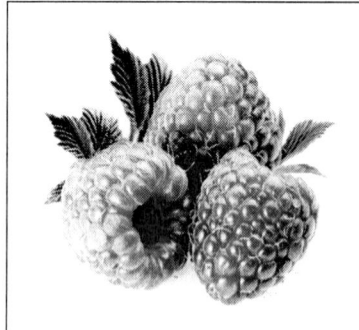

> *The easiest way to reduce the amount of trans fat in your diet is to cut down on packaged foods and eat fresh foods, particularly fruits & veggies. When dining out try to avoid fried foods and eat as many broiled or baked foods as you can!*

INFLAMMATORY FOODS: WHAT AFFECTS FERTILITY

As I explained to you earlier, one of the more outstanding health revelations of recent years has been the role that inflammation can play in so many different diseases, including not just heart disease, high blood pressure, diabetes and cancer, but also infertility.

Some of this inflammation comes from chemicals manufactured by fat cells in your body - but that's not the only source. We now know that certain foods also have the ability to create or exacerbate production of inflammatory chemicals as well. Perhaps more importantly, studies have also shown there are foods *with the power to calm down or neutralize inflammation* and maybe even undo some of the damage caused by the inflammation we've already experienced.

In fact, together, these *good* and *bad* foods form the *yin and yang* of good nutrition! And much like the Chinese concept that says we must balance our opposing forces of yin and yang energy in order to achieve optimum health, so too must we balance our diet by making certain to always eat enough anti-inflammatory foods to balance out the inflammatory factors in our body.

So how do you know which foods fall into which categories?

One method uses a rating system called the IFRS - short for Inflammatory Food Rating System. Developed by nutritionist Monica Reingold it classifies over 1500 of the most common foods according to their inflammatory potential. For those of you who are interested in learning more about this, I go into much more detail, and include the inflammatory ratings for the most common fertility foods, in my book *Eat, Love, Get Pregnant*.

But for right now it's important to note that in general foods high in animal fat, such as red meat and ham, and particularly those high in trans fats, which also includes most commercial baked goods, are believed to be high on the inflammatory scale and likely to encourage the production of chemicals that work against fertility. Meanwhile, "good fats" such as those from fish oil, flax, walnuts, and avocados are believed to have anti-inflammatory properties which can help encourage fertility and even undo some of the damage caused by a diet high in inflammatory foods.

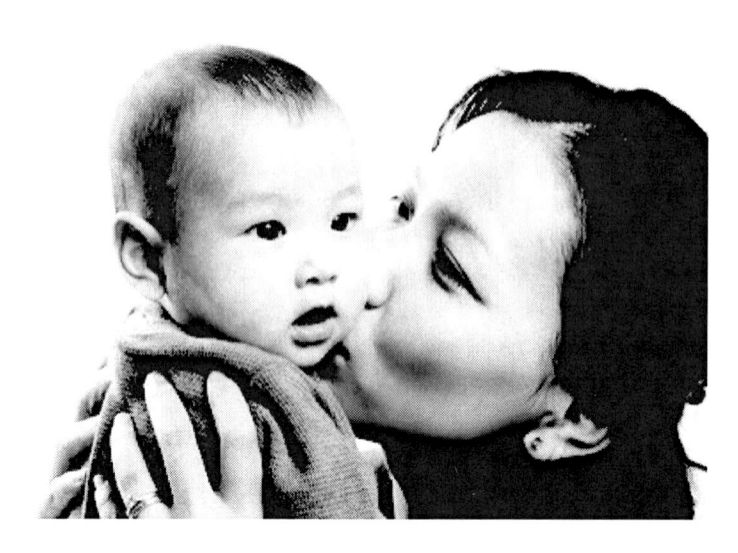

Anti Inflammatory Fertility Foods

Foods that are high in anti-inflammatory properties can help encourage your fertility while also helping to undo some of the damage caused by foods that are inflammatory.

The best anti-inflammatory foods are cold water fish such as salmon, tuna or mackerel, nuts such as walnuts, cashews and almonds, flax seeds, fruits such as avocados, cantaloupe and blueberries and vegetables such as kale, onions, and yams.

REDUCE JUST THIS ONE FAT – AND WATCH YOUR FERTILITY SOAR!

While avoiding trans fats is one way to get pregnant faster, studies also show that avoiding saturated fats is another way to boost your fertility. These are the mostly animal-based fats that come primarily from sources like red meat, processed foods, full fat dairy products, poultry skin and egg yolks. How can avoiding saturated fat help you get pregnant faster?

Much like trans fat, saturated fats can increase insulin resistance, making it harder for your body to clear sugar from your blood. But more than that, saturated fats can also increase the production of triglycerides, a byproduct of saturated fat that is stored in your cells after you eat that big juicy steak or steamy hamburger and fries. Besides increasing your risk of heart attack and stroke, triglycerides can also impact your pancreas, which is the organ that actually produces insulin. When your pancreas cells are affected, insulin production becomes erratic, and sugars can't be cleared as effectively from your blood. The end result is various types of hormone imbalances, including those that effect egg production and release.

Indeed, in one recent study published in the journal *Human Reproduction*, doctors suggested that a diet high in saturated fats can directly impact the production of key reproductive hormones, and slow down the overall functioning of the ovaries. There is also some evidence to show that these "bad fats" can reduce the number of egg follicles (the seeds from which your eggs are made) and also impact egg production and release, which is a common fertility problem for many women.

SATURATED FATS, PREGNANCY AND FERTILITY TREATMENTS

Of even greater concern: If you do manage to get pregnant while consuming a lot of these 'nasty' fats, your risk of developing gestational diabetes during your pregnancy also increases. Continue to eat these fats after your baby is born and you will find a decrease in the quality of your breast milk capable of adversely impacting your baby's development. Moreover, some very new and interesting research also published in the journal *Human Reproduction* suggests that the saturated fat you do eat may go directly to your eggs which in turn prevents them from being fertilized - even with the help of sophisticated fertility treatments such as IVF. Indeed, after analyzing eggs that failed to fertilize, the researchers found the majority contained higher-than-normal levels of saturated fat!

The good news however, is that by reducing your intake of "bad fats" and whenever possible replacing them with the "good fats" we talked about earlier, you can have your cake and eat it too – or , at least some of it!

EAT ICE CREAM AND GET PREGNANT FASTER: THE SURPRISING NEW FINDING ABOUT FAT AND FERTILITY!

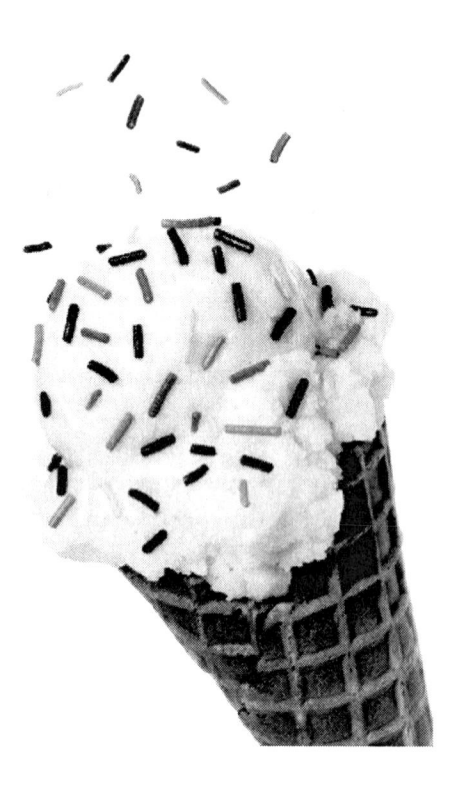

If you've ever been on a weight loss diet – or even thought about losing weight – then you know the importance of avoiding high fat dairy products. Indeed, items like whole milk, ice cream or full fat yogurt can really pack on the pounds!

Moreover, as you just read, high fat dairy foods are also high in saturated animal fat, which you now know can cause inflammatory reactions within the body that, for the most part, are bad for fertility.

This are all reasons researchers were so surprised to discover what I like to refer to as "The Ice Cream Paradox" - research which shows that high fat dairy products such as ice cream and whole milk appear to break the saturate fat rule by increasing fertility in some women. Indeed, as part of the recent Nurses Study data analyzed by Harvard researchers we learned that one or two daily servings of whole milk and foods made from whole milk— such as ice cream, full-fat yogurt, or cheese – appear to have some *protective* effects on ovulation. Ironically, the otherwise healthier skim and low fat milk products seemed to have the *opposite effect*.

Certainly, this contradicts not only common sense, but also current nutritional guidelines which tell us that foods high in animal fat are bad for our heart, blood pressure and yes, even our fertility. At the same time, however, when you look a little deeper at the differences between high and low fat dairy products, the Harvard findings begin to make a little more sense.

More specifically, estrogen and other reproductive hormones are stored in fat – not only in humans, but also in animals, particularly cows. So when milk – or milk byproducts such as ice cream or cheese – are fully fatted, they contain an abundance of these hormones.

But remove the fat from the milk – and the resulting milk products – and you no longer have these extra hormones. For older, post menopausal women this can be a good thing, since too much estrogen in the post menopausal years can increase the risk of certain cancers.

Today, however, a number of researchers believe that for some women in their *childbearing* years – particularly those with ovulatory problems or a natural estrogen deficiency - the extra hormone boost you get from high fat products may be helpful. This includes women who are very thin, or particularly those who exercise a great deal. As you read earlier, being too thin or working out too hard and too long can frequently disrupt estrogen production and make getting pregnant more difficult.

When an estrogen deficiency or ovulation problem does exist then the hormone boost from full-fat dairy products may be enough to tip the scales from infertile to fertile. According to the Harvard research, the high fat dairy products most likely to encourage conception include whole milk and ice cream. The foods most likely to have a negative impact on fertility for these women include sherbet, frozen yogurt and low fat yogurt, all of which appeared to *contribute* to ovulatory dysfunction – or at the very least did nothing to improve ovarian function.

What's more the finding was also dose-responsive: The more low fat dairy products a woman consumed, the more difficulty she had getting pregnant. Conversely, the more full-fat dairy products these woman consumed - to a point - the less likely they were to have problems conceiving.

WHO NEEDS ICE CREAM - WHO DOESN'T ?

Certainly this research is still considered preliminary. Moreover, remember that it applies only to women who are not making enough estrogen on their own – including those who may be underweight. And when this is the case, adding more whole milk and ice cream to your diet is something that may help you.

At the same time, if you are overweight, you may actually be producing too much estrogen, which can also contribute to a hormone imbalance linked to infertility. If this is the case, I believe increasing your intake of whole milk and ice cream could do you more harm than good.

The bottom line: If you are not overweight and want to try high fat dairy products as a way to encourage your fertility, feel free to do so – but be sure to do so in moderation. One serving per day of full fat milk is more than enough to see the desired result, along with two half cup servings of full fat ice cream per week –which works out to about a pint of ice cream lasting up to two weeks.

More importantly, if you do add these foods to your diet, be certain to compensate by reducing the number of calories you get from other foods – and reducing your intake of saturated fats from other sources, such as red meat. You should also reduce your intake of snack foods high in trans fat such as potato chips, French fries or donuts. Moreover, once you do become pregnant, make certain to switch back to low fat dairy products, to help control excessive weight gain during pregnancy – which is important for you and for your baby.

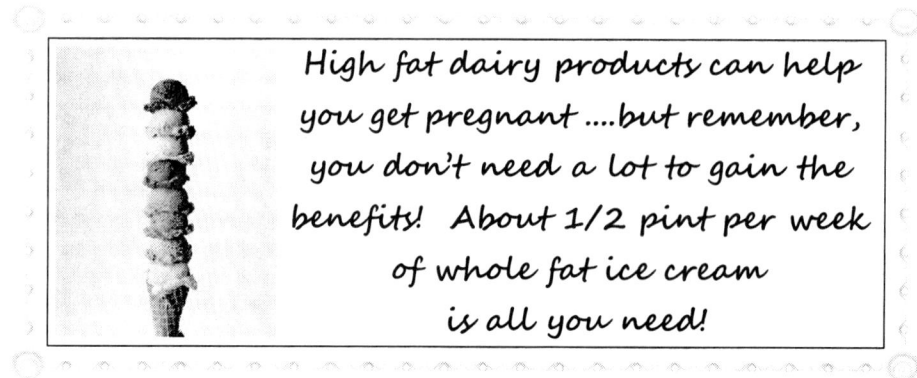

High fat dairy products can help you get pregnant ....but remember, you don't need a lot to gain the benefits! About 1/2 pint per week of whole fat ice cream is all you need!

SUPER PROTEIN FERTILITY POWER!

For many years I, and many other fertility experts, have known the secret power of protein to impact conception in a positive way. In fact, throughout years of counseling fertility patients on what to eat, I have always believed one of the best ways to insure a healthy ovulation is to increase protein intake by approximately 10 - 12 percent while trying to conceive.

How can this help? Studies show that when protein intake is high, ovulation occurs more regularly. Conversely, drop your protein intake too low and you will likely see a disruption in your menstrual cycle - one that will definitely impact your ability to get pregnant.

Also important: There are isolated studies suggesting that dietary protein can impact blood sugar and increase sensitivity to insulin – which as you read earlier can also impact ovulation.

Moreover, once you do get pregnant increasing protein intake is even more important, for you *and your baby*. According to the American College of Obstetricians and Gynecologists, consuming and adequate amount of protein during pregnancy can increase your developing baby's birth weight and that may protect against premature delivery, as well as increase your baby's health overall.

NOT ALL FERTILITY PROTEINS ARE CREATED EQUAL!

When it comes to choosing your protein sources you have several dietary options to consider. And this is important since not all forms of protein are equally healthy or equally effective for increasing fertility.

Certainly, I have always believed that lean red meat is among the best protein sources if you are trying to get pregnant, followed by white meat poultry and fish. And to some extent I still believe this is true. That said, considering some of the newer research on the impact of inflammatory compounds found in animal fats – and the mercury issues that have arisen related to excess fish consumption - several years ago I updated my recommendations to include consuming smaller portions of red meat, poultry and fish, and make up the difference by increasing

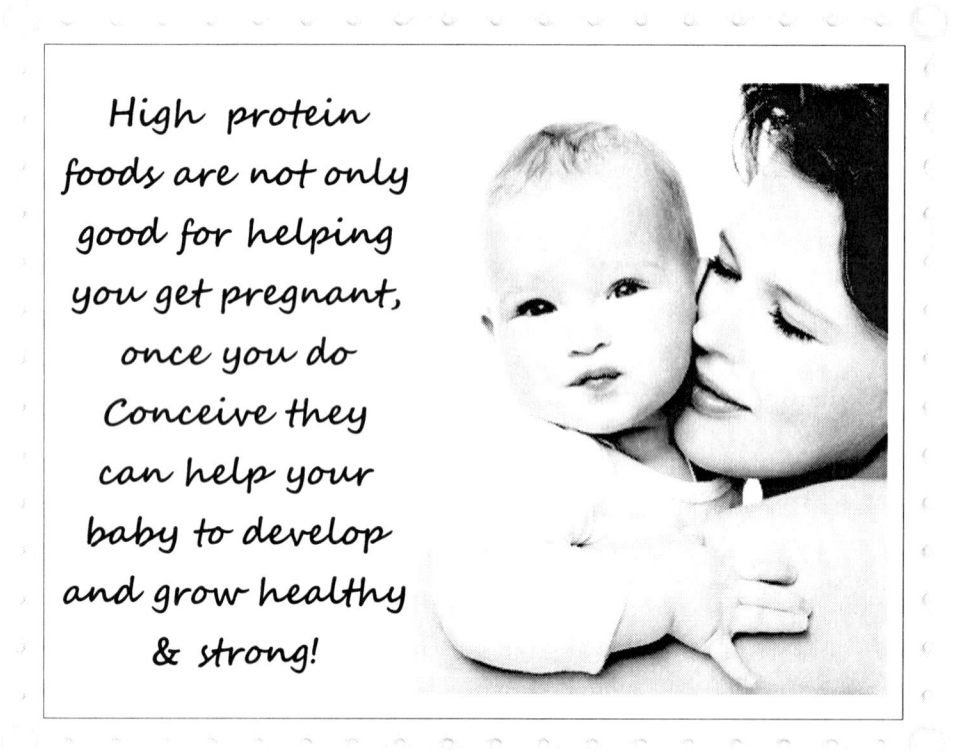

> High protein foods are not only good for helping you get pregnant, once you do conceive they can help your baby to develop and grow healthy & strong!

your intake of plant-based proteins – an idea that was recently echoed by the Harvard studies on ovulatory infertility.

According to their research women with the highest plant protein intake had a reduced incidence of ovulatory-based infertility while women who consumed high amounts of animal protein had an increase in ovulatory based infertility.

More specifically the Harvard study found that when total calories were the same, women who ate one serving per day of red meat, chicken or turkey had a one-third higher risk of ovulatory infertility than women who ate less. Protein from either fish or eggs did not appear to have any detrimental effects.

Perhaps most important, the study found that women who added just one serving per day of plant –based proteins including beans, tofu, soybeans, peanuts or other nuts - appeared to have some modest protection against ovulatory infertility problems.

CHOSE YOUR PROTEINS WISELY

While I agree with the Harvard findings in terms of the health benefits of increasing your intake of plant based proteins, where my recommendations differ is in the source of those plant-based proteins. More specifically some evidence shows that consuming large amounts of soy protein can actually be detrimental to fertility, particularly when an estrogen imbalance may be the root of your conception problems.

Now certainly, if you spend even a little time researching infertility on the Internet then you will probably find many sites filled with anecdotal stories of women who claim to have regulated their menstrual cycles and improved their fertility profile by consuming large amounts of soy – with some claiming that soy supplements are as good as fertility drugs such as Clomid when it comes to encouraging egg production and ovulation.

The factor believed to be responsible for the success of soy are two weak forms of plant estrogen known as daidzein and genistein.

But as encouraging and well meaning as these anecdotal reports are, I must caution you concerning what a number of medical studies conducted over the past 25 years have to say on the subject. Most have found that soy has either no impact on ovulation, or a slightly *detrimental* effect, actually reducing fertility.

- In one meta-analysis published in the *Journal of Nutrition* in 2002 researchers found that increasing soy intake resulted in increased menstrual cycle length and a decrease in estradiol, progesterone and sex-hormone binding globulin – all key biochemicals necessary for conception.

- In a study published a few years earlier in the *American Journal of Clinical Nutrition* researchers found that a high soy intake actually suppressed both LH and FSH – which as you read earlier are key hormones necessary for egg production and ovulation.

- More recently, a study published in the *European Journal of Nutrition* found that soy foods had no impact on fertility and offered no increase in pregnancy odds.

> Soy is a good source of protein, but eat it only in moderation. For some women, the weak plant estrogens found in soy may contribute to a hormone imbalance that can sometimes cause a delay in getting pregnant.

Of course all these studies appear to conflict with the Harvard findings, which, as you read earlier, report women who ate a diet high in soy based foods were protected against some forms of ovulatory-related infertility.

So, where does the truth lie? At the moment, I don't think anyone knows for certain. And ultimately it may turn out that soy foods can be helpful for certain types of fertility problems, and harmful – or have no impact – on others.

However, when you are in your reproductive prime, my concern is that the estrogens found in soy – no matter how weak – may, in some women, actually contribute to a hormone imbalance that could harm more than help your fertility. Of course if you know you have a ovulation-related fertility problem and your ovaries are not making adequate amounts of estrogen, then, much like ice cream and high fat milk products, soy may help you get pregnant faster.

If, however, you are ovulating on time, and you don't appear to have an estrogen deficiency, my recommendation is to include soy as one form of plant based protein – but only one form. By that I mean employ the principal on which all sound nutritional programs are built and vary your diet so that it includes a multitude of different sources of not only protein, but also healthy fats and slow burning carbohydrates. In this way you – and your fertility – will reap the benefits of what all these foods have to offer.

THE NEW FERTILITY PROTEIN: LUPIN!

If, in fact, you want to reduce your intake of soy – but still consume more vegetable-based protein - you might want to investigate the benefits of products made from lupin, another type of legume that is garnering some rave reviews in the healthy eating communities. Grown in Australia and now being milled into flours for bread, rolls and other baked goods, lupin is not only high in plant protein – higher than soy – it is also high in two types of fiber, both insoluble (like oats) and soluble(like apples). Since fiber is key to helping control blood sugar, lupin-based products may be a valuable fertility food to add to your daily diet!

If you can't find products made from lupin flour, or lupin flour itself, then check out a brand new product known as Lupin 8. A soluble, flavorless powder that can be used in everyday cooking, Lupin 8 combines the health and dietary benefits of lupin kernel flour (LKF) resulting in a product that is high in dietary protein, fiber, omega-3s, folate, niacin and is rich in antioxidants – which as you will read later in this book are key to fertility.

Another bonus: Lupin 8 also helps you feel full – increasing satiety so you don't feel as hungry. For those who are looking to lose some weight to increase fertility Lupin 8 can help you do that. In fact, lupin flour has been shown to have a positive inflluence on glycemic control, a factor that can also play a role in moderating sugar levels. And that can also help boost fertility.

For a super powerful fertility protein breakfast add Lupin 8 to your morning cereal . For lunch, add it to soups, stews, casseroles or homemade bread – you won't taste it and it won't change the texture. Or combine it with whole wheat flour, dark chocolate and walnuts for a home-made fertility-boosting brownie! (Check out our recipe at FertilityDietGuide.com!)

THE FERTILITY FOOD GROUPS: A FINAL WORD

While the three "fertility food groups" mentioned in this chapter – proteins, carbohydrates and fats – are important components of your fertility food plan, remember, they do not work alone.

Indeed, vitally important is the food grouping you will learn about in the next chapter – that being fruits and vegetables.

Perhaps most important to remember is that the ultimate "fertility diet" contains a balance of all the food groups and the nutrients they represent.

In fact, I can't emphasize enough the importance of eating a well-balanced diet while you are trying to conceive, and to continue eating that way once you get pregnant. Indeed, many of the same nutrients that can help you conceive a baby, will also help ensure a healthy pregnancy, one where you feel great and your baby grows, thrives and is healthy too!

I also want to take just a moment to remind you that diet should also remain a focal point of your partner's pre-conception game plan. Later in this book you'll find an entire chapter devoted to ways in which Mother Nature can help him to boost his fertility and your chances for getting pregnant – including foods that have been specifically shown to improve sperm count and motility.

But for right now remember that many of the same foods that make up your healthy pre-conception diet should also be a part of his meal plan as well! So shop together, cook together, eat together – and soon you'll be making a baby together as well!

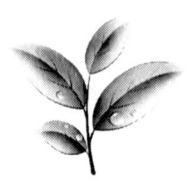

Chapter Eight

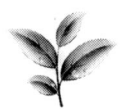

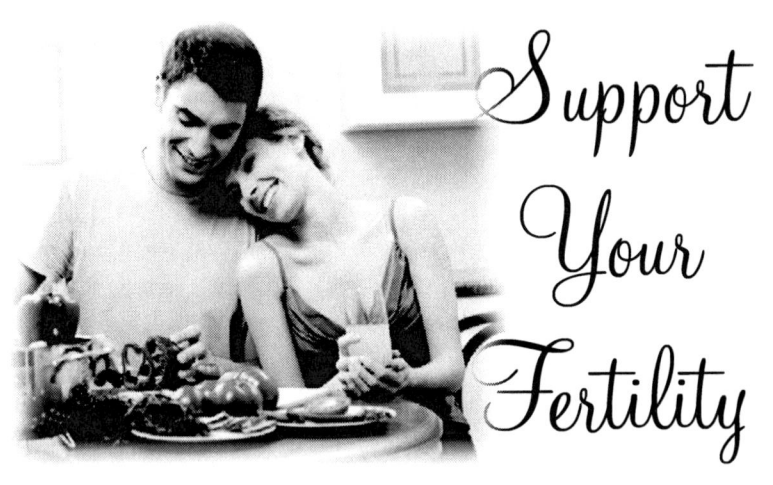

Support Your Fertility

With The Amazing Powers Of Fruits, Veggies, Nuts & Seeds!

There is perhaps no greater culinary sensation then biting into a juicy ripe peach on a hot summer's day – or a crisp red apple when there's a nip of fall in the air! The same can be said for a handful of nuts – or basket of steaming veggies. Indeed, dipping into Mother Nature's bounty offers taste sensations that are hard to beat.

But eating these – and other fruits, vegetables, nuts and seeds - offers more than just a taste treat. In fact, an abundance of medical studies now show that when it comes to getting pregnant, frequent dips into Mother Nature's bounty is one of the most important ways to boost fertility and conceive quicker and easier! How and why can these foods help you?

As you just read in a previous chapter, fruits and vegetables fall into the nutritional category known as "carbohydrates. However, since nearly all are "slow burning" *complex* carbohydrates, they can easily offer you all the blood sugar and hormone balancing benefits of other foods in this same group, including whole grains.

But from both a general health – and a fertility – standpoint, the benefits of adding some *specific* fruits, vegetables as well as nuts and seeds, into your daily diet goes far beyond simply protecting you from insulin resistance and related fertility problems.

First, they are a powerful source of both healthy fiber, and many of the key vitamins that impact fertility – and you'll learn more about that a little later on.

But there are also important, additional ways in which natural compounds found in these foods can have a direct affect on your fertility, influencing not only hormone activity, but also ovulation, and the subsequent growth, development, and implantation of healthy eggs. For all these reasons I'm devoting an entire chapter to filling you in on the most important ways that these natural fertility boosters can help you get pregnant faster.

GETTING PREGNANT: HOW FRUITS & VEGETABLES AFFECT FERTILITY

While almost every fruit and vegetable on the planet offers at least one or more specific health benefits, when it comes to getting pregnant perhaps the greatest advantage involves protecting you from "free radicals" - a type of adulterated oxygen molecule that forms via exposure to certain lifestyle factors. This includes a diet high in saturated fat, exposure to tobacco smoke (including second hand smoke) chemical toxins from pesticides or household chemicals, even overexposure to the sun.

Moreover, free radical damage can also occur via the simple act of aging. But if you're thinking you don't have to worry for a few more decades, guess again! Studies show that, at least in terms of free radical production, " aging" can began as early as your mid-twenties! In fact that's the time frame when free radical damage really begins to take hold.

But what exactly is a free radical – and how can it harm your fertility? First, a quick and easy chemistry lesson! Normally, healthy oxygen molecules contain an inseparable pair of tiny particles called "electrons." Think of them like a pair of love birds who simply must be together all the time!

For free radical oxygen molecules, however, one of those electrons are missing. And so, the lonely free radical molecule is always on the hunt, trying to find it's electron mate.

And while this may sound like a bit of sad "science romance", the truth is the lonely free radical is a ruthless hunter – a kind of tiny molecular "assassin" which roams through your body targeting any healthy cell it can find. In an attempt to disable it, and get inside to "steal" it's missing electron, it creates something called "lipid oxidation" – which is a type of biochemical stress that begins to eat away at a cells outer membrane.

This process generates the production of yet another free radical which is then off on its journey to attack other cells – which in turn causes still more damaging free radicals to be created.

But that's not the only way free radicals are generated. Indeed, environmental exposures – including spending too much time in the sun – as well as chemical pollutants and toxins from things like cigarette smoke, overexposure to household or even personal care chemicals, even just simple air pollution, can all cause free radicals to be generated in the body.

So what does all this have to do with your fertility – and your ability to get pregnant?

Once a free radical gets inside a healthy cell, it begins immediately to attack and alter the factors necessary for healthy cell function - including damaging the DNA, the very essence of each cell's life function.

When enough DNA damage to enough cells occurs, it paves the way for a number of diseases to set in – including cancer, diabetes, Alzheimer's, Parkinson's and yes, some forms of infertility.

Indeed, one study published in the *Journal of Human Reproduction* in 2007 suggests that oxidative cell damage within a woman's body has such a direct impact on conception that when levels are high, pregnancy can sometimes be impossible to achieve!

In another study published in the same journal in 2008 doctors found that when the follicular fluid surrounding a woman's egg was exposed to oxidative stress, those eggs became damaged, and were less likely to be fertilized.

But that's just the beginning. Indeed, dozens of studies now show that in one form or another free radicals – and their resulting oxidative stress cell damage - can impair fertility in myriad ways including:

- Impacting the ability of your eggs to mature and develop.
- Interfering with your ability to ovulate on a regular basis.
- Causing or exacerbating changes in the lining of your uterus, making it difficult for your embryo to attach and grow.
- Impacting the lining of your fallopian tubes, keeping your fertilized egg from reaching your uterus.
- Creating a hormonal imbalance significant enough to interfere with fertility on many levels.

Most recently, damage from free radicals has been proven to be a significant factor in "unexplained" infertility. And, it's not just women who are affected. Indeed, research shows sperm production is also impacted by free radical damage, thus increasing the risk of male fertility problems.

Finally, if you suffer from any fertility robbing conditions such as endometriosis or PCOS, the additional cell damage occurring from free radicals can exacerbate your condition, and in the process make getting pregnant that much harder.

But while both free radicals and the resulting oxidative cell stress can have an enormous negative impact on both your overall health and your fertility, it doesn't have to be this way! Indeed, you have the power to change this aspect of your body chemistry, and in the process not only improve your fertility profile, but also protect yourself from some of the most significant killer diseases of our time. And one of the easiest and most important ways to do that is through your diet.

Protect Your fertility From Free Radical Damage - & Get Pregnant Faster!

When it comes to protection from free radical damage, there is, perhaps, no greater warriors willing to come to your defense than fruits and vegetables. How can they help?

First, they are loaded to the brim with natural compounds known as antioxidants! Much like the name implies, an "antioxidant" is a molecule that prevents "oxidative damage" from occurring.

How? Once ingested, antioxidant molecules literally float through your body searching out or scavenging free radical molecules. When they find them, they latch on tight, and literally surround each molecule and work their way inside. This disarms and disables the original free radical molecule and creates a weaker new molecule, much less able to attack healthy cells while also helping to prevent new free radicals from forming.

Moreover, antioxidants also work to protect the normal healthy cells in the body, in part by reinforcing their outer membrane, making it much harder for free radicals to get inside and cause the kind of damage that disrupts fertility.

Lastly, in a situation where more is definitely better, antioxidants also help encourage the body to produce more of its own supply of antioxidant compounds, including lipoic acid. And this in turn helps to squash even more free radical production, and more importantly free radical damage.

The result: With fewer free radicals able to cause damage, and fewer free radicals being made overall, it paves the way for better health and better fertility! And that, in fact, is exactly what several studies have found.

But what's also key is that antioxidants work together in kind of "protection network". In doing so they initiate a chain reaction of events that ultimately stops free radicals from harming your cells. For example vitamin E disarms a free radical, but in the process produces a vitamin E radical – which then requires Vitamin C to disarm. The same is true for many other antioxidants, all of which must work together in a harmonizing balance if you to keep the level of free radicals under control.

It's also the reason why eating foods high in only *one antioxidant* won't give you nearly as much protection as eating a balanced diet high in a number of different antioxidants. This balance is not only important to maintaining your overall health, but particularly your fertility.

Indeed, in research published in the *Journal of Human Reproduction* in 2008, findings suggest that a diet high in many antioxidants can favorably influence not only how quickly and easily an egg can be fertilized, but whether the resulting embryo will survive and thrive – or be lost to an early stage miscarriage. And I can tell you from my personal patient population that many women who were referred to me because of repeated miscarriages were able to stop the cycle of loss and give birth to a healthy baby, simply by changing their diet!

But it's not just pregnancy loss that is affected by antioxidants. Indeed, these powerful nutrients also have the ability to neutralize a host of the fertility-robbing factors - and in the process not only help you get pregnant right now, but also protect your fertility for the future.

EXTRA POTENT FERTILITY FOODS: THE ORAC SYSTEM

Although virtually every fresh fruit and vegetable is a healthful eating choice, when it comes to antioxidant protection, there are some which clearly go to the head of the class. So how do we know which ones to choose? It all comes down to something called the ORAC Score. ORAC stands for "oxygen radical absorbance capacity" - which is a very complicated way of saying it represents how quickly and easily any given food "mops up" the free radical spills taking place in your body. Based on this ability, foods are assigned a certain number of *points* – and these *points* are what make a foods "ORAC Score". While it may sound a bit mathematical and even complicated, in just a few moments I'll explain how simple it is – and how it can help you eat a healthier diet.

Understanding The ORAC Score

A relatively new concept that burst on the nutrition scene in the early 1990's, the ORAC system was developed by Dr. Guohua Cao, a physician with the US National Institutes On Aging. Since that time many top universities and scientists have come on board to further define the ORAC concept and apply it to foods we eat.

The ORAC Scale is now considered to be among the most precise ways to measure the antioxidant potential of a food, supplement or compound, and as such rate it's antioxidant power. Based on that rating, each food is supplied an ORAC score – a type of point value that coordinates with its antioxidant potential.

Today, the current recommendation is for each of us to eat foods totaling between 3,000 and 5,000 ORAC points per day. And while that may seem like a lot, the truth is, cutting edge nutritionists – and doctors such as me – believe that in today's pollution-packed, chemically treated "environment", to be truly healthy – and to get pregnant fast – you should consume up to 30,000 ORAC points per day!

Now before you say "impossible", let me assure you that by choosing just a few high ORAC scoring fruits and veggies per day, you can easily reach that number – and even go beyond. For example, a ½ cup of blueberries can be as high as 9,700 ORAC points, while a single Granny Smith apple will give you nearly 8,000 ORAC points! Green tea is 3,000 ORAC points a cup, while squeezing a lemon in a glass of water will net you 3,200 ORAC points! Add a cup of chopped onions to your salad and take in 1,600 ORAC points! And, the news you've been waiting to hear: One ounce of dark chocolate has a whopping 5,600 ORAC points!

And so, you see, it's not hard to garner the protection you need – and eat some fabulous foods in the process! Later in this chapter you'll find some specific super fertility foods to include in your diet, many of which have a very high ORAC Score. But to find a full listing of the ORAC scores of the top fertility fruits and vegetables I invite you to visit FertilityDietGuide.com .

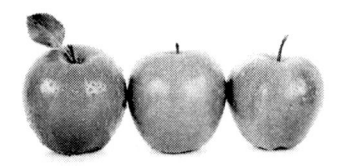

> ### SCORING POINTS TO GET PREGNANT FASTER!
>
> To reach your 30,000 ORAC points
> a day & get pregnant fast try:
>
> 1 Granny Smith Apple - 8,000 points
> 1 ounce of dark chocolate - 5,600 points
> 2 cups of Green Tea - 6,000 points
> 1 cup of chopped onions - 1,600 points
> 1 cup of water with lemon juice - 3,200 points
> 1 cup blueberries : 12,000 points

THE PHYTO NUTRIENTS THAT BOOST FERTILITY !

As important as antioxidants are to your fertility, they are just one component of a complex network of natural compounds known as "phytonutrients" - natural, health-giving chemicals found in *great abundance* in the plants that yield a good many fruits and vegetables.

Indeed, one unique thing about plants – of all types – is that they don't possess the same kind of biochemical warning system about impending dangers that both humans and animals do. Indeed, the adrenalin-fueled "fight or flight" response that is genetically programmed into your DNA works to both alert you to danger and help you escape it.

While plants don't have this unique advantage, Mother Nature did not leave them in the lurch! Instead, they possess a very special kind of *natural chemical protection* from danger – and it involves a complete network of protective natural compounds known as phytonutrients. In fact the sole purpose of these phytonutrients is to protect plants from assault by insects, fungus, and many of the very same environmental threats that can harm you, including the damaging rays of ultra violet light from the sun. And here lies the key as to how phytonutrients can protect you as well.

Indeed, phytonutrients are the compounds that offer your body a highly efficient natural repair system – one that is able to correct cellular damage caused by oxidative stress and other free radical activity, be it from the environment, your diet, or almost any cause at all. And in much the same way that these compounds keep plants from being destroyed by environmental assaults, so too can they protect you as well.

In fact, for many years, researchers believed that the health benefits of eating fruits and vegetables came solely from their vitamin content – specifically the antioxidant vitamins such as C, E and beta carotene. And in fact these nutrients are still important – and you'll learn more about how and why in the next chapter on fertility nutrients.

But over the past decade, and particularly in the last five years, researchers have uncovered an extremely important – and some say even startling fact: The real protection from fruits and vegetables may actually come not just from vitamins, but from their phytonutrient content.

In one of these studies researchers intentionally caused damage to a strand of DNA – in much the same way that the environmental influences, for example, might harm your cell's DNA. They then treated the broken strand with several different types of phytonutrients as well as vitamin C. Using a computer to analyze the results they found that the combination of phytonutrients did a better job of repairing cell damage than the vitamin C alone. Interestingly, this finding was also echoed in a study on sperm. In research published in the journal *Teratogenisis, Carcinogensis and Mutagenisis* researchers found that certain phytonutrient compounds were able to help repair damaged sperm, making them better able to fertilize an egg!

Moreover, studies have also begun to show that many of these same natural compounds also impact egg development and fertilization. So, clearly women also have much to gain from foods high in these compounds.

So what should you and your partner be eating? Certainly, a well rounded diet containing many different fruits and veggies can go a long way in ensuring that your intake of many important phytonutrients - as well as antioxidants - remains high.

However, in terms of optimizing your health as well as your fertility, there are several key foods that we now know can play an especially important role. Choosing foods highest in these nutrients *can* give an extra special boost to your ability to get pregnant.

Moreover, incorporating these foods into your pre-conception diet will not only improve your chances of conceiving, but when you do get pregnant you'll be giving your baby the very best and most nutritious start to life.

To discover the foods you should begin incorporating into your diet ASAP, what follows are some of the key fertility phytonutrients, how they can specifically help you get pregnant – and, of course, the fruits and vegetables that contain them in the greatest amounts! Eat them every day and I promise that your chances for a quick and easy pregnancy will increase dramatically!

> *While all fruits and vegetables are good for fertility, certain ones – those containing high levels of the free-radical fighting anti-oxidants – have specific effects, directly influencing hormone production necessary for conception!*

The Phytonutrients:
What To Eat To Get Pregnant Faster!

While there are literally thousands of phytonutrients, found in fruits, vegetables, nuts and grains – and all of them good for your health - when it comes to boosting fertility, most of them can be grouped into just three important categories. They are: Phenolic acids, flavonoids, and carotinoids. While each group contains several key individual phytonutrients, for the most part they work as a team to not only optimize your general health, but also have some specific effects on your fertility and your ability to get pregnant.

What follows is a quick run-down of some of their more outstanding health - giving and fertility boosting effects and the foods that contain them.

Group # 1 : Phenolic Acids –

These compounds help protect the body from pollutants, repair damage caused by cigarette smoke and air pollution, and offer protection from heart disease. One particular type of phenolic acid making huge headlines right now is "reservatrol. It's actually manufactured by plants in response to environmental stress, so it's not hard to see why it is so closely associated with overcoming the effects of oxidative stress on cells. Foods high in this compound not only protect your heart, and every cell involved in conception, but also help ensure good flow throughout your body but particularly to your ovaries and your uterus - which can be key to conception.

To increase your intake of polyphenols add these foods to your diet:

- Red or purple fruits such as grapes, raspberries, strawberries, pomegranates and cranberries.
- Citrus fruits but particularly red grapefruit.
- Wine made from red grapes.
- Walnuts and pecans.

GROUP # 2 : FLAVONOIDS -

These are the nutrients that studies show can have a direct impact on blood pressure, plus support the heart and aid capillaries in maintaining good circulation –which is key to egg production and ovulation.

- One type of flavonoid known as quercertin (found in grapes and cherries) helps keep tiny particles found in blood from sticking together and forming clumps, which may help some women reduce their risk of miscarriage.

- Another type of flavonoid known as catechins – found in green tea – pack a heavy punch against cancers of the reproductive system, as well as protecting you from heart disease.

- Still another type of flavonoids is known as "isoflavone", which contain a type of plant estrogen helpful to many women.

But it is really the impact of two more specific flavonoids - anthocyanin and proanthocyanidins - found in fruits like blueberries, that may help your fertility the most. How?

They work to reduce the production of cytokines, inflammatory compounds produced by various cells in the body, but particularly fat cells. As you just read in an earlier chapter, the more fat cells your body has, the more cytokines you produce, so the more flavonoid compounds you need to counteract the damage.

In terms of your fertility, studies show that inflammatory compounds can also exert subtle negative effects on everything from egg production and ovulation, to egg transport inside your fallopian tube, to creating a hostile environment for sperm.

This is one reason why being overweight can make it harder to become pregnant. In addition, whether or not you are overweight, these same inflammatory compounds can also play a role in insulin resistance and PCOS, as well as endometriosis – all three conditions that impact fertility.

To increase your intake of flavonoids consume more:

- Tea, and particularly green tea which contains three times the flavonoid content of black tea. Also eat more grapes, cocoa, lentils, black eyed peas, peaches and nectarines which are also good general sources of flavonoids.

- You can increase your intake of quercertin by eating more red grapes, cherries, kale, lettuce, apples, pears, nectarines, peaches, broccoli and onions, as well as drinking more tea.

- Gain the fertility-boosting effects of anthocyanin and procanthocyanidins by adding more blue-red fruits to your diet including blueberries, raspberries, strawberries, loganberries, cherries, currants, pomegranates, grapes and cranberries.

- Increase estrogen levels naturally with foods rich in isoflavone including soybeans, tofu, tempeh, and soy milk – but here I must add a word of caution. While for some women the estrogen boost garnered from soy foods can be helpful for fertility, for others it can have the opposite effect, creating a hormonal imbalance that makes it harder to get pregnant. So, unless you have been diagnosed with low estrogen, or a low-estrogen condition such as PCOS, go easy on this last group of foods and get the bulk of your flavonoids from foods in the other categories. While eating soy foods in moderation won't cause you any harm, don't make them your sole source of flavonoid nutrients.

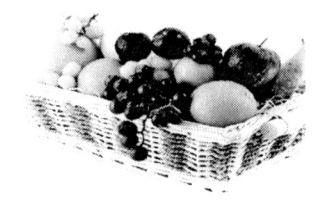

GROUP # 3: CAROTINOIDS -

This mighty group of compounds – the best known of which is beta carotene - is another powerful source of antioxidants and has been shown to offer protection against a wide range of diseases, from Alzheimer's to cancer.

But from a fertility standpoint, these phytonutrients - which include compounds such as lycopene, lutein, and zeaxanthin - may be among the most important to include in your diet.

Why? First, carotinoids are what your body uses to make vitamin A , a nutrient that is essential for the healthy growth and development of an embryo. In fact when a serious vitamin A deficiency exists it's almost impossible to create a healthy embryo.

Moreover, research published by the European Society of Human Reproduction and Embryology demonstrated how several compounds within the carotinoid family are essential to healthy follicular fluid – the semi-liquid substance which surrounds your egg and aids in growth and fertilization. Because follicular fluid appears to get its supply of beta carotene from the bloodstream, it stands to reason that when levels are low, eggs may not fertilize as quickly or as easily.

Equally important, animal studies have shown that beta carotene impacts the release of LH – luteinizing hormone, the brain chemical which helps to signal the release of your egg and actually allow ovulation to occur.

Moreover, a healthy corpus luteum (the shell your ovulated egg leaves behind) is naturally rich in beta carotene. Since this is the major source of progesterone, the hormone that helps prepare your uterus for a healthy conception, fortifying it with additional beta carotene may also help optimize hormone production necessary for a healthy implantation.

When it comes to male fertility, one particular member of the carotinoid family – a compound known as "lycopene" - has been shown to be especially important for manufacturing healthy sperm. You'll read more about this in the chapter on male fertility.

To increase your intake of carotinoids eat:

- Carrots, butternut squash, tomatoes, sweet potatoes, cantaloupe, kale and mangoes.
- To add more lycopene to your diet eat more tomatoes, watermelon, guava, plus red and white grapefruit.
- To maximize levels of lutein eat more avocados, oranges, and leafy green vegetables.
- For more beta carotene try apricots, papayas, plantains, broccoli, celery, pumpkin, spinach and winter squash.

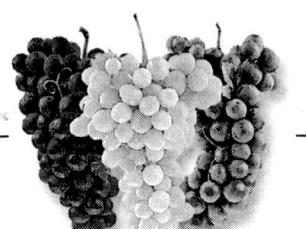

THE COLORS OF FERTILITY

Taking advantage of all the important phytonutrients found in fruits and vegetables is easier than you think! In fact, all you need do is add more colorful foods to your plate every day! Indeed, studies show that many of the most important phytonutrients identified to date are the same compounds that give fruits and vegetables their vivid, natural colors.

So the more "colors" you have on your plate, the more likely it is that you will be receiving a good variety of powerful, fertility-boosting phytonutrients.

What To Eat To Get Pregnant !

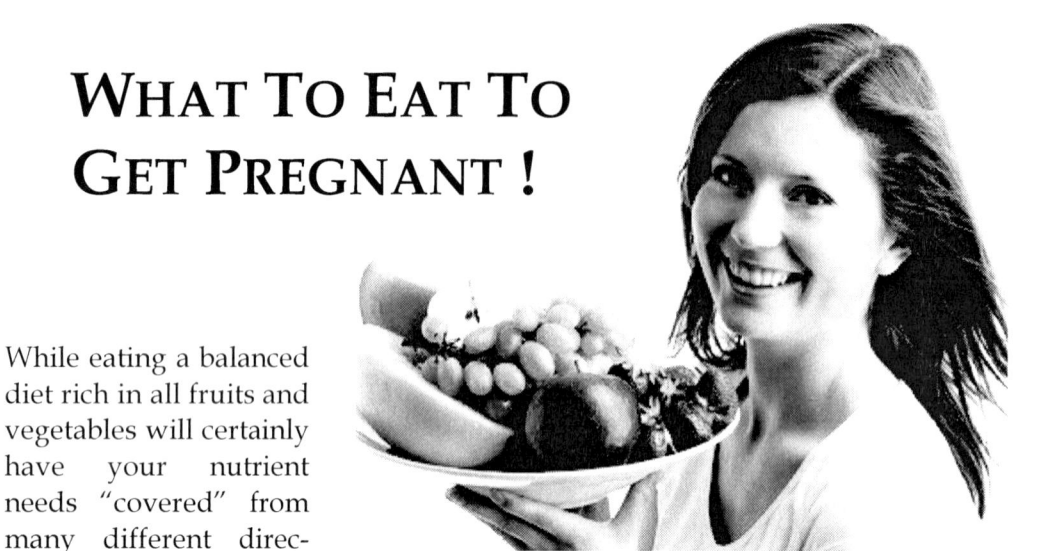

While eating a balanced diet rich in all fruits and vegetables will certainly have your nutrient needs "covered" from many different directions, throughout years of counseling fertility patients I have found that certain specific foods offer an extra "heaping portion" of nutrients that are especially good for fertility. I like to call them my Super Fertility Food Boosters - each one with a high Orac score and loads of the important phyto nutrients you just read about. Being certain to include them in your diet can a long way in boosting your fertility and helping you get pregnant faster!

Six Super Fertility Food Boosters

Fertility Super Boost # 1 :   Blueberries

It's hard to pick up a magazine or open your lap top without seeing a news story about the powerful, health-giving benefits of blueberries. As you just read, these tiny berries are packed with a powerful phytonutrient known *anthocyanins* – a natural compound that is actually responsible for giving this fruit it's deep rich color. But it also does much more than that. This powerful natural chemical helps reduce the impact of inflammation body-wide and in doing so benefits nearly every segment of reproduction. This includes making and ovulating healthy eggs, helping sperm and egg meet, keeping your fallopian tubes clear for the easy transport of your embryo to your uterus, and finally, keeping the lining of your uterus healthy so that your implantation and your pregnancy can be healthy and strong.

And if that were not enough, studies show that adding just a half cup of blueberries to your daily diet can lower cholesterol, fight high blood pressure, reduce the risk of memory loss and brain motor function disorders, and even protect you from cancer!

That said, it's also important to note that not all blueberries are alike.

Although all varieties offer health and fertility advantages, there is now significant evidence to suggest that organically grown blueberries may pack a significantly greater phytonutrient punch, and offer greater antioxidant protection than blueberries that are grown in the conventional way.

Moreover, scientists have also discovered that where blueberries are grown – particularly the area of the world, and the climate - can also impact the nutritional content of these fruits.

Among the blueberries offering the biggest bang for your nutritional buck is wild berries grown in Alaska. According to research conducted by National Institutes of Health scientist Maureen McKenzie, PhD, thanks to certain genetic adaptations, the Alaskan blueberry is able to thrive even in the harsh climate of the frozen tundra. Not coincidentally, these adaptations involved a dramatic increase in natural antioxidant production – up to seven times that found in blueberries grown in warmer climates. And that extra protection is passed on to all those who eat the berries!

If you can't get your hands on Alaskan blueberries, there are blueberry supplements – most notably Aurora Blue – made from pure Alaskan berries. Even with processing, it still maintains an ORAC score (the measure of a product's antioxidant potential) four times that found in wild Maine blueberries, and seven times that of blueberries grown in most other locations.

FERTILITY SUPER BOOST # 2: CRUCIFEROUS VEGETABLES

If you want to get pregnant faster and easier you might want to munch on some broccoli, cauliflower, Brussels sprouts, kale, cabbage, and bok choy. An interrelated group known as "cruciferous vegetables" these green veggies are packed with phytochemicals, vitamins, minerals, and fiber that not only protect your heart, but also act as powerful cancer-fighting warriors.

But in terms of your fertility it is their powerful antioxidant punch that does you the most good!

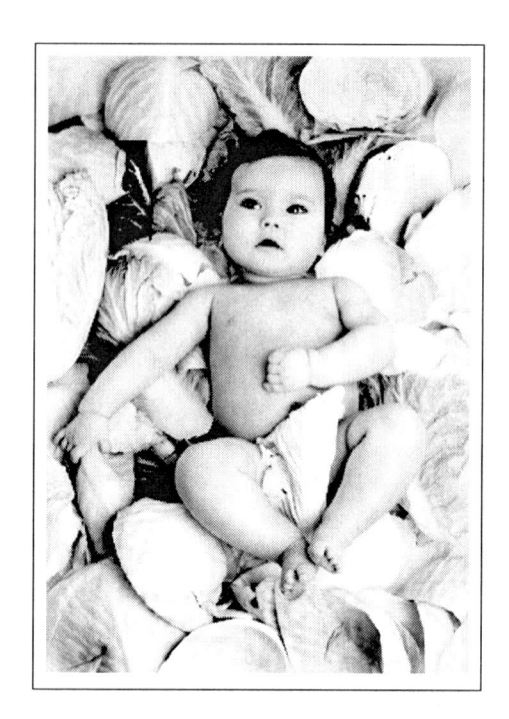

In one study funded by the National Cancer Institute, researchers found that body-wide oxidative cell stress (including that which adversely impacts fertility) dropped by 22% after just a few weeks of a diet high in cruciferous vegetables. Now if you think you can get the same effects by popping a vitamin supplement, guess again. The study also showed that those who took a vitamin supplement instead of eating the veggies saw nowhere near the same level of decrease in oxidative stress.

But that's not the only way in which these crunchy greens can aid your fertility. Indeed, studies have also shown that natural compounds found in these vegetables may help promote healthy estrogen metabolism – a hormone essential for almost every stage of reproduction.

More specifically, researchers have found that two natural chemicals found in cruciferous vegetables – compounds known as I3C and DIM – help promote optimal estrogen metabolism.

But the news gets even better: These vegetables are not only healthy they are also smart! And here's why: There are two pathways through which the body metabolizes estrogen. One way results in an healthy metabolic byproduct known as 2-hydroxyestrone. The other way results in the production of a more toxic by product, a chemical known as 16 alphahydroxyesterone. And in fact, several studies have now reported that women who metabolize estrogen into this compound are more susceptible to breast cancer. Other research indicates fertility may also be affected.

Now, here comes the vegetable link: The compounds I3C and DIM appear to help shift the way estrogen is metabolized in the body, encouraging greater production of the healthy metabolites and lower production of the more toxic ones. This not only reduces the risk of breast and cervical cancer in women, but also prostate cancer in men.

And while research on the link to fertility is still in its early stages, I and many of my colleagues, particularly in Europe, agree that the positive healthful changes in estrogen metabolism brought about by eating these vegetables will also make a difference in the creation of healthier eggs. This, combined with their powerful antioxidant effects means that a diet high in cruciferous vegetables cannot only improve your chances for getting pregnant, it may even help you cross the line from infertile to fertile!

While three to four ½ cup servings a day can offer the best protection, even eating just one to two servings a day can be helpful. The highest nutrient values can be achieved if you choose fresh veggies and eat them raw or lightly steamed. That said, you can still gain benefits from frozen veggies, as well as from cooked veggies – but you will need to eat a bit more to reach the optimal nutrient levels. And remember, you can and will see a difference in as little as three weeks!

> *Studies show that the compounds found in broccoli, cauliflower and cabbage may help promote healthy estrogen metabolism – and that means your eggs will be healthier and more plentiful!*

FERTILITY SUPER BOOST # 3: ONIONS AND GARLIC

When I was in medical school, the running joke in the gynecology department was that onion and garlic were the most effective method of birth control - because if you ate them every day no one would want to get close enough to get to know you!

But the truth is, these two powerful foods may , in fact, have the opposite effect – because at least on a biochemical level, they contain compounds that might just help you get pregnant!

Both vegetables belong to the family of phytonutrients known as "allylic sulfur compounds" - a group that also includes leeks, scallions and chives, and other "bulb" vegetables. But it is onions and garlic that alone, or especially together, that pack the biggest punch in terms of protecting your health and your fertility.

First, studies show that compounds found in these vegetables are potent anti-cancer fighters - helping to protect against colon, stomach, breast and in particular ovarian cancer. In fact, studies show adding these vegetables to the diet, even after cancer has been diagnosed, can help slow the growth of some types of malignant tumors.

But in terms of your fertility, these foods can also play a key role in helping to repair damaged DNA, as well as regulating the life cycle of a cell. Indeed, one way in which fertility can become impaired is via exposure to environmental toxins and pollutants – factors which ultimately break down cell walls and alter DNA. Thus, it stands to reason that any natural compounds which can halt this process can't help but boost your fertility.

But the protection doesn't stop here. In a study published in the *Journal of Nutrition* in 2003, researchers found that extracts made from garlic powder also had a potent effect on levels of cytokines – the inflammatory chemicals that, as you read earlier, can impact fertility on many levels, particularly in women diagnosed with endometriosis or PCOS.

My suggestion is to use onions and garlic as a garnish or in salads, at least a few times a week. To help neutralize breath odors: Toss in a sprig or two of parsley or watercress!

FERTILITY SUPER BOOST # 4: GREEN TEA

Although the facts surrounding the impact of green tea on fertility are still considered a bit controversial, increasingly research is showing that it can have a favorable impact on getting pregnant. One reason of course, is it's powerful antioxidant activity. Indeed, tea of any type is high in a phytonutrient known as polyphenols, a type of "flavonoid" with robust antioxidant activity.

But the polyphenols found in green tea are present in amounts as much as three times greater than what is found in black tea – meaning it's antioxidant power is greater as well. And many experts now believe that this power can be a defining factor in those seeking to get pregnant.

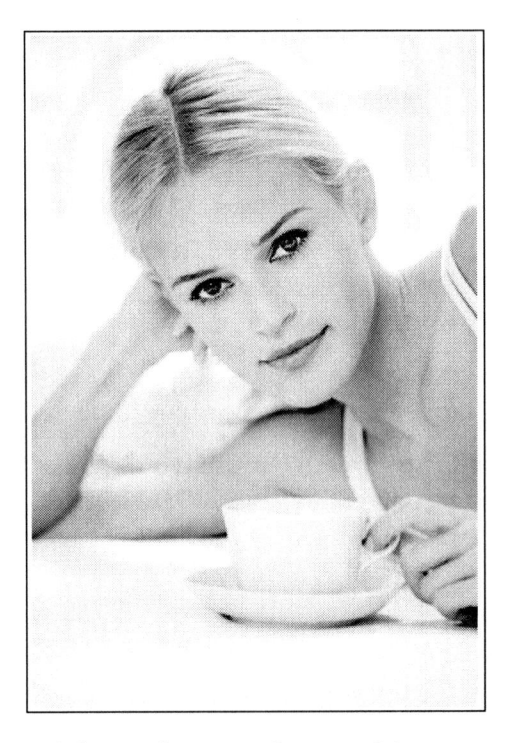

A second chemical that is plentiful in green tea – a natural compound known as hypoxanthine – is actually the same chemical found in the follicular fluid that surrounds your egg in your ovary, helping to foster growth, development and eventually ovulation. As such, a number of researchers theorize that drinking green tea may have beneficial effects on egg production and growth.

Indeed, in one now-classic study published nearly a decade ago, researchers from Kaiser Permanente Health System found that women who drank as little as one-half cup of caffeine-rich green tea daily nearly doubled their chances of conceiving! The same effect was not seen with other caffeine-rich beverages.

More recently a Stanford University study of 30 women, aged 24 to 46 who had not been able to conceive for up to three years, found that a supplement containing green tea and several other herbs and vitamins improved conception odds considerably. Indeed, one-third of the women taking the supplement were able to conceive within five months, compared with no pregnancies in the placebo group. What we don't know however, is whether green tea alone would have had the same effect.

That said, if the findings of a new European animal study translates to humans, green tea may indeed, be the catalyst that increases fertility. In research published in April 2008, researchers from the University of Bologna reported that when used in conjunction with IVF, a compound found in green tea known as EGCG increased pregnancy rates significantly, mostly by increasing the number of eggs available for fertilization.

Interestingly, however, when concentrations of EGCG were elevated too much, the percentage of eggs produced actually went down.

What does this mean for you? As with most factors that impact your health, moderation is the key! While it seems clear green tea can have beneficial effects on fertility, overdoing may not be a good thing.

My suggestion: Up to seven cups of green a week is likely to benefit your overall health and may improve your fertility - but until we have more information I would limit it to that amount.

FERTILITY SUPER BOOST # 5: NUTS!
ALMONDS, WALNUTS, CASHEWS AND MORE!

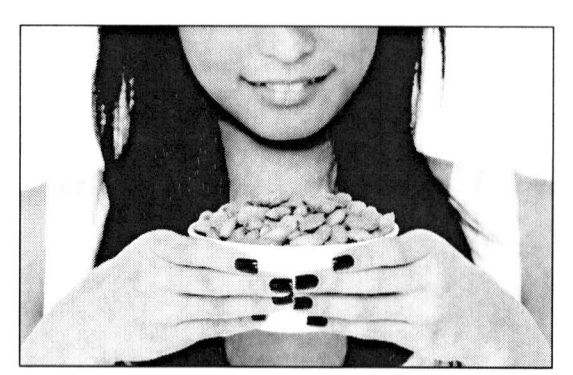

Although foods that are high in fat are generally not good for your health, that tenet changes dramatically when it comes to nuts. Indeed, there are almost 300 different types of nuts, and while they are high in fat (and calories) it's the type of fat they contain that makes them a healthy choice – and even a super fertility food. How can they help you? Nuts contain mostly monounsaturated and polyunsaturated oils – the "good fats" that can help lower cholesterol and have anti-inflammatory effects on your cells. Many nuts, but walnuts in particular, are a potent source of healthy Omega-3 fatty acids – which can help build a stronger cell membrane and protect it from free radical attack. For those of you who may be dealing with inflammatory conditions that impact fertility – such as endometriosis and PCOS – the healthy fats found in nuts can make a huge difference in not only your symptoms, but also in helping you conceive.

And if you love almonds – well you are in luck! Not only do they contain healthy fats, they are also one of the richest sources of antioxidants! According to researchers from Tufts University, after testing the skins and kernels of eight varieties of California almonds, they found the phytonutrients contained in these nuts offered the highest level of free radical damage protection of any flavonoid group! In fact, ounce for ounce you're getting the same level of phytonutrient protection found in broccoli, black and green tea, and red onions!

In addition, nuts, as well as seeds are also high in a natural compound known as "phytosterols" - a type of plant based fat that recently gained lots of attention for its ability to lower cholesterol. You've probably already heard the term "sterols" in regard to "healthy" margarine such as a Bencol or Smart Balance. But what you might not know is that a recent analysis of 27 different varieties of nuts as well as certain seeds (see Fertility Boost # 6) have among the highest concentrations of healthy sterols.

And here's the really big surprise: Besides reducing cholesterol, these same plant sterols also help decrease the risk of some cancers, as well as enhance the immune system – and therein may lie a very quiet but powerful link to fertility. What is that link?

First, when your immune system is strong, your body defends itself against the ravages of several fertility-robbing infections. But perhaps more importantly, now classic research conducted at Mt. Sinai Medical Center in New York City by my colleague, fertility expert Dr. Norbert Gleicher found that problems in the immune system may be to blame for many cases of infertility in women. Indeed, in his research women who were prone to fertility problems had a significantly higher level of autoimmune antibodies, not only in their blood, but also in the fluid that surrounds a fertilized egg.

In fact, in one study of women with abnormal levels of autoimmune antibodies who had undergone IVF, Dr. Gleicher found pregnancy rates were only 1/5th of those women who had normal levels of blood antibodies.

Also important to remember: Nuts are also very high in protein, which, as you read earlier in the book, is key to healthy ovulation and egg production. But unlike meat and other animal sources which can be loaded with saturated fats, the protein found in nuts is healthier overall.

Lastly, nuts are also a potent source of fiber, which means they can help balance blood sugar, reduce the risk of insulin resistance and in doing so also help keep ovulation on track. Of course they can also be high in calories – so you don't want to overdo it! A hand full of mixed nuts and seeds a day is plenty to give your fertility a boost! Plus, if you eat them instead of a typical "junk food " snack – like some chips or cookies – you'll keep your calorie intake balanced and do a good deed for your body and your fertility !

One other important note: Some nuts, particularly peanuts, are high in isoflavone – which means that, like soy, they can be a somewhat significant source of plant estrogens. If you have an estrogen deficiency – if you are past 35 for example, or if you have PCOS – then peanuts can give your estrogen levels an extra boost that might help you get pregnant. If, however, your estrogen level is already very high in relation to your level of progesterone (one tell-tale sign can be raging PMS before every menstrual cycle) then the estrogens found in isoflavone might tip your fertility balance in the wrong direction.

While eating a small hand full of nuts a day probably won't " rock your estrogen boat", if you do find that symptoms of PMS occur or increase, then it might be affecting your fertility as well, in which case you should cut back and eat less.

Also, you may want to keep your partner from dipping into the peanut bowl – particularly with an icy glass of beer , at least while you are trying to get pregnant. Why? The latest studies show that the isoflavone found in both beer and peanuts can have a detrimental effect on sperm that could make getting pregnant much more difficult! You'll learn more about this and many other effects of diet on sperm a little later in this book.

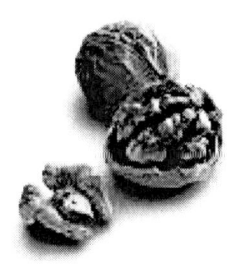

FERTILITY SUPER BOOST # 6: PUMPKIN SEEDS, SUNFLOWER SEEDS AND WHEAT GERM

When I was a small boy growing up in Denmark, my mother frequently fed my brother, my sister and I snacks made with both wheat germ and a variety of different seeds. At the time we all wanted more cookies and pies – but in a classic case of " Mother Knows Best", I now know that Mom had our best health interests at heart! Indeed, adding foods like wheat germs plus sunflower, pumpkin and sesame seeds to your diet can not only protect you from both cancer and heart disease, it might just increase your fertility as well.

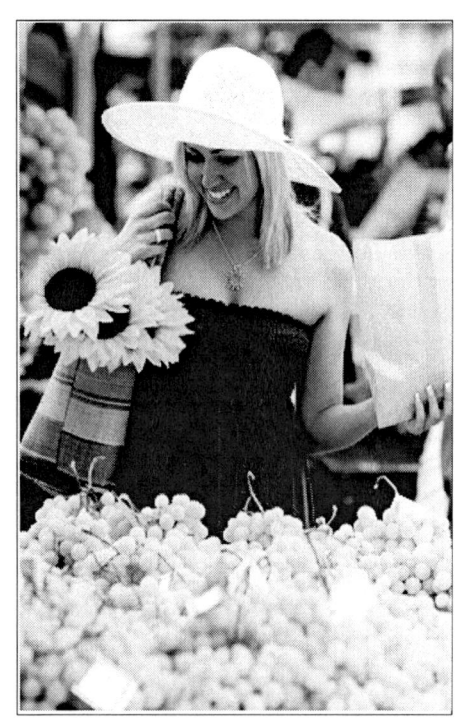

How? First they are powerful plant sterols, which as you just read can impact your immunity and ultimately your fertility. But these seeds also contain relatively high concentrations of Omega-3e fatty acids – which can boost fertility in a variety of ways, including stimulating the production of sex hormones in both men and women.

Moreover, pumpkin seeds, high in vitamin E and zinc, can be particularly beneficial for male fertility. Research shows that just ¼ to ½ cup a day can boost the overall health of a man's reproductive system and increase the concentration of healthier sperm in each ejaculation.

If you are prone to miscarriage – or just want to ensure an extra healthy implantation, be sure to add more wheat germ to diet. High in both vitamin E and selenium, research shows these two nutrients are essential to reducing the risk of miscarriage. Wheat germ, as well as sunflower and sesame seeds are also high in vitamin B6, which is essential to not only produce female hormones, but to maintain proper ratios of estrogen and progesterone necessary for a quick and easy conception! (And you'll read more about these and other fertility nutrients in the next chapter).

Food & Sex: How To Turn On Your Fertility!

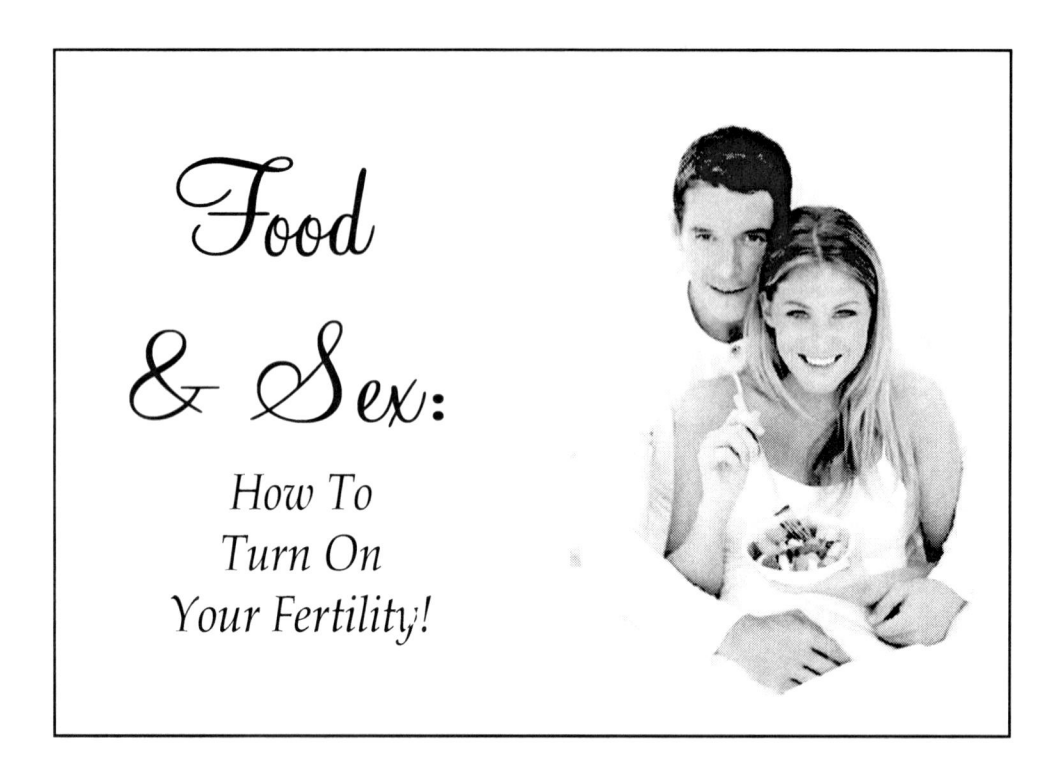

While the idea of foods acting as aphrodisiacs is as old as, well, love itself, the belief is more than just folklore passed from one generation to the next. Indeed, like most beliefs that appear to survive the test of time, there is some truth behind the premise – and such is the case for many of the foods believed to increase both our sexual appetite and our virility and fertility.

So what are the foods that "science" has shown make a difference? Here's a quick look at some of the delicious dishes believed to make a difference, and why they work! While I can't promise that eating these foods will make a difference in the bedroom, I can promise you'll have a deliciously good time finding out!

1. **PLUMS-** The secret here is the anti-clotting nutrients found in the skin and meat of this fruit. According to an article in the *British Journal of Nutrition*, plums may prevent plaque build up in arteries – and that in turn means better circulation to your entire reproductive system. And that means more enjoyable sex – and maybe better fertility!

2. **ALMONDS** – Since Biblical times, the almond was considered a sign of fertility, with the scent of this sweet nut rumored to arouse passion in women. Modern science tells us that almonds are super high in vitamin E and magnesium – minerals tied to both fertility and sex drive.

3. **BANANAS** – This fruit doesn't just resemble a male fertility symbol, it's loaded with nutrients that can actually make a man more potent! First, it contains sperm loving nutrients such as potassium, magnesium and B vitamins. But it also contains minerals and some enzymes which are believed to enhance a man's libido.

4. **CHICKPEAS** – The magic in this legume is the amino acid L-Arginine, which is a potent source of nitric oxide. This widens blood vessels for better circulation and helps to create natural lubrication which in turn makes sex feel better – and may help sperm move more easily through your reproductive system.

5. **CHOCOLATE** – The crown prince of aphrodisiac foods, chocolate contains a variety of compounds that can impact mood and increase the function of the pleasure-loving centers of the brain. In fact, chocolate is known to increase production of phenylethylamine, the chemical precursor to "dopamine" – a natural feel good chemical that is released during orgasm. This same chemical has also been shown to induce feelings of excitement and sexual attraction

6. **OYSTERS** – Perhaps the oldest "aphrodisiac" food in recorded history, the mighty oyster has long been rumored to hold sexual powers. But now science has given us at least a few reasons why! First, the oyster's slightly sweet – slightly salty scent is said to be scientifically similar to that produced by female pheromones - the natural scent that turns men on. But more importantly, oysters are a potent source of zinc, which is key for testosterone production as well as playing an important role in both male and female libido. As a lean source of protein, many men credit oysters – and their zinc content – for keeping them virile well into their golden years. Rumor has it that the famous lover Casanova ate 50 oysters a day to keep his sex drive in good working order!

7. **RED WINE -** Too much alcohol can dampen fertility and make it harder to conceive. But a study from the University of Florence in Italy revealed that a glass of wine with dinner may help increase vaginal lubrication making sex more pleasurable and conception possibly easier.

8. **ASPARAGUS –** In 19th Century France bridegrooms were served three courses of asparagus-rich dishes as a prenuptial fare – and apparently for good reason! This veggie is loaded with potassium, fiber, vitamin B6, vitamins A and C, thiamin and folic acid – a combination that appears to boost the production of histamines, a natural chemical that is necessary to achieve orgasm in both men and women.

A FINAL WORD:
EAT HEALTHY, BE HAPPY, DON'T WORRY!

While these last two chapters contain what I believe is good advice about the foods I hope you will add into your diet - *and some warnings about the foods I hope you will eat less of -* the real take home message, from me to you, is to simply eat as healthfully as you can, and not worry.

While your diet can certainly play an important role in helping you get pregnant, if you are filled with worry and fear about what you are eating, the resulting stress will only negate what a good diet can do for you. As you read earlier, stress can be a major contributing factor to fertility problems, so I don't want you to add to your anxiety with worries about what you are eating! In fact, I urge you to take a deep breath and let go of any fears and anxieties you may have about not "doing the right thing" – be it with your diet or anything else related to getting pregnant. Certainly, it's a good idea to heed precautions when and how you can. But what's more important is that you remain confidant and secure in your ability to get pregnant, and not put your energies into worry or fears about not getting pregnant.

In fact the most important things you can do to help prepare for pregnancy is to eat healthy, relax your body, and try to avoid both emotional and physical stress. In short, be happy, don't worry, eat healthy!

Chapter Nine

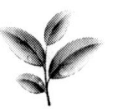

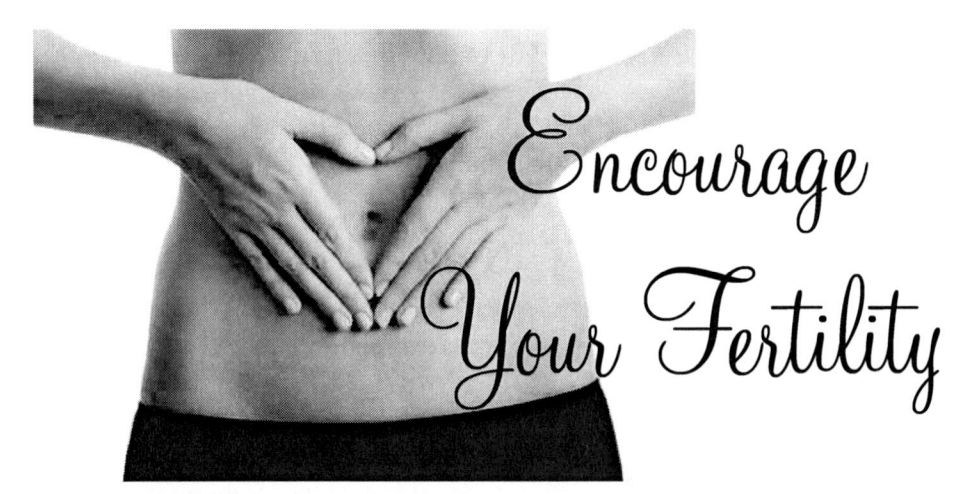

Encourage Your Fertility

With Power-Packed Vitamin Supplements

While the concept of "healthy eating" is the topic of so many of today's good living headlines, the link between good food and healthy fertility is something I have long "prescribed" for my patients. And I have seen firsthand how powerful it can be.

At the same time I also know how difficult it sometimes is to eat as healthfully as we should. This is particularly true when so many factors in our busy lives – including environmental pollutants, stress, even our lack of sleep - continually place such a drain on our nutrient supply.

As such, I have always believed that vitamin supplements can go a long way in filling in the gaps to help ensure your fertility stays healthy and strong – even in the throes of a hectic, busy life.

Even more important, however, is that there is some outstanding new research to show that specific vitamins, alone and in combination, have some specific fertility –boosting powers. In short, even if you are eating healthfully, adding certain specific supplements can enhance the power of good eating by a significant margin – and in the process support and boost your fertility as well.

Certainly, in my own medical practice, where I have helped thousands of couples conceive and deliver healthy babies, I have seen first-hand the power of these nutrients to not only increase fertility but to help bring into the world healthier, stronger, even smarter babies. In fact, based on my own personal research as well my personal experience with patients, I continued to recommend nutritional supplements to my patients even when there was only a glimmer of evidence proving the impact.

Today, I am proud to say that much of what I have always believed to be true about the power of vitamins has been *proven* true in study after study – with some of the research conducted at the biggest medical centers and universities in all parts of the world.

A little later in this book you'll find important information on supplements to boost your partner's fertility. But right now I want to concentrate on what I like to call the ***Female Super Nutrients*** – supplements that I believe can be helpful in encouraging, supporting and boosting *your* fertility, and insuring the health of your baby right from the moment conception takes place! It is my hope that you will use this information to custom tailor a supplement program that is specific to your personal fertility needs – and in this way bolster your ability to get pregnant quickly, easily and naturally!

At the same time, however, I want you to keep in mind that supplements are exactly that – *supplements,* which means " in addition to" your daily diet.   While it's true that certain nutrient supplements have amazing restorative powers, it's also true that the most positive and beneficial effects come when your diet and lifestyle are healthy as well.

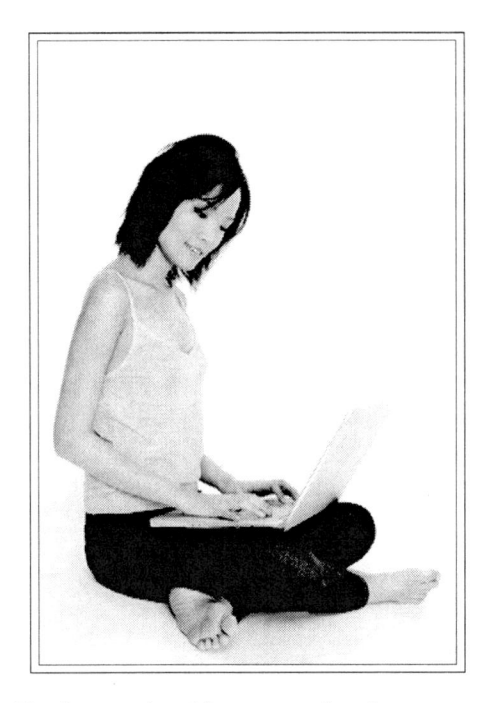

Is Your Fertility In Nutritional Jeopardy? Take This Quiz and Find Out

For some of you reading this book, eating healthy in conjunction with taking a prenatal vitamin or any good multi vitamin may be all that's necessary to ensure your pre-conception nutritional needs are being met.

For others, however, this may only be the start. Indeed, I would guess that in today's fast paced, hectic world a good many of you reading this book will have nutritional needs above and beyond what even a good multi or prenatal vitamin can supply.

To determine if you need to boost your pre conception nutritional status take this fun and easy quiz. Answer True or False to each of the following 18 statements–then check the Answer Key on the next page to know your score.

Answer True Or False:

- I love anything made with white flour – and I can't go through a day without eating at least one sandwich, some cookies or a donut before bedtime!
- I can't get through the day without a caffeine buzz – be it from coffee, soda or a "high energy drink".
- Most of my snacks and desserts contain high fructose corn syrup.
- I smoke cigarettes – or I am exposed to second hand smoke in my home or workplace.
- I consume more than two alcohol drinks per day.
- I recently used oral contraceptives for a year or more.

- I live or work in a major urban area.
- I sleep six hours or less per night.
- I am a "frequent flyer" and find myself on an airplane every few weeks.
- I have been diagnosed with fibroid tumors, excessive menstrual bleeding or anemia.
- I have been diagnosed with endometriosis or a hormone imbalance.
- I have been diagnosed with Poly Cystic Ovarian Syndrome, insulin resistance or type 2 diabetes.
- I have terrible PMS!
- I never know when my period is going to arrive – it's highly irregular.
- My job is stressful.
- My friends say I seem tense.
- I almost never exercise.
- I feel tired all the time and have a lack of energy.

If you have answered "TRUE" to between three and seven questions then you could definitely benefit from extra vitamin supplements.

If you answered "TRUE" to between eight and twelve questions then besides a multi vitamin I strongly urge you to pay close attention to the Super Female Fertility Nutrients - and add specific vitamins and minerals in therapeutic doses according to your needs

If you have answered "TRUE" to 12 or more questions then you should also seek the help of a registered nutritionist to help assess your full nutritional profile and make sure all your needs are being met.

The Seven Super Nutrients

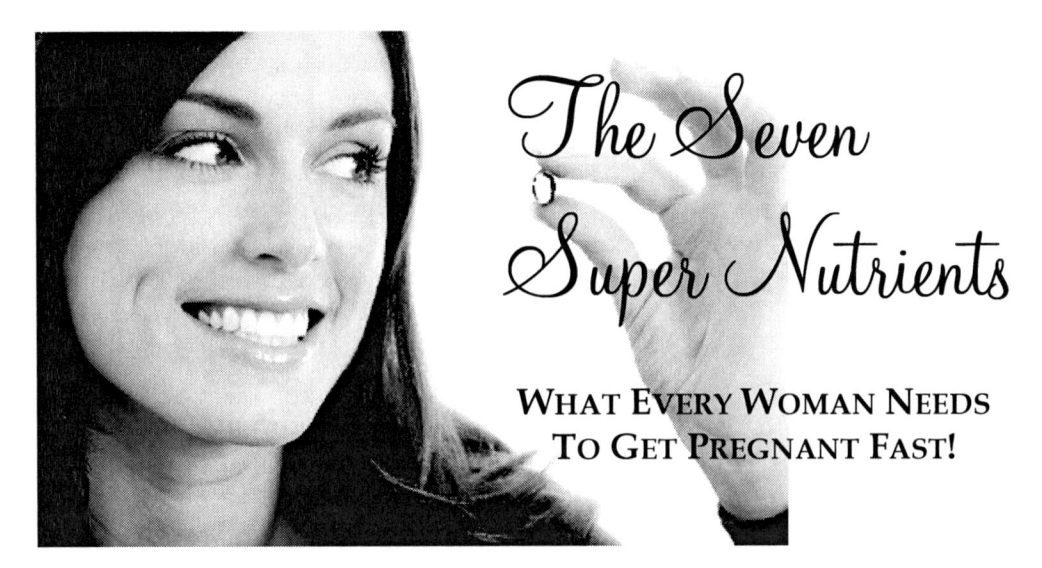

What Every Woman Needs To Get Pregnant Fast!

Super Female Fertility Nutrient #1 : Folic Acid

When it comes to both boosting your fertility and protecting your baby's health right from the start, there is perhaps no nutrient as important as vitamin B 9 - otherwise known as folic acid. Necessary for the production of red blood cells, folic acid also holds special significance for those trying to conceive.

Indeed, in one study involving more than 18,000 women those who took a vitamin supplement high in folic acid dramatically reduced their risk of developing ovulation-related fertility problems. Moreover, the effect was dose-related. In short, the more folic acid a woman consumed, the lower her risk of fertility problems.

There is also evidence showing folic acid helps an embryo to survive – an idea which seems to dovetail perfectly with evidence showing folic acid may help reduce the risk of early miscarriage. And, in fact, this is the finding of one major collaborative research project between the National Institutes of Child Health and Development (NICHD) in the United States and the Karolinska Institute in Sweden. Publishing their findings in the *Journal of the American Medical Association,* researchers suggested that the earlier in your pregnancy you begin taking folic acid, the greater your chance of avoiding miscarriage. If you start taking folic acid before you conceive, you'll be that much farther along in protecting against miscarriage when you do get pregnant.

Moreover, taking taking folic acid during your pre conception time also benefits your baby in other ways. How? We have long known that when used during pregnancy, folic acid supplements reduce a baby's risk of neural tube defects, a serious congenital malformation that is also a leading cause of infant death. Indeed, the NICHD reports that the simple act of adding folic acid to your diet during your reproductive years can dramatically decrease your baby's risk of developing both brain and spinal cord defects. In fact, even adding just 100 mcg of folic acid a day is enough to reduce your baby's risk of birth defects by some 22%.

By taking folic acid during your pre-conception time, you can doubly insure that your baby will have enough of this important nutrient right from the very moment of conception. In fact, since you could easily be pregnant four, six or even eight weeks before you know it by waiting until your pregnancy is confirmed to start this nutrient could actually deprive your baby of it's important benefits in the first critical six to eight weeks of life.

What's most important to realize is that many factors deplete folic acid, making it easy to fall short of this nutrient. Certain oral contraceptives, cholesterol medications, and drugs used to treat Poly Cystic Ovarian Syndrome and type II diabetes, as well as common pain relievers like aspirin and ibuprofen, and most antibiotics, can all deplete folic acid – even if your diet is healthy. For this reason it's imperative that you begin taking folic acid supplements as soon as you decide you want to get pregnant!

Taking vitamins before you conceive means your baby will get the best possible start in life ... right from the moment of conception!

Folic Acid Fertility Snapshot

Recommended Daily Allowance: 400 mcg daily before pregnancy; 800 – 1000 mcg daily after pregnancy.

ACOG Recommendations: 800 mcg daily

My Personal Recommendation : To enhance your fertility and give your baby the best possible start in life, I recommend a supplement containing 800 to 1,000 mcg of folic acid daily beginning as early as six months prior to when you want to get pregnant.

Foods High In Folic Acid Include: Fortified breakfast cereals (up to 400 mcg per serving); half cup of boiled spinach (100 mcg); four spears of asparagus (85 mcg); ½ cup chopped broccoli (50 mcg); one ounce of dry roasted peanuts (40 mcg); ½ cup Romaine Lettuce (40 mcg); two tablespoons wheat germ (40 mcg); six ounces tomato juice (35 mcg); ¾ cup orange juice (30 mcg); ¼ cantaloupe (25 mcg) ; one medium banana (20 mcg).

Signs Of Folic Acid Deficiency: Irritability or depression (folic acid is essential to the healthy functioning of the central nervous system and without it you may become irritable, sluggish, forgetful or depressed); general weakness; sore tongue; headaches; heart palpitations.

Factors That Deplete Folic Acid:
Medications: Topical or systemic corticosteroid drugs (such as hydrocortisone, prednisone, Beclomethasone); **NSAIDs** (ibuprofen, naproxen,); **Aspirin; most antibiotics; oral contraceptives** containing Ethinyl Estradiol and Desogestrel, Ethinyl Estradiol and Levonorgestrel, Ethinyl Estradiol and Norethindrone, and Ethinyl Estradiol and Norgestimate; **cholesterol drugs** Cholesetyramine and Colestipol; **Meformin** (for diabetes); **ulcer medications** such as Cimetidine, Famotidine, Nizatidine, Ranitidine Bismuth Citrate, Ranitidine Hydrochloride and Methotrexate used to treat Lupus. In addition, both anemia, and celiac disease (gluten sensitivity) can deplete folic acid. Because folic acid helps control "homocysteine", high levels of which may increase your risk of heart attack, if a blood test shows homocysteine levels are high, then you may need additional folic acid.

Want Twins?

TRY ADDING MORE FOLIC ACID TO YOUR DIET!

For many women who have struggled to get pregnant, the news that they are carrying twins comes as a delightful surprise. In fact, I have always believed that if you have been trying to have a baby for quite some time, especially if you are over 35, twins can be a true blessing, helping you to "catch up" with your family planning with just a single pregnancy.

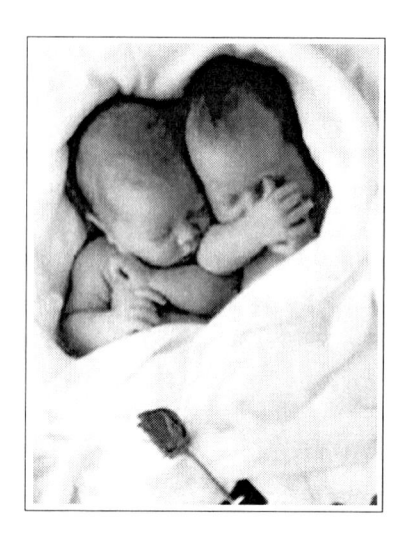

Moreover, if you must rely on fertility treatments to help you get pregnant, then the cost alone may preclude you from having more than one procedure. When this is the case, having twins can be even more of a blessing.

And now, research published in the journal *Lancet* revealed taking extra folic acid in the weeks before conception may help encourage twins! And I must say that on a personal level, this was something I had always found to be true in my practice as well. In fact, many fertility experts often asked what was my "secret" to helping so many women who wanted twins, to have twins! My answer was always "Extra vitamins"! And now research has proven this really can work.

Moreover, it's not just effective in IVF! The Lancet study backed up previous findings published by of a group of Hungarian researchers. They studied a large population of Chinese women and found that those who took up to 1mg (or 1,000 mcg) of folic acid daily, were more likely to have twins via natural conception as well.

So, does this mean that every woman who adds extra folic acid to her diet will conceive twins? Definitely not. Having twins via natural conception is still rare, and most often influenced by heredity. That said, if twins do run in your family, then taking extra folic acid in the weeks and months before attempting conception just might increase your chances of having twins!

SUPER FERTILITY NUTRIENT #2: BETA CAROTENE/VITAMIN A

If you've ever shopped for a multi-vitamin, then you probably know that most contain vitamin A – also known as Retinol. This is a fat soluble vitamin that most folks know as the nutrient that aids vision.

But when it comes to fertility, vitamin A is also an essential nutrient, and it's necessary for the creation of a healthy embryo. In fact, without adequate vitamin A it's almost impossible to create an embryo that is healthy enough to implant in your uterus and grow into a strong and healthy baby.

One way to ensure your body has adequate vitamin A is, of course, to take a supplement. But there is also another way to make certain your body has an adequate supply of vitamin A – and it involves taking supplements of a nutrient known as "beta carotene."

Found in many fruits and vegetables, but particularly those with an orange or yellow color (such as carrots, squash or cantaloupe) beta carotene is known as a "precursor" nutrient, because *the body uses it to make vitamin A* - in a ratio of about two-to-one. This means your body needs 2 mcg of beta carotene to make 1 mcg of vitamin A.

So, why not just take vitamin A directly? Well as you read in the previous chapter, beta carotene belongs to a group of nutrients known as "carotinoids. And together, this very special group of compounds play an enormously important role in fertility, over and above what vitamin A can do for you on it's own.

First, several carotinoid nutrients are essential to developing healthy follicular fluid. This is the liquid that surrounds and nourishes your egg, helping it to grow and develop. When follicular fluid is inadequate, your egg simply won't develop. But there's still more. Because once your egg *has* developed and is ready to be ovulated, beta carotene levels help signal the release of LH or luteinizing hormone. This, as you remember from Chapter 1, is the brain chemical that prompts your egg to leave your ovary and pop into your fallopian tube, where it can meet your partner's sperm.

So , these important activities alone are certainly enough reason to maintain a healthy level of beta carotene.

But there's still one more step in the fertilization process that uses this essential nutrient. Once your egg is ovulated, the "shell" it leaves behind is called the "corpus luteum" - and it immediately begins to manufacture progesterone. This is the hormone that, together with estrogen, helps turn the lining of your uterus into a soft, spongy "nest" or "womb" where your newly fertilized egg can implant, develop and grow. The more spongy your uterine lining is, the better the chance that your fertilized egg *will* attach and begin growing – and the more likely it is that your pregnancy will be successful. Conversely, the thinner your uterine lining is, the weaker it is – and the less likely it is that your pregnancy will continue. In fact many women who are plagued with recurrent miscarriages are actually deficient in progesterone – meaning their uterine lining never becomes thick or strong enough to "hold" onto a fertilized egg.

So, how does this all tie in with beta carotene? Well the corpus luteum shell is made up largely of beta carotene! Moreover, when levels are insufficient, progesterone production may suffer - and when it does, your fertilized egg may not ever get a chance to implant fully and grow.

The good news: Keeping levels of beta carotene high may help insure adequate progesterone production. In fact, for many women with PMS - a condition wherein progesterone is frequently low – eating foods high in beta carotene, or taking beta carotene supplements may help re-balance hormones and alleviate symptoms.

Perhaps the most important reason to use beta carotene instead of a vitamin A supplement is that once you are pregnant, excess levels of vitamin A have been shown to increase the risk of some birth defects. In fact, the American College of Obstetricians and Gynecologists (ACOG) recommend that once you are pregnant, vitamin A supplementation should not exceed 770 mcg daily (or 2,567 IUs)

Since you might be pregnant up to eight weeks before you know it, it's a good idea to watch vitamin A intake before pregnancy as well as during pregnancy. With beta carotene however, you won't have this problem – so that's another reason to make this your vitamin A supplement during your preconception time.

Indeed, when you analyze all the benefits, it seems that getting your vitamin A from a carotene supplement - instead of a vitamin A supplement - offers the best possible advantage for your fertility! This may be particularly true if you have had one or more miscarriages in the past

When shopping for a beta carotene supplements, however, do be certain to choose a product that contains *the full complement* of carotinoid nutrients and not just beta carotene alone. Not only will all the compounds work together to bolster your fertility, there is evidence that doing so may be healthier for your body overall.

If, however, you choose to take a vitamin A supplement, make certain that it does not exceed the ACOG recommendation of 770 mcg per day – or 2,567 IUs.

Important To Note: While vitamin A from supplements can build in the body and eventually cause a toxic overdose, beta carotene appears to not have this effect, so generally supplements are safe. However, at very high doses (30 mg or more) there are some risks, so make sure to speak to your doctor before adding supplements of this nutrient.

VITAMIN A – BETA CAROTENE SNAPSHOT

RECOMMENDED DAILY ALLOWANCE: Vitamin A : 700 mcg daily (or 2,333 international units.

There is no RDA for beta carotene.

RECOMMENDED BY ACOG DURING PREGNANCY: Up to 770 mcg daily or 2,567 international units of Vitamin A (Retinol).

MY PERSONAL FERTILITY RECOMMENDATION: Supplements containing up to 25,000 international units of beta carotene, daily in a supplement that also contains other carotenoids including lycopene, lutein, and alpha lipoic acid.

FOODS HIGH IN BETA CAROTENE INCLUDE: Carrots, sweet potatoes, yams, apricots, winter squash, pumpkin, cantaloupe, and mangoes. Other good sources include dark green leafy vegetables such as kale, collard greens, spinach, leaf lettuce and broccoli. Interestingly, your body can use the beta carotene in these foods best when they are cooked, chopped or pureed.

Foods High In Vitamin A Include : Whole or fortified milk, fish liver oils, tuna, shrimp, salmon, liver, eggs, some varieties of cheese.

Signs of Vitamin A/Beta Carotene Deficiency: Night blindness, rough dry skin, decreased sense of smell, fatigue, skin blemishes; sometimes PMS may also be a sign of a beta carotene deficiency.

Factors That Deplete Vitamin A/Beta Carotene : The most prominent cause of a vitamin A deficiency is overindulgence in alcohol. Because even a mild deficiency can begin damaging the lining of the stomach, it becomes difficult to absorb this nutrient (and others) from food, setting the stage for an even greater deficiency. Drugs that can deplete vitamin A include Orlistat and Olestra (for weight lose); Tetracycline antibiotics; cholesterol lowering medications cholestyramine (Questram) and cholesterol (Colestid); Neomycin.

Signs of Vitamin A Overdose : Headaches that last abnormally long, fatigue, muscle and joint pain, dry skin and lips, dry or irritated eyes, nausea or diarrhea, and hair loss. While vitamin A is considered safe in the dietary form, it is possible to get too much from supplements.

Signs of Beta Carotene Overdose: As a supplement, beta carotene is generally recognized as safe by the FDA, but taking more than 30 mg a day can result in a temporary yellowing of the skin, particularly on the palms of the hands and soles of the feet. This disappears once the supplement is stopped.

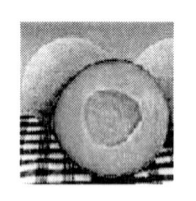

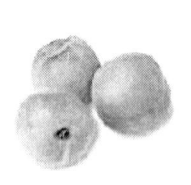

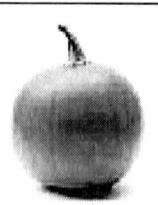

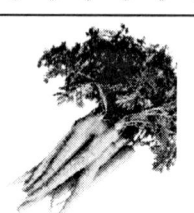

Cantaloupe, nectarines, pumpkin & carrots are a few of the many fruits & vegetables high in beta carotene. Generally, the more orange in color, the more beta carotene a fruit or vegetable will have!

SUPER FERTILITY NUTRIENT # 3: VITAMIN B6

As part of the group of nutrients known as B complex, doctors have long believed that vitamin B6 (pyridoxine) plays an important role in many aspects of women's health. In fact, this water - soluble vitamin first isolated and "discovered" in the 1930's, performs a wide variety of functions involving over 100 enzymes linked to key chemical reactions within the body . Vitamin B 6 is also necessary for red blood cell function, and both your nervous system and your immune system rely heavily on this nutrient to function properly. Vitamin B6 is also necessary to convert a compound known as "tryptophan" into niacin, also key for optimum health.

But while doctors have long known the importance of Vitamin B 6 to your *general* health, it wasn't until researchers began to make connections between this nutrient and PMS (pre menstrual syndrome) that we began to fully understand and appreciate the impact this vitamin appears to have on fertility.

More specifically, research began to show that vitamin B6 has a direct connection to the production of both serotonin and dopamine, two brain chemicals related to not just mood and behavior - including depression - but also able to influence activity of key reproductive hormones. Indeed, when levels of either serotonin or dopamine are out of balance, you can not only experience an increase in anxiety and depression, but also a decrease in hormone activity necessary to get pregnant. In fact, by impacting levels of both FSH (follicle stimulating hormone) and LH (luteinizing hormone), serotonin may even have a direct influence on the daily activity of your ovaries – affecting everything from egg production and maturation, to egg release, and the subsequent production of progesterone necessary for a healthy pregnancy.

That said, when a B6 deficiency exists, serotonin production is compromised, and so is at least some of the brain chemistry necessary for egg growth and ovulation.

For many women, the most outstanding symptom of B6 deficiency is a whopping case of PMS – for which studies show Vitamin B6 can help. I have found that many women who do suffer from severe PMS – and the subsequent hormonal imbalances – also have a problem getting pregnant. And when this is the case I and many other fertility experts believe that vitamin B6 can help.

But it's not just the connection to PMS that makes B6 an important fertility nutrient. Indeed, vitamin B6 also impacts the way your body controls blood sugar levels - and here lies another link to fertility. What's the connection?

Generally speaking, Vitamin B6 is one of the nutritional safeguards that helps keep blood sugar within a normal range. In fact, when you diet, or when your caloric intake is generally low, your body relies on vitamin B6 to convert stored carbohydrates or other nutrients into glucose so that blood sugar levels remain normal. Conversely, when there is a shortage of vitamin B6, sugar levels have a problem remaining stable, and levels can begin to fluctuate out of control – and that is the point where your fertility can be disrupted. How?

As you read in earlier chapters, when your sugar can't get into your cells (a condition known as 'insulin resistance') it initiates an entire cascade of hormonal activity that ultimately impacts ovulation - and sometimes can even keep eggs from growing and developing. For some women this can become a chronic problem, frequently resulting in a condition known as Poly Cystic Ovary Syndrome (see Chapter 17).

But even if you don't have PCOS, insulin resistance can affect you on a transitory, level, often experienced as monthly symptoms of PMS. In fact, if you've ever experienced food cravings or ravenous hunger in the days before your period is due , chances are your blood sugar was a little bit "off" causing you to experience a type of *temporary* insulin resistance.

Certainly, this doesn't carry the same negative impact on fertility as it does when true insulin resistance is present all the time. However, it makes sense to connect the dots here and see that for some women, these temporary bouts could have an effect on egg production on a month-by-month basis. Moreover, since we know that taking extra vitamin B6 during the premenstrual time can mediate or even alleviate many of the symptoms – including those linked to temporary insulin resistance - for me it has always seemed a logical and linear assumption that B6 would also play a role in improving ovarian function as well. And for many of my patients who had these problems, and had problems getting pregnant, increasing their intake of B6 did indeed appear to help.

As I previously reported in my best selling fertility book *"Getting Pregnant: What You Need To Know Now"*, studies conducted as early as 1979 revealed that women who were diagnosed with "unexplained infertility" appeared to benefit from taking between 100 mg and 800 mg of vitamin B6 daily. While the study was small and in no way was considered conclusive, I can personally tell you that I have helped many women diagnosed with *unexplained infertility* to conceive within several months via a combination of dietary changes and increasing their intake of B complex vitamins and particularly B6.

One more key fact you should know: As essential as Vitamin B6 is to your health and your fertility, your body cannot manufacture this nutrient on its own. It must be obtained from dietary sources, or from supplements – which is another key reason why you must include vitamin B6 in your pre conception nutrient program.

Q: *Is there any difference between a regular multi vitamin and a prenatal vitamin – and which is best for fertility?*

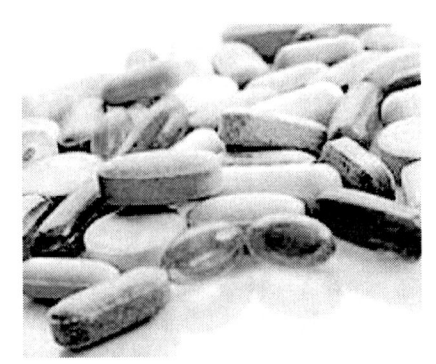

A: Many years ago, high levels of folic acid were only available by prescription. As such, prescription prenatal vitamins were the only way a woman could get an adequate prenatal supply of this nutrient. However, now that higher levels of folic acid are available over-the-counter, a good multi vitamin can be as good or sometimes even better than a pre natal vitamin. As long as your vitamin product contains the basics detailed in this chapter, it's perfectly okay to take a multi. Just be certain it contains the "magic" number of at least 400 mcg of folic acid - key for fertility.

VITAMIN B6 : FERTILITY SNAPSHOT

RECOMMENDED DAILY ALLOWANCE: 1.3 mg per day

RECOMMENDED BY ACOG DURING PREGNANCY: 2 to 2.5 mg daily

MY PERSONAL FERTILITY RECOMMENDATION: 200 mg daily (in conjunction with a B complex or prenatal vitamin).

FOODS HIGH IN B6 INCLUDE: Fortified breakfast cereals - ¾ c (up to 2 mg per serving); Baked Potato - flesh and skin, one medium (up to .70 mg); Banana, one medium (.68 mg); Garbanzo beans, canned, ½ c (.57 mg); Chicken breast, cooked, ½ breast (.52 mg); Oatmeal, instant, fortified, one packet (.42 mg); Pork loin, lean only, cooked, three oz (0.42); Sunflower seeds, kernels, dry roasted, one oz (.23 mg).

SIGNS OF B6 DEFICIENCY: Early signs of deficiency are sometimes "silent" and without a blood test, you might not know anything is wrong. However, for many woman symptoms of PMS, including cyclical anxiety and depression and sometimes unexplained infertility can be a sign that more B6 is needed. In the later stages of deficiency you may experience dermatitis (skin inflammation), glossitis (a sore tongue), deeper depression, and mental confusion. A deficiency can also cause anemia.

FACTORS THAT DEPLETE VITAMIN B6: Heavy alcohol consumption (it promotes the destruction and loss of vitamin B6 from the body); use of the asthma medication theophylline; a poor diet. You may have a greater need for vitamin B6 if you suffer from PMS, insulin resistance, type II diabetes, or Poly Cystic Ovarian Syndrome.

SIGNS OF OVERDOSE: Although vitamin B6 is a water-soluble vitamin, meaning any excess not needed by the body is excreted in the urine, taking a high dose supplement for an extended period of time may result in a painful neurological condition known as sensory neuropathy. Symptoms include pain and numbness of the arms and legs, and in severe cases, difficulty walking. Typically these symptoms only develop when your intake of vitamin B6 exceeds 1,000 mg per day for a period of time, and it is taken alone and without the balance of the " B complex vitamins.

SUPER FERTILITY NUTRIENT # 4: VITAMIN B 12

Part of the family of B complex vitamins, B12 is the nutrient that is essential for the production of healthy red blood cells – the "transport wagons" that carry life-giving oxygen to every muscle and organ in your body. When B 12 is in short supply, it can result in "anemia " - condition characterized by fatigue. Your body feels tired because there simply aren't enough red blood cells to provide the oxygen and other nutrients you need to thrive.

But from a fertility standpoint, even a very mild deficiency of vitamin B12 can have some extremely detrimental effects, frequently interfering with ovulation, and in general making it much more difficult, or sometimes even impossible to conceive.

Because B12 is also crucial to normal cell division within a fertilized egg, if you do happen to get pregnant when your nutrient stores are low, your embryo may not develop normally, or at all. Moreover, B12 is also crucial to a healthy uterine environment and without it your embryo may not implant normally or be able to grow.

In fact research has even linked a B12 deficiency to recurrent miscarriage, and that link involves "homocystine" – a natural compound that, in high amounts, can promote the development of blood clots. Normally, B12 is one of the nutrients that help keep homocysteine levels in check. But when levels go down – homocysteine goes up – and the risk of developing blood clots increases. In many women those clots develop in the blood supply leading to the uterus , thereby blocking nourishment to the embryo. The result is frequently a miscarriage – and unless the deficiency is discovered and treated , every pregnancy thereafter has the same, sad result.

What makes all of this truly significant is that it's entirely possible to be deficient in B12 and not even know it. Why? First, mild deficiencies often produce no obvious symptoms. But more importantly , a number of common factors can mask even a significant deficiency. These include a diet high in folic acid which is recommended for getting pregnant.

Moreover, many women who are deficient in Vitamin B12 are frequently misdiagnosed as having an iron deficiency and given iron supplements instead of B12. Additionally, if you are a vegetarian or even a woman who tends to eat very few animal products, it's also easy to develop a B12 deficiency.

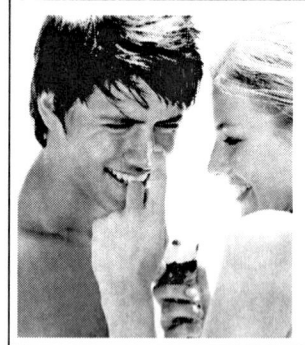

> ### B12 : NOT JUST FOR WOMEN!
>
> Vitamin B12 isn't just important for female fertility, it's also important for male fertility! Not only does a B-12 deficiency reduce sperm motility and sperm count, taking 1000 mcg of B12 daily can boost sperm count & increase sperm motility - even if a deficiency does not exist!

And lastly, if you suffer from even mild digestive disorders, or particularly conditions such as Crohns or celiac disease, levels of B12 can plummet before you know it.

But the really comforting news here is that for most women eating a healthy, balanced diet will levels of B12 within the normal range. If, however, a deficiency does occur, correcting it is relatively easy via increasing your intake of foods rich in B12 – such as leafy green vegetables – and taking a B12 supplement.

And once you do, it can completely turn your pregnancy odds around – and quickly! In one research study published in the *Journal of Reproductive Medicine* women with a history of up to seven consecutive miscarriages were treated with vitamin B12 for several weeks. Once a normal level of this nutrient was achieved, all the women were able to successfully conceive and deliver healthy babies. For several, the B12 resulted in an immediate pregnancy, with a full term delivery of a healthy baby within nine months!

Indeed, correcting even a mild B12 deficiency not only gives your fertility an immediate boost, it also helps insure your pregnancy is healthy and that your baby has the best possible chance to grow to grow and thrive.

For this reason I strongly recommend that you consider taking B12 supplements beginning at least a few weeks prior to when you want to get pregnant. If you are already have having problems getting pregnant, ask your doctor about a test to measure your levels of B12 – and certainly do so before starting any fertility treatments Sadly, a vitamin B 12 deficiency is often overlooked even by fertility specialists, causing many couples to experience months or even years of failed fertility treatments when in reality all they really needed was vitamin B 12.

VITAMIN B12 : FERTILITY SNAPSHOT

RECOMMENDED DAILY ALLOWANCE: Adults, aged 19-51 : 2.4 mcg daily.

RECOMMENDED BY ACOG DURING PREGNANCY : 2.6 mcg

MY PERSONAL FERTILITY RECOMMENDATION : 500 mcg daily

FOODS HIGH IN B12 INCLUDE: Three ounce servings of : Clams (84 mcg) mussels (20 mcg) ; salmon (2.4 mcg) beef (2.1`mcg); chicken and turkey (0.3 mcg); egg (0.6 mcg); milk – eight ounces (0.9 mcg); brie cheese (one ounce – 0.5 mcg).

SIGNS OF B12 DEFICIENCY: General weakness and fatigue; light headedness and dizziness; palpitations and rapid heartbeat; shortness of breath; sore tongue with a red 'beefy' appearance; nausea or poor appetite; weight loss; diarrhea; yellowish tinge to the skin and eyes. Note, however, that symptoms tend to develop slowly and may not be recognized immediately. Long term deficiencies can result in numbness and tingling in the hands and feet; difficulty walking; muscle weakness; irritability; memory loss; dementia; depression; psychosis.

FACTORS THAT DEPLETE VITAMIN B12: A diet high in folic acid; vegetarian diet; conditions that impact the movement of food through the digestive system such as diabetes, scleroderma, or diverticulitis; eating disorders such as bulimia or anorexia. Medications that deplete B12 include most birth control pills, ; sulfa drug antibiotics; cephalasporins; certain myacin drugs; penicillin derivatives such as Amoxicillin; tetracycline derivatives such as doxycycline and minocycline; Metformin (used to treat diabetes); ulcer drugs such as Cimetidine, Famotidine, Nizatidine, Ranitidine. If you are diagnosed with an intestinal disorder that is preventing you from absorbing even the B12 that is in supplements, talk to your doctor about intra muscular B12 injections, or sublingual tabs, which dissolve under the tongue and do not have to be digested in the stomach as a tablet would.

SIGNS OF OVERDOSE: No toxic or significant adverse effects have been reported even with high doses as high as one mg (1000 mcg) daily by mouth or 1 mg by intra muscular (IM) injection. This is particularly true via oral dosing of B12, since so little is absorbed.

SUPER FERTILITY NUTRIENT # 5: VITAMIN C

Vitamin C has always been known as the "healing" vitamin – the nutrient that aids in the production of collagen, the natural compound that indeed helps wounds to heal. But on a more popular level you probably know Vitamin C for its ability to fight off colds and flu!

What you might not know however, is that Vitamin C is also a powerful fertility nutrient, aiding conception and helping to encourage a healthy pregnancy in myriad ways.

But how exactly does it work? First, this nutrient has an affinity for the tissue of the reproductive organs. In women, it likes to accumulate in the ovaries, in men, in the testes. So immediately we know that maintaining adequate levels must be key to proper functioning of these organs. A little bit later in this book you'll learn more about the role of vitamin C in male fertility. But right now I want to concentrate on the role of this nutrient in female fertility – and how it works to keep your ovaries healthy.

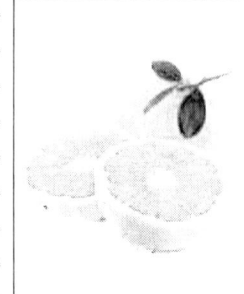

> Research shows that when vitamin C intake is high you give your eggs some special "fertility armor" to fend off free radical damage. This results in not only healthier eggs, but a healthier – and quicker conception overall! This is even true when having fertility treatments!

In much the way that your bone continues to breakdown and build up throughout your lifetime, so too does ovarian tissue go through a similar "remodeling" process. Eggs are made, they pop through the ovary, the ovary tissue heals itself, and the next cycle another new egg is made. While several key compounds are involved in this process – including the hormone estrogen – the healing that allows the rebuilding to occur and ovulation to continue with each cycle – is very dependent on vitamin C. In fact, without it, the natural cycle of ovarian function could not go on.

But that's the not the only link this nutrient has to conception. Vitamin C also acts as a powerful antioxidant helping to protect your developing eggs from free radical damage. As you read in a previous chapter, free radicals are formed during many natural body processes – including egg development and ovulation. Without the body's natural free radical protection, eggs would be damaged almost as soon as they come out! Many could not survive the ovulation process. But by keeping vitamin C levels optimized you can insure that your body always has the nutrient resources necessary to protect your eggs from free radical damage, and help guarantee that they remain healthy and protected while they grow and develop.

GIVE YOUR EGGS A VITAMIN BATH
AND GET PREGNANT FASTER!

But there is still more protection from Vitamin C to be had! Studies gleaned from in vitro fertilization procedures have shown that Vitamin C is also present in follicular fluid – the semi-solid liquid that surrounds your egg and aids in growth and development. When vitamin C is in short supply, so is follicular fluid – and that can dramatically curtail the growth and development of a healthy egg.

Conversely, when vitamin C levels are adequate, follicular fluid is plentiful – and that means your eggs have a much better chance of not only developing, but also being fertilized. In fact, studies show that taking vitamin C supplements can actually enhance the egg-making benefits of clomiphene citrate, or Clomid, a drug commonly used to help women produce more eggs during a cycle.

Perhaps more importantly, when it comes to getting pregnant, the level of vitamin C itself found within follicular fluid also appears to make a dramatic difference in how quickly you conceive. In one study of women undergoing IVF treatment for infertility, doctors actually measured the level of vitamin C in follicular fluid from each of the eggs they extracted. What they found: Those women who took 500 mg of vitamin C daily had the highest levels of this nutrient in their follicular fluid.

Moreover, the researchers also found that the eggs of the women who had successful pregnancies were much higher in antioxidant capacity that those eggs which failed to be fertilized. Again, this tells us that when you take vitamin C you give your eggs some special "fertility armor" to fend off free radical damage. This results in not only healthier eggs, but a healthier conception overall!

VITAMIN C CORRECTS COMMON FERTILITY PROBLEM

In a study published in the journal Fertility and Sterility in 2003, a group of Japanese doctors offered important evidence showing that vitamin C can correct what is known as a "luteal phase defect" - a common endocrine disorder that causes a deficiency in progesterone during the second half of the menstrual cycle. As you recall, progesterone is manufactured by the shell your ovulated egg leaves behind and it works to help create a spongy lining inside your uterus so your fertilized egg can implant and grow. Without adequate progesterone, implantation may not occur. Or, if it does the lining of your uterus may be so weak that miscarriage results. In fact, studies show that luteal phase defect is the cause of miscarriage in up to 35% of women who experience chronic pregnancy loss.

The good news is that taking vitamin C supplements can completely turn this problem around! In the Japanese study doctors found that just 750 mg of vitamin C daily increased progesterone levels by up to 53%. More importantly it also significantly increased the rate of pregnancy while reducing the rate of miscarriage. And this might be of special interest to those of you who find it's taking longer than normal to get pregnant. Why?

It has been my experience that many women who believe they cannot get pregnant are actually conceiving, but miscarrying very early on – sometimes before the pregnancy can even be measured on a test. When this is the case, vitamin C may be especially helpful in preventing that early miscarriage and insuring you sustain a healthy and normal conception.

So, while we are far from having conclusive evidence that vitamin C can, on its own, increase fertility, there is certainly enough research to suggest that taking vitamin C supplements can improve not only your chances for getting pregnant, but also ensure that your resulting embryo is strong and well developed enough to thrive.

Certainly, in my own practice, I have seen this important nutrient make a significant difference in the ease with which many of my patients were able to get pregnant. For some, it was the key factor that tipped the scales from infertile to fertile! For others it was the success factor in fertility treatments that had previously failed. And for some lucky women – those in their 40's and long past their reproductive prime - simply taking vitamin C in consort with the other nutrients and a healthy diet, was enough to allow them to have a natural conception – even after other doctors told them their only hope was donor eggs!

Vitamin C Fertility Snapshot

Recommended Daily Allowance: Adults, aged 19-51 – 75 mg daily.

Recommended by ACOG During Pregnancy: 60 mg daily before pregnancy; 80 mg daily after conception.

My Personal Fertility Recommendation: 500 mg twice daily.

Foods High In Vitamin C include: Orange juice (6 ounces, 75 mg); Grapefruit juice (6 ounces – 60 mg); Orange, (1 medium ,70 mg) ;Grapefruit (½ medium, 44 mg), Strawberries (one cup, whole 82 mg); Tomato (1 medium, 23 mg); Sweet red pepper (½ cup, raw chopped 141 mg); Broccoli (½ cup cooked, 58 mg); Potato (one medium baked, 26 mg).

Signs of Vitamin C Deficiency: Bleeding and bruising easily; hair and tooth loss; joint pain and swelling.

Factors That Deplete Vitamin C : Smoking; alcohol; birth control pills, exposure to air pollution; inhalant medications used to treat asthma, corticosteroids, regular use of aspirin, diuretics such as Bumetanide, Ethacrynic Acid, Furosemide and Torsemide.

Signs of Overdose/Toxicity: Because vitamin C is water soluble, generally the body excretes what it cannot use. So, there is very little risk of a toxic overdose. That said, there have been some reports of kidney stones as well as diarrhea and other gastrointestinal disturbances with exceedingly high levels of vitamin C supplementation. As such the FDA has put a cap on 2000 mg or two grams of vitamin C a day as a safe "upper limit", tolerated by almost everyone.

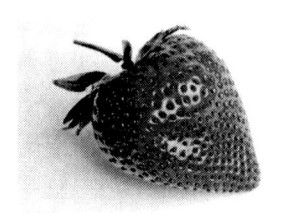

Not All Vitamin C is Alike!

If you've ever spent even a few minutes in the vitamin aisle of your pharmacy or health food store, then you probably already know there are many variations of vitamin C. In addition to synthetic vs. natural, there are also several types of "C" available including L-ascorbic acid, calcium ascorbate, magnesium ascorbate, and ester C.

So, how do you choose which one is right for you?

First, it's important to note that most experts contend both synthetic and natural C supplements react the same way in the body. According to the Linus Pauling Institute at Oregon State University, "Natural and synthetic L-ascorbic acid are chemically identical and there are no known differences in their biological activities or bio availability."

That said, there can be some differences in the various types of vitamin C, especially regarding how they react in your system. Some forms can be decidedly gentle on your tummy, while others may be exceedingly harsh, particularly at therapeutic dosages.

To help make choosing easier, here's what you need to know about each of the four types of Vitamin C available.

- **L-Ascorbic Acid -** This is pure vitamin C and in its raw form has a sharp taste. It is also highly acidic and the form most likely to cause an upset stomach in high amounts. If you take this type, take it with food in order to reduce the risk of stomach upset.

- **Calcium Ascorbate –** This version of vitamin C binds the nutrient to a calcium molecule, which offers a buffering action in the stomach that reduces the normal acidic effects. It is easy on the digestive system plus offers you a bonus boost of extra calcium!

- **MAGNESIUM ASCORBATE** - In this formulation, ascorbic acid is bound to magnesium, making it super gentle on the stomach. This form of vitamin C is also very easy to absorb, and it works great if you normally have problems with excess gas. It is also considered a supplemental form of magnesium, so if you use this type be certain to also take calcium supplements, (see Chapter 10) since it's important that these two minerals remain in balance.

- **ESTER C** - This is a patented form of the ascorbic acid-calcium combination – a blend that makes it extremely non-acidic and ultra easy to absorb. It is considered by many to be the top of the line in terms of vitamin C supplementation and is often recommended by nutritionists when you are seeking maximum rapid absorption. It is also the type favored if you are taking large doses of C. Because, however, it is also the most expensive type of vitamin C, if cost is a factor, you can simply look for calcium ascorbate products which I believe will give you similar benefits.

TABLET VS POWDER C

There are advantageous to both types and which one you chose is often a matter of personal preference. Among the differences: Powdered vitamin C (which you can mix into any beverage) does not require digestion, so it's rapidly absorbed . It also does not contain any "extra" ingredients such as binders or fillers required to make a tablet, so if you are sensitive to these factors, then a powdered form is best for you.

At the same time, because there are no buffers a vitamin C powder can be more harsh on your stomach. While a tablet may take longer to break down and absorb, it's more likely to be buffered so it's kinder on your stomach. Tablets also come in time-release formulas so if you are spreading your vitamin C supplementation throughout the day, this form can be helpful since you only need to take one dose once a day

IMPORTANT NOTE : Regardless of what type of vitamin C you choose, take your supplements with a fruit juice or filtered water. The metals in tap water (particularly copper and iron) may oxidize the vitamin C before it gets into your blood stream and dramatically reduce the effectiveness.

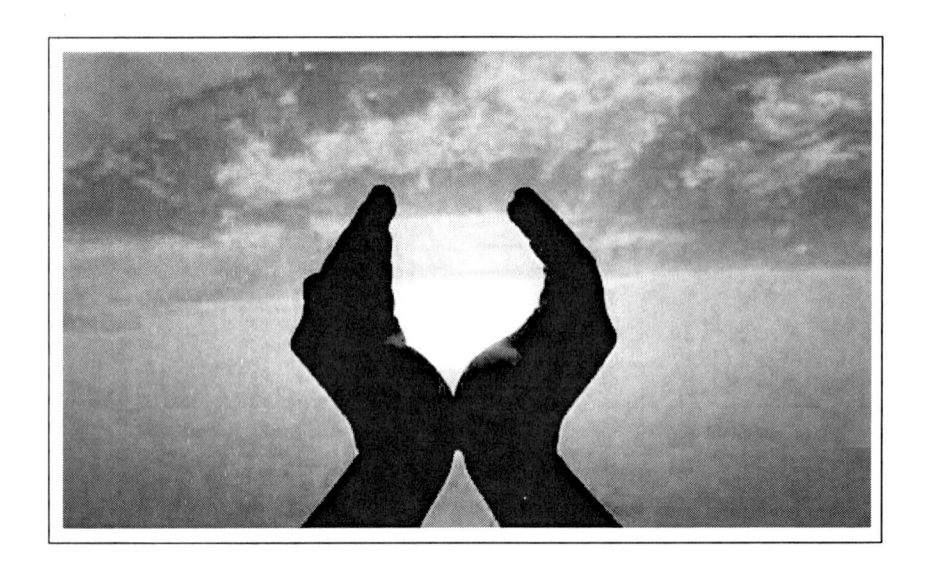

SUPER FERTILITY NUTRIENT # 6 : VITAMIN D -

Vitamin D is a fat-soluble nutrient that plays a vital role in not only your fertility but many aspects of your overall health. It's frequently known as the "The Sunshine Vitamin" - and with good reason. Your body makes the most important form of this vitamin from exposure to the sun! And, it's the only nutrient that is made this way. How does this occur?

When you feel the soothing warmth of the sun hitting your skin, you are also experiencing a localized chemical reaction that results in the production of a natural compound known as 7-dehydrocholesterol. This compound heads straight from your skin cells to your liver where it is rapidly converted into what is called a "bio active" form of vitamin D – meaning a form of the vitamin your body can immediately use.

As a nutrient, vitamin D works different from every other vitamin as it is the only one that functions as a hormone. In fact, many experts believe that D was incorrectly classified as a vitamin and should, in fact be considered a hormone. But whatever category you place it in, maintaining a proper level is key to good health. What exactly does vitamin D do ?

Among its most important jobs is regulating and controlling blood levels of calcium. More specifically, when the level of vitamin D falls too low, your blood supply cannot maintain adequate levels of calcium. To make up the difference, your body begins pulling calcium from your bones – which in turn creates a deficiency in your skeleton and in the process increases your risk of fracture. This is actually part of what happens in a bone thinning disorder known as osteoporosis .

But it's not just low calcium that's a problem. When your intake of calcium is high but your intake of Vitamin D is low, a problem known as calcifications or "calcium build up" can occur, in the arteries, in the kidney and even in the joints. If you have a bit of osteoarthritis this buildup can exacerbate joint pain and swelling.

But while regulating calcium is important, it's not the only job for vitamin D. Indeed, this nutrient also impacts brain chemistry directly related to your mood. While you may have always known that spending time in the sun made you feel better, you might not have known why. Today it's clear that the extra vitamin D garnered from time spent in the sun plays a key role in orchestrating some of the brain chemicals linked to mood disorders. So, spending time in the sun may actually help alleviate symptoms of mild depression in some people.

In fact, the ability of vitamin D to impact your overall health is now considered so powerful , many believe it helps reduce the risk of high blood pressure, heart disease, and even some cancers. Most important, you are trying to get pregnant, vitamin D can have a positive effect on your fertility *and make conception quicker and easier.*

HOW VITAMIN D AFFECTS FERTILITY

Among the most important factors linking Vitamin D to fertility is that it has a direct impact on the reproductive organs – the gonads in men and the ovaries in women, where it works to regulate how estrogen is utilized to help egg follicles mature and grow. Vitamin D also plays a role in how estrogen acts in the uterus, particularly in regard to development of the lining. But that's not the only way in which vitamin D can impact your ability to get pregnant.

One way in which your body maintains proper levels of FSH and LH – the hormones that promote both egg production and release - is linked to blood levels of calcium. Without proper amounts of vitamin D, calcium levels can go out of sync – which in turn can impact the production of both FSH and LH, and of course, keep you from getting pregnant.

In fact, one group of Yale researchers studied 67 women who had problems

> **Q:** *I was diagnosed with PCOS ...and I'm wondering if Vitamin D will have any impact on my ability to get pregnant?*
>
> **A:** The answer is a resounding YES! A new study has found that women who have lost their menstrual due to extreme PCOS were able to resume normal periods *and* get pregnant after just a few months of high potency Vitamin D therapy! You can augment the power of your vitamin supplements by getting 20 minutes of sun exposure daily.

conceiving – and found that 93% of them were low in vitamin D. According to researcher Dr. Lubna Pal, " Of note, not a single patient with either ovulatory disturbance or poly cystic ovary syndrome demonstrated normal Vitamin D levels; 39 per cent of those with ovulatory disturbance and 38 per cent of those with PCOS had serum 25OHD levels consistent with deficiency. "

If that were not enough to get you to run right out to the nearest health food store and stock up on vitamin D supplements, consider this: When calcium levels go down, the rate of PMS climbs! More importantly, however, the reverse is also true! According to a study conducted by University of Massachusetts researcher Elizabeth R. Bertone-Johnson, ScD, and published in the *Archives of Internal Medicine,* when the intake of both calcium and vitamin D is high, the risk of PMS is significantly reduced. In fact, they found women who ate just four servings a day of calcium-rich low fat dairy or yogurt, or drank orange juice fortified with calcium and vitamin D, were 40% less like to experience PMS!

So what's the connection to getting pregnant? First, when PMS is under control you will simply feel better with far less stress – which in turn means that all hormone activity will be better balanced. But more importantly, since PMS is a condition underscored by a reproductive hormone imbalance, reducing your risk *of this* problem automatically helps insure better hormone balance, and a quicker and easier pregnancy.

VAGINAL INFECTIONS, VITAMIN D AND FERTILITY

There is still one more important reason to keep vitamin D levels high: It can protect you from a fertility robbing V zone infection! Indeed, the very latest research shows that Vitamin D deficiencies may be linked to a higher rate of bacterial vaginosis (BV) an intimate infection that occurs when natural bacteria found in your V zone begins growing out of control. It's a problem that impacts up to 30% of all women in their childbearing years – and it can have fertility robbing consequences.

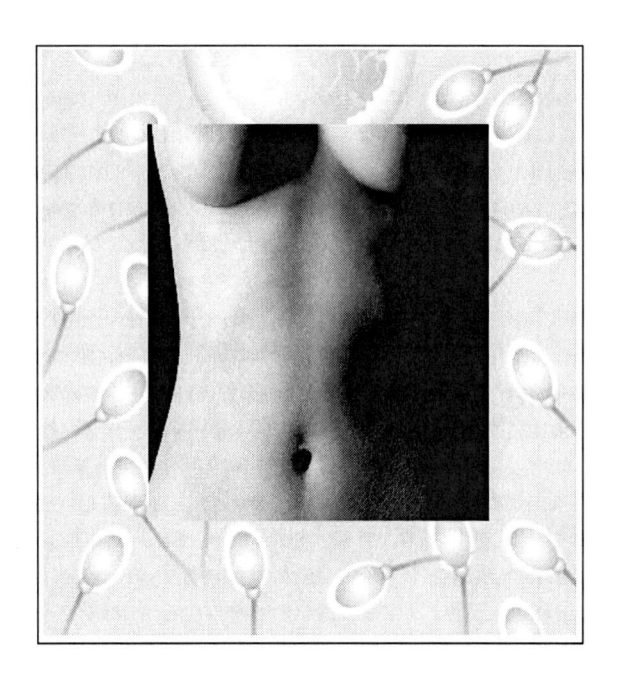

If left untreated, for example, this infection can lead to a much more serious condition known as PID – pelvic inflammatory disease. This involves infection that spreads into the fallopian tubes, ovaries and even the uterus and not only directly and immediately impacts your ability to get pregnant, but also creates scar tissue that can interfere with conception in the future.

But even if your BV infection is localized, pathogens or germs linked to this condition can harm your partner's sperm and keep it from fertilizing your egg. If you do happen to get pregnant, a BV infection could lead to miscarriage, and is linked to premature labor and low birth weight babies.

The good news : You can dramatically reduce your risk of developing any of these problems by simply keeping your vitamin D levels high.

How can this help?

While doctors aren't completely sure, many believe that vitamin D helps give a boost to the immune system, which in turn helps keep the natural bacteria found in the V zone from growing out of control.

Vitamin D Deficiency:
It Can Happen To You!

As important as we know vitamin D is today, for generations, few people paid much attention to it - simply because it was so easily made via exposure to sunlight. Moreover, because in pre-computer and pre-technology days, so much of our working time and our leisure time was spent outdoors there was little worry about vitamin D deficiency.

In the latter part of the 20th century however, and particularly now, in the 21st century life began to change. The development of the computer and all its subsequent technologies turned us from an outdoor society to an indoor one – dramatically decreasing our sun exposure in the process.

Add to this the fear of skin cancer linked to too much sun exposure – as well as the risks of premature skin aging - and we not only started spending less time in the sun, when we were out of doors we frequently coated our skin with potent sunscreens.

While they do effectively block damage from the sun, they also dramatically reduce the chemical reaction necessary for the body to make vitamin D.

The end result: We have became a nation – and in many ways a world – that is grossly vitamin D deficient. In fact, if you spend just one long winter with very little exposure to sunlight, a significant vitamin D deficiency can quickly and easily take hold.

So it's easy to see how season after season, year after year of limited or even no sun exposure can lead to a whopper of a deficiency!

The good news: Even if you have a Vitamin D deficiency, it's very easy to correct! In fact, the body responds almost immediately to any type of vitamin D stimulation – including spending just 20 minutes in the sun every day for as few as five days! If you also begin eating foods high in vitamin D (see following page) and you take a vitamin D supplement (which I highly recommend) you will not only quickly and easily overcome any deficiency, but at the same time give a whopping boost to your fertility -and your ability to get pregnant fast!

VITAMIN D FERTILITY SNAPSHOT

RECOMMENDED DAILY ALLOWANCE: ADULTS: 400- 600 IU (international units) daily – though recent research has shown this is far too low. Today most experts recommend between 800 and 1200 IUs daily.

RECOMMENDED BY ACOG DURING PREGNANCY : 5 mcg or 200 international units.

MY PERSONAL FERTILITY RECOMMENDATION: Up to 1,000 international units daily in summer, and 2,000 international units daily in winter.

FOODS HIGH IN VITAMIN D INCLUDE: There are two dietary forms of vitamin D: Cholecalciferol and Ergocalciferol. These are naturally found in a number of foods and are usually added to milk and sometimes orange juice. It's important to note, however, that other dairy products such as yogurt and cheese are usually NOT fortified with vitamin D. Other foods sources high in vitamin D include: Cold Liver Oil (highest amount); fatty fish such as salmon, mackerel, tuna, sardines and herring; D-fortified milk and cereals; eggs.

SIGNS OF VITAMIN D DEFICIENCY: Osteomalacia (a softening of bone tissue); muscle weakness and pain; at later stages you may experience osteoporosis and an increase in bone fractures.

RISK FACTORS THAT INCREASE VITAMIN D DEFICIENCY: Lack of sun exposure; dark skin; aging; using sunscreen; inflammatory bowel disease; liver disease.

MEDICATIONS & VITAMIN D: Certain drugs can increase the level of Vitamin D in your blood or change the way it is metabolized. If you are taking any of the following medications do not take vitamin D supplements in high therapeutic doses until you consult with your doctor: **Estrogen**; **Thiazide** (a type of diuretic); **antacids** (chronic use can alter the level, metabolism and availability of vitamin D; **calcium channel blockers** (to treat high blood pressure); **Cholestyramine** (a specific type of cholesterol lowering medication); **Phenobarbital, Phenytoin, and Other Anticonvulsant Medications** (they may accelerate the body's use of vitamin D); **Mineral oil** (it interferes with absorption of vitamin D); weight loss products such as **Orlistat**.

MEDICATIONS THAT DEPLETE VITAMIN D: Inhalant and topical corticosteroid drugs; Phenobarbital; Phenytoin; Cholestyramine and Colestipol; mineral oil; Cimetidine, Famotidine, Nizatidine, Ranitidine Bismuth Citrate, Ranitidine Hydrochloride.

SIGNS OF OVERDOSE/TOXICITY: Most people tolerate even high levels of vitamin D well, however, signs that you are taking too much include: Excessive thirst; metallic taste in the mouth; loss of appetite; bone pain; fatigue; sore eyes; itchy skin; vomiting; diarrhea; constipation; frequent urination.

If you have the following conditions do not take vitamin D supplements unless you consult with your doctor first: High blood calcium or phosphorus levels; heart problems; kidney disease.

IMPORTANT TO NOTE: You cannot develop an excess of vitamin D from sun exposure, and you are highly unlikely to overdose on food sources of vitamin D.

Q: *If I want to get my vitamin D from the sun, can I still wear sunscreen while I am outdoors?*

A: You should definitely wear sunscreen if you are going to be outdoors in the sun for any length of time. This one simple step can reduce your risk of skin cancer dramatically. That said, most sunscreens will prevent absorption of up to 90% of vitamin D. In fact, the popularity of sunscreens is one reason why so many people are now Vitamin D deficient.

To get the best of both worlds try for 20 minutes a day of sun exposure daily *without* sunscreen - which won't harm you. The rest of time you are out of doors, apply the sunscreen lavishly!

Take a Beach Vacation & Get Pregnant Faster!

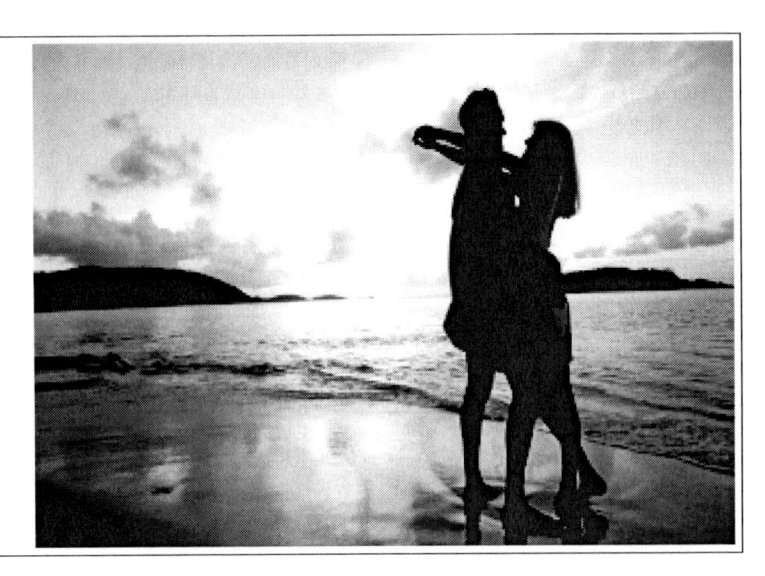

For decades – or longer – gynecologists and even some fertility experts have been advising couples to "take a vacation and you'll get pregnant!" This is often the the first line of suggestion when a couple is suffering with unexplained infertility – where there appears to be no physical reason standing in the way of pregnancy.

The goal behind the suggestion has always been primarily relaxation. Indeed, as you have already read, stress and the hormones secreted when you are stressed can have a direct and immediate impact on fertility in both men and women. And I'm happy to say that for many couples, taking a vacation – and having some relaxing time together – turns out to be the quickest route to getting pregnant.

Now, however, research shows there may be yet another, truly scientific reason behind why so many couples do get pregnant when they go away, particularly on a vacation to a warm or sunny climate. And that is, the fertility-enhancing effects of Vitamin D, garnered from that time spent in the sun.

Indeed, vitamin D is known to have an important and sometimes immediate effect on your ovaries, as well on the production of brain hormones intrinsic to getting pregnant. But perhaps even more interesting is the potential effect the sun may have on your partner.

In one very early study on sunlight and male fertility, a group of researchers measured levels of testosterone (the male hormone key to sperm production) in a group of men both before exposure to sunlight. They then exposed the men's chests to daily UVB light for five days – each day just long enough to cause a slight reddening of the skin. At the end of five days they re-measured testosterone levels. What did they find? Exposure to the UVB light (the same kind you get from the sun) caused a whopping 120% increase in testosterone production!

More importantly, they re-measured the levels again eight days later – during which the men got no UVB exposure – and their testosterone levels once again dropped down to pre-testing level.

> ### VITAMIN D: NOT FOR WOMEN ONLY!
>
> *While Vitamin D is critical for female fertility, it's not just for women! Indeed, studies show that Vitamin D can also have powerful restorative effects on sperm! It works by increasing levels of testosterone, the male hormone that is responsible for setting the sperm making process in motion!*

Now to be totally fair, I have to add that no one has ever attempted to duplicate the results of this study, so we cannot say for certain that sun exposure will increase a man's fertility.

However, I can tell you that much the way vitamin D helps orchestrate egg development in your ovaries, it similarly plays an equally important role in your partner's testes, where sperm is made. Adding a bit of epidemiological fuel to this sun power is data showing that in countries where the latitude is the highest and sun exposure varies dramatically during the year, researchers documented conception rates are highest in late summer (following a season in the sun) and birth rates are highest the following spring!

So, will a vacation in the sun help you get pregnant? There is no guarantee. But, if you combine the romance of the moonlight with the power of vitamin D from the sun....it could happen!

VITAMIN E AND FERTILITY : SOME SPECIAL ADVICE

Throughout the years we have seen the popularity of Vitamin E wax and wane . At its height it was considered the "ultimate" vitamin that protected us from heart disease, cancer, and even infertility.

As time went on and more studies were conducted, Vitamin E lost a bit of its luster. Some of the earlier health claims were disputed and some new concerns arose. And there for a while the "popular" nutritionists seemed to shun the idea of recommending anything more than a minimum daily requirement.

So where are we now? Clearly, the vitamin E pendulum has swung both ways, but the result has brought us to a comfortable middle ground in terms of the power of this nutrient. What has been proven: Vitamin E, particularly when taken with Vitamin C remains a powerful antioxidant – and therein lies the link to your fertility. As with other antioxidant vitamins it is a strong warrior in the battle against free radical damage, plus it also has anti-inflammatory effects. So, for those of you battling borderline insulin resistance, or even if you're just slightly overweight, vitamin E can help control some of the inflammatory factors that might otherwise interfere with your fertility.

But there's another, perhaps even more important link between vitamin E and getting pregnant – and it centers on your cholesterol levels. More specifically, vitamin E helps prevent the "bad" cholesterol (known as LDL or low density lipoprotein) from undergoing "oxidation" – a process which eventually causes it to form plaque, which are clumps of fats that clog your arteries and eventually can cause blood clots to develop. Indeed, when vitamin E is present in adequate amounts, LDL harmlessly passes into your artery wall and moves along. Since no plaque is made , no clots will form. Vitamin C helps the whole process run more smoothly by helping vitamin E to accomplish all this.

So, how does this tie in to your fertility? Some interesting animal research has shown that when cholesterol levels are abnormal, eggs are dysfunctional – which means they cannot be fertilized. Indeed, in one study published in the *Journal of Clinical Investigation* researchers not only noted this effect, they also found that by simply treating the mice with a cholesterol-lowering medication, they were able to restore normal egg production and fertility.

As such, I have always believed that keeping vitamin E levels up to par is one way to help keep cholesterol levels more balanced – which in turn may help egg production.

But perhaps the most powerful link between vitamin E and fertility is not seen in a woman's body, but in a mans. Indeed, numerous studies have shown that vitamin E plays an intrinsic role in keeping sperm healthy – so much so that when levels are low, male fertility can really suffer. Later on, in my chapter on male fertility, you'll learn more much about this vitamin can help your partner and how much he needs to take.

For you, however, my recommendation is a minimum of 100 units of vitamin E daily. If you have any problems with cholesterol (or if you're okay but you have a strong family history of this condition), then you can safely take up to 600 units a day – as long as you are not taking any blood thinners. If you are, or if you suffer from a very heavy menstrual flow, then talk to your doctor before going above the Recommended Daily Amount of 30 units a day.

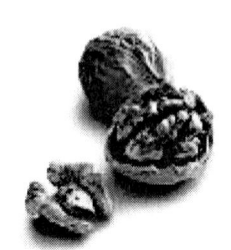

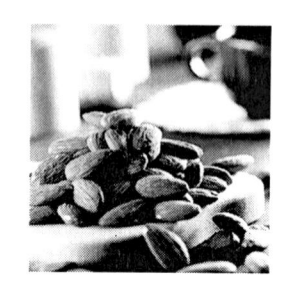

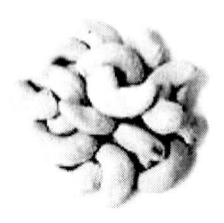

Eat Nuts - Get Pregnant!

Don't forget that most nuts are a powerful and important source of vitamin E - as well as containing other important nutrients that can help you get pregnant!

So to boost vitamin E levels and your fertility, reach for a handful of walnuts, cashews or almonds every day!

VITAMINS AND YOUR FERTILITY: SOME FINAL WORDS OF ADVICE

As I mentioned to you at the start of this chapter, my long held belief is that eating healthfully is the real key to maintaining a strong nutrient profile. And even though this chapter offers up much information on the power of individual nutrient supplements to boost your fertility, I hope you will remember that a vitamin pill is not a substitute for a good diet. Why?

While we have some very good research on the power of these nutrients to help and even heal your body, compared to the nutrient blessings of whole foods, what supplements can provide is somewhat limited. Indeed, while the vitamin C extracted from an orange, for example, can be a key player in your good health, there are dozens, if not hundreds of other compounds found inside the whole orange itself that will benefit your health in many more ways . While some of these compounds are identified, many remain Mother Nature's secret!

It is my guess that , certainly, within time, we will come to unlock all the nutrient goodness in each of the foods we now know house the healthiest vitamins – like A, C, D, E and B Complex. And in time there may be supplements so complete that they actually do provide you with all the benefits of eating a whole food. But at the moment, that time has not yet arrived, so it's important that you use vitamin supplements as an "adjunct" to a healthy diet – and not in place of healthful eating! By doing so I promise you will reap nutritional and reproductive rewards more fruitful than you can imagine!

Moreover, as we go forward through the next few chapters you'll also discover that in addition to vitamins there are other important compounds that work with these nutrients to support your fertility – including minerals that can help you get pregnant faster, as well as some natural supplements that science shows us will make a difference. But once again let me caution you that first and foremost is eating a healthy diet and living a healthy lifestyle. When you are doing that, you maximize your ability to get pregnant and have a healthy baby . And that means everything in relation to your fertility – including not just your hormones, but also fertility treatments, should you ever need them – will work better, faster and more effectively.

Chapter Ten

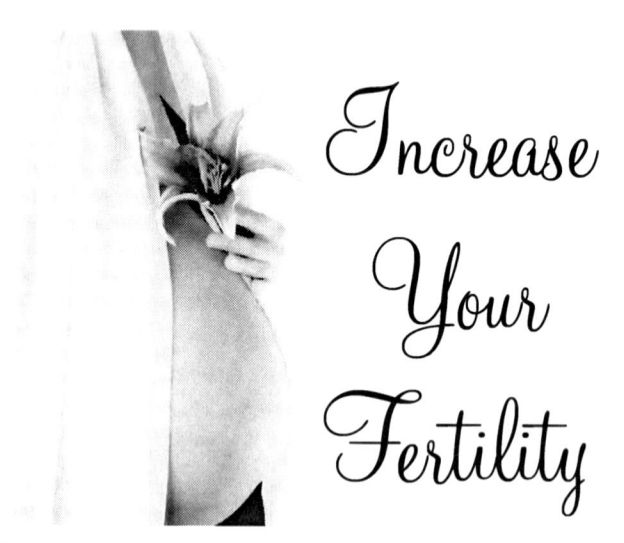

Increase Your Fertility

With Mother Nature's Mineral Secrets

There is no question that over the past two decades, and particularly in the past 10 years, there have been astonishing developments in the world of high tech fertility treatments. Today, couples have options and opportunities, some of which were not available even as little as five years ago.

And while I am always grateful to know how many couples these technologies have helped, I am sometimes a little bit worried that in the process many couples will overlook some of the important natural treatments that might be of equal – or even greater value. Nowhere is this more true than when it comes to minerals.

In fact, for many people, minerals are almost a *forgotten* category of supplementation – even though they play a significant role in both your overall health and especially, your fertility.

What's more it's not just a woman's body that can benefit from minerals. As you will learn a little later in this book, these compounds can give an enormous boost to male fertility, influencing almost every aspect of the sperm making process. When mineral support is adequate in both you and your partner, you *will* be able to get pregnant faster and easier.

At the same time, however, even a slight mineral deficiency – or more importantly a mineral imbalance – can have the opposite effect. And the results can be close to devastating on your fertility. In fact, when even a slight mineral deficiency exists in either you or your partner, it could significantly delay getting pregnant.

Now if you think it can't happen to you …well guess again. Because studies show that developing a mineral deficiency significant enough to impact fertility happens far more often – and far easier – than anyone thinks. Environmental assaults combined with less-than-perfect dietary habits, have come together in our brave to new world to cause deficiencies where and when we least expect them.

THE ROAD TO PREGNANCY IS PAVED WITH MINERALS!

The good news is that by paying attention to all the essential minerals, and learning how to create the right balance in your body, you can not only protect your fertility, but give it a significant boost! Where do you begin?

First, you always start with a healthy diet - one rich in fruits and vegetables. This will give you a good foundation of mineral support. Next, you should be taking a multi-vitamin supplement containing minerals. This will help fill in the dietary gaps and go a long way towards ensuring you are closer to meeting your daily mineral requirements.

That said, however, there is also considerable research to show that some key minerals linked to fertility may not be found in either your "typical healthy diet " or even your typical multi-vitamin. Or, if they are, they may not be in the amounts necessary to make a difference in how quickly you get pregnant. Which is why I have long recommended that all my fertility patients begin taking therapeutic doses of several key minerals. I like to call them my "Fertility Soldiers" – because they not only fight deficiencies that harm fertility, but they also help reinforce and support many of the natural physiological functions involved in getting pregnant, including egg production and release.

To this end I have put together the following guide featuring the six key minerals I believe can increase your fertility and make a significant difference in how quickly and easily you get pregnant. Not only will you discover what you need, but also how much you'll need to optimize your chances for a quick and easy pregnancy! And while I do recommend supplements, I also want you pay close attention to the food sources listed for each mineral as well, and make an effort to include them in your diet as often as possible. Together with the supplements in the recommended amounts, you will have all your bases covered and in doing so optimize your fertility.

What's important to note, however, is that while all minerals interact and work together, certain specific minerals must be taken in conjunction with others in order to prevent some key deficiencies from occurring. So in this respect do pay attention to the recommended "pairings" listed in the categories listed below. Doing so will help ensure that you not only get the right amount of each mineral necessary for fertility, but that you also get the correct balance of minerals for optimal health.

MINERAL # 1: CALCIUM

For most folks, the mineral "calcium" brings to mind tall glasses of milk and deep dishes of ice cream – and the ability to help make bones strong. And it's true that calcium is key to not only helping to keep *your b*ones strong and healthy, but during pregnancy it also helps insure your baby's skeleton grows healthy and strong as well. So, from this respect it's vital that your calcium needs are met and even exceeded beginning the moment you decide to get pregnant.

But in addition to helping you and your baby have strong, healthy bones, calcium can also influence how quickly and easily you get pregnant.

Indeed, several studies have shown that when calcium is in short supply, the production of estrogen naturally decreases. Since the ability to get pregnant not only depends on estrogen, but also that the amount in your body is maintained at a specific level, it's easy to see how calcium can impact your ability to get pregnant at many points along the way – from influencing egg growth and development to ovulation, even gestation and growth of a newly formed embryo inside your womb.

And while it's important for all women trying to get pregnant to maintain adequate calcium levels in the pre conception period, it may be especially important if you suffer from PMS. Why?

As you read in the previous chapter when calcium levels go down, symptoms of PMS can worsen. But more importantly, since the underlying problem responsible for PMS is a hormone imbalance, using calcium supplements to control symptoms can also benefit the underlying hormonal issues – and your fertility – as well.

If you are diagnosed with PCOS – poly cystic ovarian syndrome – then keeping calcium levels high may be especially important for you as well. Why?

First, calcium plays a key role in the regulation of many hormones, including insulin. Since PCOS is related to insulin resistance, (read more about this in Chapter 17) keeping calcium levels high is one way to help improve your insulin profile.

Equally important: In PCOS estrogen production is frequently compromised. So, any further reduction caused by a lack of a calcium could increase your risk of infertility further - even when PCOS is believed to be under control.

Certainly every woman trying to get pregnant should strive to obtain as much calcium from dietary sources as possible. But to ensure that you are meeting your daily requirements, I believe all women trying to get pregnant should take a calcium supplement. While most multi vitamins contain at least *some calcium*, for the most part you will need a separate calcium supplement to meet your daily fertility requirements.

Moreover, be certain your calcium supplement contains at least some vitamin D for maximum absorption. Indeed, as you just read in the previous chapter, it is vitamin D that helps your bones absorb and use calcium and keeps blood levels balanced.

Your Calcium Fertility Snapshot:

Daily Fertility Calcium Requirements: Up to 1,200 mg daily for women in their childbearing years and up to 1,600 mg daily during pregnancy.

My Personal Calcium Recommendation: 1,600 mg daily while you are trying to conceive.

Best Food Sources: Eight ounces of plain, low fat yogurt (415 mg); eight ounces of skim milk (402 mg); fortified orange juice (200 mg); three ounces of salmon (180 mg); ½ cup of cooked spinach (120 mg); one serving of kale (94 mg); one serving of bok choy (74 mg).

Calcium And Your Pregnancy

In addition to helping to strengthen both your bones and build your babies skeleton, calcium along with the mineral magnesium, play key roles in helping blood vessels to relax - which in turn can be highly beneficial to maintaining a healthy blood pressure. Because some women develop a condition known as pre eclampsia in their final stages of pregnancy - a condition that involves a dangerous and sudden rise in blood pressure - getting your pressure under good control before you get pregnant can go a long way in insuring you and your baby will remain healthy throughout your pregnancy.

In addition calcium plays a role in controlling muscle movements and nerve impulses involved in the labor and delivery process. So, by insuring you meet or exceed your calcium levels prior to getting pregnant you will be setting the stage for not only a healthier pregnancy but also an easier labor and delivery!

FERTILITY MINERAL # 2: MAGNESIUM

While it's important to maintain a balance of all nutrients, nowhere is this more crucial than when it comes to magnesium. As one of the dominant minerals inside every cell, its effect can be seen body wide – and that includes your reproductive system.

One way to insure that your magnesium needs are met is, of course to take supplements. There is, however, one caveat you cannot ignore: Magnesium supplementation must be balanced with calcium in order to gain the benefits of both minerals.

Indeed, calcium and magnesium are a little like a happily married couple – they balance each other perfectly, while their opposing characteristics help keep each other in check! For example, while calcium excites nerves, magnesium calms them; while calcium causes muscles to contract, magnesium allows them to relax; while calcium helps blood clot (necessary for healing wounds), magnesium keeps the blood flowing freely in those situations where clotting can be dangerous.

Under normal circumstances your body does a pretty good job of keeping the ratio of calcium to magnesium balanced. Since magnesium must remain the dominant mineral inside every cell, calcium is kept at bay just outside the cell wall. In these positions they function as a team to keep many aspects of your physiology in check.

Unfortunately, this can all change the minute stress enters the picture. What happens? As part of the body's natural defense system, the moment you experience stress calcium is shuttled inside each of your cells. Once there it totally dominates magnesium – and for the moment, that's a good thing. In an effort to help you "fight or flee" your stressors, it is calcium that allows nerves to become over excited, muscles to tighten, blood pressure to rise and your heart to beat faster - all designed to help you move quickly and again, either fight or flee.

Once you are out of harm's way, and your stress levels drop, calcium takes it rightful place just outside your cell, allowing magnesium to once again gain control. This causes blood pressure to drop, muscles and nerves to relax, and your body to return to its normal pre-stressed state.

But what happens when stress is chronic and present in your life all the time? First, too much calcium is continually being shuttled into your cells, which in turn dramatically tests and strains your calcium- magnesium ratio. This in turn makes it harder for magnesium to "bounce back" as the dominant partner after each stress response subsides.

Moreover, the more stress you have in your life, and longer you have it, the more likely your body is to begin responding to even small irritations with a major stress reaction. In fact, did you ever notice that when you are "on edge" things that don't normally bother you are suddenly making the hair stand on the back of your neck stand up? Well this is because your stress is now chronic - meaning your natural "alarm" system has a hair trigger response. And once this begins happening, so much calcium is continually pouring into your cells it can become almost impossible for magnesium to once again gain cell dominance. And the effects of this can be seen body-wide. They include not only a chronic increase in blood pressure, but also an increase in blood "stickiness" - the first stage of blood clot formation and an increased risk of not only stroke and heart attack, but also miscarriage. Indeed, studies show that when magnesium levels are chronically low, the rate of miscarriage increases significantly and one reason is the potential for blood clots to form in the placental lifeline between mother and baby.

Moreover, since it is magnesium that helps temper your body's reaction to stress hormones such as adrenaline, if levels drop too low, the way your body handles stress can be adversely affected. In the worst case scenario – when you are living with a constant state of tension – you can easily fall into a condition known as "adrenal exhaustion". Here, your entire hormone/endocrine system can shut down making it almost impossible to become pregnant.

Fortunately, there is something you can do to not only protect your fertility but stop all these potential problems before they even start! First and foremost, of course, is to reduce stress. But you can also give your body the help it needs to overcome your fertility-robbing stressors by making doubly sure your magnesium-calcium ratio reamins in good standing. And the best way to do that is to include magnesium in your daily supplement regimen – and to make certain that you take these supplements in the correct ratio with whatever calcium supplements you are also taking. To help ensure that you do I've included the ratio levels in the requirements section on the following page.

Soda and Your Fertility

Do you drink two or more cans of soda a day? If so your body may be already crying out for a magnesium supplement. Why?

Most sodas are high in compounds known as phosphates, which bind with magnesium, thus preventing your body from absorbing it.

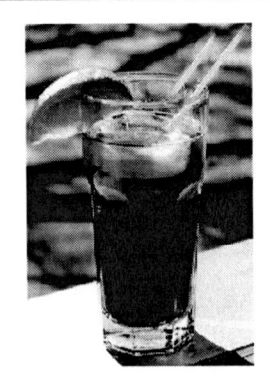

Indeed, just two cans of soda per day is enough to put your calcium-magnesium balance out of whack and your fertility in jeopardy. If your soda is sweetened with aspartame (Nutra Sweet) the effect on magnesium may be even greater and occur much sooner, since this chemical sweetener increases the binding effects. When you can, cut down on the amount of soda your drink – and avoid artificial sweetener while trying to conceive.

DAILY FERTILITY MAGNESIUM REQUIREMENT:
The minimum daily requirement for magnesium is from 300 to 450 mg – including after you are pregnant. However, remember it is important for calcium and magnesium to remain in balance, so if you are taking calcium supplements, your magnesium intake should be about half of your calcium intake.

MY PERSONAL RECOMMENDATION: Since most women now take at least 1,000 mg of calcium daily, I routinely suggest taking about 500 mg of magnesium to help maintain the proper balance. If your calcium supplement is even higher, or you eat a lot of calcium-rich foods, I suggest you fill the remainder of your magnesium needs by adding more foods rich in this mineral to your daily diet.

BEST MAGNESIUM FOOD SOURCES : Beans, black (1 cup 120 mg); Broccoli, raw, (1 cup 22 mg); Halibut - 1/2 fillet (170 mg); Peanuts one oz.,(64 mg); Okra, frozen,(1 cup 94 mg); Oysters, (3 oz – 49 mg); Plantain, raw, (1 medium, 66 mg); Scallops (6 large - 55 mg); Seeds, pumpkin and squash (1 oz, 151 mg); Spinach, cooked (one cup, 157 mg); Whole grain cereal, cooked (1 cup 56 mg).

FERTILITY MINERALS # 3: ZINC AND COPPER

When it comes to natural ways to increase fertility, no one mineral has been studied more than zinc. And while it's frequently known as the "male " fertility mineral – and you'll read more about why later in this book – the fact is that zinc also plays an important role in female fertility.

In fact, throughout history, in cultures where certain foods are believed to have "fertility powers", universally those foods have just one compound in common - zinc! Moreover, in certain ancient cultures it was believed that a quick and healthy conception required that both women and men receive special "fertility nourishment" in the months leading up to conception. Most often that nourishment included eating lots of shellfish - which we now know is very high in zinc!

But folklore aside, is there any science to show that zinc can help you get pregnant? You bet there is!

First, zinc is an essential part of the genetic material found in every egg you produce. When a zinc deficiency exists in your body, studies show it may lead to chromosomal damages inside your egg. This not only reduces your chances for conception overall, but should pregnancy occur, the lower your zinc supplies, the greater your risk of miscarriage – largely due to the defective chromosomal material in your egg.

In addition, zinc is also vital for your body to properly utilize estrogen and progesterone within each fertility cycle . So, when zinc is low these hormones may not be as plentiful or function quite as well as they should. And that too can diminish your chances for conception.

Finally, zinc also plays a key role in cell division. This is the process that allows the cell of a fertilized egg to develop and multiply into a multi-celled embryo – one that eventually attaches to your uterus and begins to grow into a healthy and strong baby. Without adequate cell division, your fertilized egg may simply fail to develop at all.

But as important a mineral as zinc can be, you can have too much of a good thing. Indeed, when zinc levels rise too high the effect on the body is not only toxic, the effect on fertility can be devastating. Additionally, when zinc levels rise too high it also interfere with your body's ability to absorb copper – which in turn causes a deficiency of this mineral, and still more harm to your fertility.

Indeed, copper is essential for your body to absorb and use iron, which as you will discover in a moment, also plays a key role in helping you get pregnant.

Moreover, copper is part of an antioxidant enzyme known as superoxide dismutase (SOD). In animal studies it was found that a shortage of SOD can cause a marked decrease in fertility – making it much harder and taking much longer to get pregnant.

While a copper deficiency in and of itself is rare, it can occur if, for example, you overdo it on zinc supplements. If you are also taking high doses of vitamin C- which have a mild effect on copper absorption – it's even easier to become copper-deficient.

The way around it is to make certain you always balance your intake of zinc and copper.

While it is less likely that you will have a problem if all your zinc comes from food sources, still, it's a good idea to include some copper-rich foods in your diet time and again.

Choosing A Zinc Supplement: What You Should Know

When it comes to choosing a zinc supplement, there are three types to choose from: zinc gluconate, zinc sulfate and zinc acetate and they differ mostly by the amount of "elemental" zinc they contain.

For example, 23% of zinc sulfate is made up of *elemental zinc,* so 220 mg of zinc sulfate contains 50 mg of elemental zinc – *which is the amount your body is actually able to absorb from the supplement.*

So, when purchasing a zinc supplement always look to the Supplement Facts panel on the bottle to check for the amount of **elemental zinc** your product contains. This is the "true" amount of zinc you are getting.

Moreover, some research shows that purchasing zinc which has undergone a process called "chelation" may make it easier for your body to absorb and use it. Chelated zinc is usually sold as "zinc picolinate."

Also be aware that besides standard zinc supplements, cold lozenges containing zinc are also a viable source of this mineral. Again, check the package label to see how much you are actually getting in each portion.

Daily Fertility Zinc Requirement

The current RDA for women of childbearing age is up 8 mg daily, with an increase to 11 mg during pregnancy, and 12 mg while breastfeeding. This should be balanced with approximately 1 mg of copper.

My Fertility Prescription: If there is a chance you are low in zinc you should talk to your doctor about increasing your daily intake to 30 mg daily, in balance with approximately 3 mg of copper.

Foods High In Zinc: Oysters, (6 medium, 76.7 mg); Beef shanks, cooked, (3 ounces 8 mg); Crab, Alaskan king, (cooked, three ounces, 6.5 mg); Pork shoulder, cooked, three ounces 4.2 mg) ; Fortified cereal , (¾ cup, 3.8 mg); Chicken leg, roasted, (1 leg, 2.7 mg); Lobster, cooked, (3 ounces, 2.5 mg); Baked beans, canned, (½ cup, 1.7 mg); Cashews, dry roasted, (1 ounce, 1.6 mg); Yogurt, fruit, low fat, (1 cup, 1.6 mg.)

Foods High In Copper: Seafood (oysters, squid, lobster, mussels, crab, and clams); Nuts and nut butters (cashews, filberts, macadamia nuts, pecans, almonds, and pistachios); Legumes (soybeans, lentils, navy beans, and peanuts); Chocolate (unsweetened or semisweet baker's chocolate and cocoa); Enriched cereals (bran flakes, shredded wheat, and raisin bran); Fruits and Vegetables (dried fruits, mushrooms, tomatoes, potatoes, sweet potatoes, bananas, grapes, and avocado); black pepper.

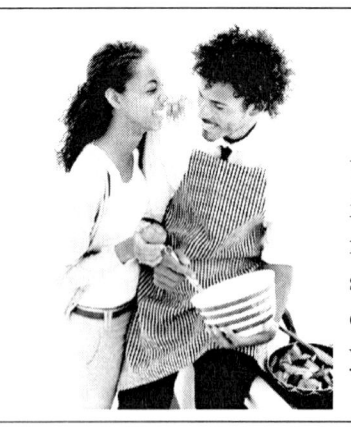

ZINC:
The Sperm Loving Mineral

While zinc is an important component of female fertility it's absolutely essential for male fertility! Zinc is a key component for sperm production - and it's essential to produce healthy, mobile sperm! So, make sure you and your partner get your daily supply!

FERTILITY MINERAL # 4: IRON

From the moment you were a girl entering puberty until the time when, as a woman, you will enter menopause, taking iron supplements can be a key part of optimizing your health. Why?

First, iron is what is known as an essential mineral - essential because it plays a part in so many body functions. That said, it's also essential because iron carries and delivers precious life-giving oxygen to all your tissues, bones, muscles and organs. It does so by attaching to red blood cells which then carry it through your body. Without enough iron, however, your body cannot produce enough "hemoglobin"- the substance in red blood cells that enables them to carry the oxygen. And this is important, since without an adequate oxygen supply, many aspects of your fertility can suffer – from egg production and ovulation, to the implantation of a healthy embryo.

Ironically, however, it is during the reproductive years that you are most likely to be at risk for an iron deficiency. Your monthly menstrual cycle, particularly if complicated by heavy bleeding from fibroid tumors or endometrial or cervical polyps, can cause you to lose so much blood that your number of red cells actually decreases. The fewer red blood cells you have, the less oxygen-rich iron is being transported - and ultimately that means a whole lot less oxygen-rich nourishment will be getting to your cells.

Moreover, when your amount of available iron also declines, the red blood cells you do have are unable to manufacture hemoglobin - the substance which carries the oxygen to your cells. When this occurs you can develop a condition known as "iron deficiency anemia", characterized by symptoms such as weakness and fatigue, occuring because your blood can no longer supply cells with the oxygen necessary to function at peak capacity. This includes the cells of your reproductive organs, causing them to work under par as well.

In addition, m new evidence from an eight year study of more than 18,000 nurses revealed low iron can also take a direct toll on fertility. According to the research, recently published in the *Journal of the American College of Obstetricians and Gynecologists*, women who are low in iron during their reproductive years are far more likely to suffer from ovulatory infertility than women who take iron supplements. Thus researchers concluded that taking iron supplements during the childbearing years is one important way to reduce the risk of ovulatory failure.

And I have found this to be true as well. In fact, I have had many patients with what I call "borderline ovulatory infertility" go from infertile to fertile by simply adding more iron to their diet. For these women, some of whom were very thin and bordering on anemia, ovulation was frequently "hit and miss" - simply because their ovaries were not getting the nourishment necessary to produce eggs during every cycle. Once they brought their iron levels up to par, ovulation kicked in on a more regular basis, and pregnancy usually occurred within several months afterwards.

But before you reach for that bottle of iron supplements, there's something you should know: Too much iron can sometimes be detrimental to fertility. This is particularly true if you suffer from endometriosis, a common menstrual related disorder that is among the leading causes of infertility (See Chapter Sixteen)

In fact, recent research has shown that women who have endometriosis frequently have an increased amount of iron in the fluid surrounding their reproductive organs. In one study published in a leading European medical journal, doctors found that this heavy iron-rich fluid is detrimental to sperm, preventing it from completing all the steps necessary for fertilization. Essentially, the iron was disabling the sperm, making pregnancy impossible.

Other studies suggest an iron overload may even be a precipitating factor for endometriosis, encouraging the development of this condition in women who are susceptible. This is particularly important if you want to get pregnant since endometriosis is a primary cause of infertility among young women.

How Much Iron Do I Need?

For many women, adequate iron intake is easily achieved by eating a balanced diet. Many foods such as whole grain cereals and even some breads are now fortified with iron – plus there are a variety of foods which are direct sources of this mineral. In choosing what to eat, however, you should know there are two forms of dietary iron. They are known *heme,* and *nonheme.*

Heme iron is what is found in the protein of red blood cells, and the main dietary sources are animal foods that originally carried these same red cells. This includes red meats, fish and poultry. *Nonheme* iron is derived from plants, such as lentils, beans or broccoli. This is the type of iron that is added to foods or beverages that are sold as "iron enriched".

Although the human body absorbs heme iron far better than nonheme iron, absorption of either form is increased with vitamin C. So, for example, if you combine a plant source of iron with a glass of orange or grapefruit juice (both high in vitamin C), or if you a take a C supplement, your iron absorption will improve dramatically.

But as important as these foods are, for some of you dietary sources of iron are simply not enough - particularly if you suffer from heavy menstrual bleeding due to fibroid tumors or polyps. If you are cutting back on red meat to help you lose weight or reduce cholesterol levels, then dietary sources may be scant as well.

When any of these conditions prevail, then iron supplements are a "must have". In fact taking iron supplements while you are trying to get pregnant is a good idea for another reason: Once you do conceive your need for iron dramatically increases. Not only does your baby need this mineral to develop their red blood cell supply, but your own expanding blood volume during this time requires more iron as well, essential for you to nourish your own body and your baby with life-giving oxygen. As such, if your level of iron remains high while trying to conceive, there's a better chance that your body can give your baby all the nourishment necessary for a healthy start - starting from the moment of conception.

CHOOSING AN IRON SUPPLEMENT: WHAT YOU SHOULD KNOW

Unless you are anemic, with a low red blood cell count, for the most part the amount of iron found in a prenatal vitamin should be enough during the preconception time. Many multi-vitamins also contain adequate iron already built into the formula.

If however, you decide to take a separate iron supplement the most commonly prescribed type is known as "ferrous sulfate". An average dose is about 325 mg, 65 mg of which is "elemental " iron - which is iron in its purest form. This may differ slightly from the amount found in your prenatal or multi-vitamin simply because these supplements usually contain a slightly different form of iron.

Daily Fertility Iron Requirements

If your doctor finds that you are anemic, you may need to take a separate iron supplement over and above what a prenatal or multi vitamin offers. If you are not anemic, the American College of Obstetricians and Gynecologists recommends 18 mg daily of elemental iron before pregnancy and up to 75 mg a day of elemental iron after you are pregnant.

My Personal Iron Recommendations: If you eat very little red meat or if you are a vegetarian and eat very few high-iron vegetables, and particularly if you are having ovulatory problems, my personal recommendation is 325 mg of ferrous sulfate which contains 65 mg of elemental iron daily, or a prenatal vitamin with iron. If, however, you have been diagnosed with moderate to severe endometriosis, talk to your doctor before taking any iron supplements.

Moreover, it's important to note that sometimes iron supplements can cause nausea, particularly if taken on an empty stomach. To avoid this problem, I suggest you always take all vitamins, minerals and herbs *after meals*. You can also try taking your iron supplements or other vitamins later in the day or in the evening, after your main meal. Additionally don't be alarmed if you see that your stool is much darker after you begin iron supplementation - *this is normal*. Some women can also develop constipation when taking iron supplements, which can be overcome by increasing your intake of high fiber fruits and vegetables, or by taking a stool softener.

Foods Highest in Iron Content: Liver, and other organ meats; lean red meat; poultry; fish; and shellfish (particularly oysters). Non animal sources of iron include: dried beans and peas, legumes, nuts and seeds, whole grains, dark molasses, and green leafy vegetables. In the U.S., grain products such as breads and cereals are fortified with iron to help increase amount in our diet.

> *If you have a heavy menstrual period or if you eat very little read meat or beans then you most likely need an iron supplement!*

Fertility Mineral #5 : Selenium

If you're like many of my former patients, you probably believe that antioxidant protection comes mainly from vitamins. And it's true, that certain vitamins, particularly A, C and E are power-packed with antioxidant protection – which is not only good for your overall health but great for your fertility.

But what you might not realize is that the mineral known as selenium is also a powerhouse source of antioxidant protection that can play a key role in helping you get pregnant!

Indeed, as you just read in the chapter on vitamins, antioxidants wear many hats and play many roles in a variety of steps leading to conception. Moreover when levels are high your chances for a quicker and easier conception increase.

But when it comes to specific fertility boosting powers of selenium, the antioxidant component is just part of the story. Indeed, several studies have shown that if your level of selenium falls too low, a variety of reproductive problems can occur. This includes a reduced chance of getting pregnant, as well as an increased risk of miscarriage if you do conceive. In fact, in one study published recently in the *British Journal of Obstetrics and Gynecology* doctors found that women who suffer recurring miscarriage are frequently diagnosed with low levels of selenium. For many, pregnancy loss was occurring so early on, they didn't even realize they were getting pregnant, and instead believed they were simply infertile.

What was really interesting about this study, however, was that in most of these women their blood level of selenium was considered "normal." It wasn't, in fact, until doctors measured levels of selenium in hair samples (which some believe may be a more accurate reflection of nutrient deficiencies) that they found these women were indeed deficient in this mineral.

The point is that even if your doctor takes a blood test for selenium deficiency and your levels seem normal, you could still have a deficiency capable of impacting your fertility. As such I have always advised my patients to make certain their multi vitamin contains at least the minimal dose of selenium as a way of ensuring against related fertility and pregnancy problems.

And by the way, it's not just women whose fertility can benefit from selenium – it's also an important mineral for sperm health as well. You'll learn more about how and why a little later in this book.

HOW MUCH SELENIUM DO I NEED?

Since this mineral is present in many foods, if you're already eating a healthy diet, you are well on your way to meeting your selenium requirements.

That said, there are also a number of common factors that deplete selenium – and could be placing you or your partner at risk for deficiency. These include:

- Smoking cigarettes – or exposure to second hand smoke.
- Moderate alcohol intake
- Birth control pills
- Any type of gastro intestinal mal absorption syndrome (such as Crohn's disease or ulcerative colitis).
- Regular use of aspirin or other blood thinners

If any of these factors are present in your life, or were in the very recent past, then chances are your fertility could definitely benefit from a selenium supplement.

One word of caution: Selenium supplements may reduce the effectiveness of certain cholesterol drugs including "statins". If you are taking a cholesterol medication talk to your doctor before adding a selenium supplement.

DAILY FERTILITY SELENIUM REQUIREMENTS

For women over the age of 16, 55 mcg daily is the suggested requirement; this increases to 60 mcg daily during pregnancy, and 70 mcg daily during breastfeeding.

MY PERSONAL SELENIUM RECOMMENDATIONS: 60 mcg to 70 mcg daily.

FOODS HIGHEST IN SELENIUM : Brewer's yeast, wheat germ, liver, butter, fish (mackerel, tuna, halibut, flounder, herring, smelts) and shellfish (oysters, scallops and lobster), garlic, whole grains, sunflower seeds, and Brazil nuts . Because selenium is destroyed during some types of food processing, one of the best ways to ensure you get adequate amounts of dietary selenium is to eat as many whole, unprocessed foods as possible.

FERTILITY MINERAL # 6 : CHROMIUM PICOLINATE

As trace minerals go, chromium piconlinate is usually not on the "Top Ten" list of nutrient "must haves"! In fact, many multivitamins might not even contain any of this mineral at all!

But if you're trying to get pregnant, and particularly if you are already having any type of ovulatory problems, then a chromium picolinate supplement could turn out to be one of the most important minerals you can take. How and why can it help you? The answers, at least in part, are linked to chromium's effect on insulin resistance - which as you read earlier is often linked to ovulatory problems and certain types of infertility.

But how does chromium make a difference?

When we eat, glucose from our food is transported from our bloodstream into our cells where it is used to supply energy for our entire body. What transports the glucose is insulin, a hormone which acts like a "knock on the door" asking cells to open up and let the sugar in. When insulin resistance occurs, cells have difficulty "hearing" insulin's "knock". And that means it takes much longer - and much more insulin – to clear the sugars from our blood. Chromium picolinate speeds up the entire process by increasing a cell's sensitivity to insulin. In fact, working much like the diabetes drug Metformin, chromium encourages cells to respond to insulin's "knock" and let the sugars in.

Indeed, in one study published recently in the journal *Fertility and Sterility*, doctors found that overweight woman who took 1,000 mcg of chromium picolinate daily for two months improved their insulin sensitivity by 38%. Although the dosage is higher than what is frequently recommended, still the results led researchers to conclude that chromium can prove very useful in treating insulin sensitivity in a way that most people can easily tolerate, even with long term use.

In a second study also published in *Fertility and Sterility*, a lower dose of chromium taken for a longer period of time - (200 mcg daily for 4 months) did not appear to impact insulin resistance, but did significantly decrease blood sugar levels during an oral glucose tolerance test – the blood screening used to diagnose diabetes.

Moreover, according to William Cefalu, MD, chief of the division of nutrition and chronic diseases at the Pennington BioMedical Research Center, Louisiana State University System, " Emerging research suggests that 200-1,000 µg of chromium as chromium picolinate may play an important role in carbohydrate metabolism."

So what does all this have to do with fertility? Well clearly, chromium supplements are most useful to women diagnosed with PCOS – a ovulatory related fertility-robbing condition which has its basis in insulin resistance. (See Chapter 17).

However, one of the really "tricky" things about PCOS is that it doesn't always present with obvious symptoms. In fact, for some women, particularly those with mild forms of this condition, the only sign that something is wrong is that it's taking longer than usual to get pregnant. For some, in fact, discovering they can't get pregnant is the single factor that leads to a diagnosis of PCOS.

Moreover, it is also my personal belief that many more women have what is known as 'subclinical' PCOS – a condition wherein the impact of this disease is not quite strong enough to be picked up as a clinical diagnosis, yet it is strong enough to impact ovulation and reduce chances for conception.

For this reason I suggest that any woman who wants add an extra layer of fertility protection and boost her conception odds as well, consider taking a daily supplement of chromium picolinate, the form of this nutrient that is both the safest and the easiest for the body to absorb.

GOOD CHROMIUM – BAD CHROMIUM:

WHAT YOU SHOULD KNOW

If you are a fan of actress Julia Roberts you are probably familiar with the movie Erin Brockovich - a picture in which Miss Roberts played the feisty legal assistant who helped bring justice to a town whose water and land had been poisoned by chromium, deposited as a form of industrial waste.

In fact, in my first fertility book "Getting Pregnant: What You Need To Know" I caution against exposure to chromium, which is a heavy metal known to be an industrial toxin - and exposure can impact both male and female fertility in a very negative way.

What's important for you to know, however, is that there are two types of chromium – and while one type is very bad for your health, the other is a trace mineral that is essential to good health. Indeed, the substance known as Chromium VI is the ill-fated toxin which results from industrial pollution. It can be so lethal that significant exposure can lead to disease or death. Chromium III is an entirely different substance. An essential trace mineral it is key to your health and not dangerous. There are several types of chromium III but among those found to be

> **Are you :**
> * 20 pounds or more overweight?
> * Feel hungry all the time
> * Get ravenously hungry every time you exercise?
> * Have irregular menstrual cycles?
>
> If any of these things are true for you, then chromium picolinate might be the nutrient for you!
>
> Be sure to talk to your doctor about a glucose tolerance blood test as well to check for insulin resistance - which in some women can be a major stumbling block to getting pregnant!

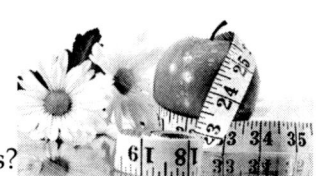

the most beneficial is chromium picolinate. As a supplement it appears to be extremely safe and well tolerated, even at levels hundreds of times above the recommended daily dosage.

Adding to this profile, in 2004 researchers presented new data at a Centers for Disease Control conference showing that chromium picolinate supplements are safe. It was here they announced that research studies conducted by the United States Department of Agriculture (USDA), The National Toxicology Program (NTP) and independent testing laboratories all concluded that supplements of chromium picolinate showed no evidence of genetic toxicity. This new research is believed to supersede some smaller animal studies which suggested adverse effects on hamster cells exposed to chromium picolinate.

Moreover, in what some view as a further boost to the safety of chromium picolinate supplements, in 2005 the FDA gave it's nod of approval to health claims made in relation to these supplements. While FDA officials caution that the relationship between insulin resistance type 2 diabetes and chromium picolinate remains uncertain, still, they conclude that enough evidence is present to suggest this mineral supplement may reduce risks .

How Much Chromium Picolinate Do I Need?

As far back as 1989 the National Academy of Sciences established the safety dosing for chromium supplements as falling between 50 to 200 mcg daily. In 2001 the Daily Requirement Intake for chromium was established at 25 mcg per day for women between the ages of 19 and 50, 30 mcg per day if you are pregnant, and 45 mcg per day if you have already given birth and are breastfeeding.

That said, however, most experts now agree that certainly 200 mcg per day of chromium picolinate is safe for everyone, and that up to 2,000 mcg per day may be necessary for some women who experience ovulatory problems related to PCOS and insulin resistance.

My personal recommendation: Start with at least 200 mcg daily and up to 500 mcg daily if you are having ovulation problems. If you are already diagnosed with PCOS, talk to your doctor about increasing your dosage as high as 1,000-2,000 mcg daily of chromium picolinate.

Foods High In Chromium

In addition to supplements, there is some chromium present in certain foods. While most supply only a small amount, (less than 2 mcg per serving) the effects can be cumulative, so the more of these foods you eat, the more likely you are to get a natural supply of chromium every day. Foods containing the highest amounts are meat, whole grains, fruits, vegetables and some spices. Foods that contain the least amount include simple carbohydrates like white bread, or anything containing sugar, fructose or high fructose corn syrup.

Here are some specific foods and their chromium content: Broccoli (½ cup – 11 mcg); Grape Juice (1 cup, 8 mcg); Whole Wheat English Muffin (1, 4 mcg); Mashed potatoes (1 cup, 3 mcg); Dried Garlic (1, tsp, 3 mcg); Dried Basil (one tbsp, 2 mcg); Orange juice (1 cup – 2 mcg); Turkey Breast (3 ounces – 2 mcg); Whole wheat bread (1-2 slices, 2 mcg); Red Wine (5 ounces, up to 13 mcg).

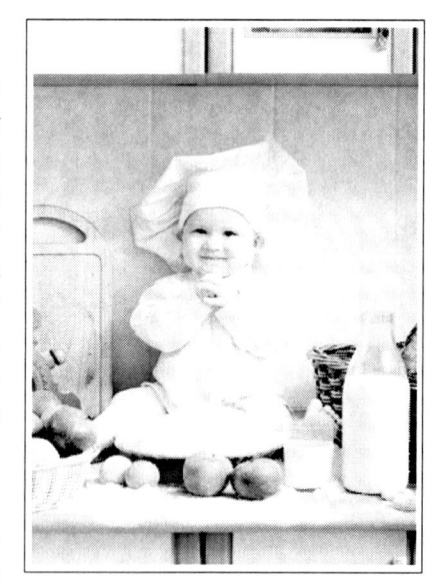

MINERALS AND GETTING PREGNANT: A FINAL WORD

Although the minerals mentioned in this chapter are believed to be among the most important in terms of your fertility, as I have stressed to you all along, balance is really the key to using nutrition to enhance your fertility.

So while each individual mineral plays an important role in helping you get pregnant, the awesome power of nutrition really comes together when each nutrient or natural compound is part of a complete picture of supplementation. Certainly, eating a healthy diet, high in fruits and vegetables, fiber, and good sources of protein are all important ways to get a balanced intake of all the nutrients necessary for good health and healthy fertility.

But supplements can be useful as well, as long as you remember that balance is key. If, for example, you read that one particular vitamin or mineral is helpful in a situation that seems to apply to you, then yes, it's important that you take enough of this nutrient, perhaps even therapeutic doses. At the same time, if you focus on just that one nutrient, to the exclusion of all others, you not only diminish its power, but you also run the risk of creating another problem by inducing a nutrient imbalance.

The point I want you to keep in mind is that good health and healthy fertility is never the result of one food, one nutrient, one vitamin, one compound or one herb. It is the result of a balanced diet and a balanced lifestyle which together work to give your body everything it needs to work optimally. And that includes optimizing your fertility.

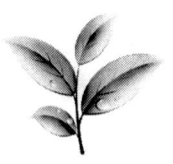

Chapter Eleven

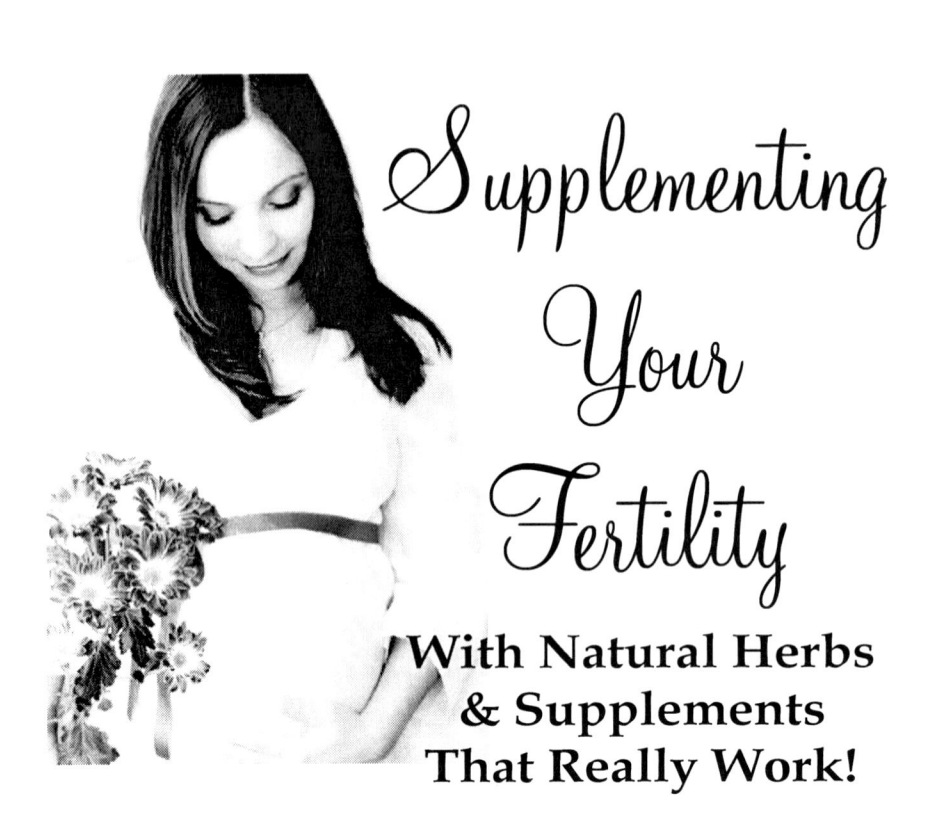

Supplementing Your Fertility
With Natural Herbs & Supplements That Really Work!

Whether you have just started thinking about getting pregnant, or certainly if you're actively trying to conceive, you've no doubt been intrigued – and maybe even a little mystified – by the abundance of "natural" fertility supplements available today.

In fact, just a quick trip down any drugstore aisle and you'll know there is certainly no shortage of natural and herbal "cocktails" claiming to enhance fertility and help you get pregnant faster. As a medical doctor who has long believed in the power of Mother Nature to gently and effectively encourage pregnancy, seeing these treatments blossom and grow into such popular options is no great surprise. In fact, while many western doctors are just now beginning to appreciate nature and all it can contribute to medicine, I have been among a legion of European - trained physicians who have always believed in the power of natural compounds to aid in many health concerns. And certainly fertility is no exception.

But what's really exciting is that some of the compounds available right now are not based on just age-old folklore. Many have been the subject of some key scientific clinical trials conducted over the past several years, research from which we have gleaned much about how these compounds work - and who they can help the most.

In fact, I am very happy to report that today there is not only a collection of herbal supplements that have been proven to make an impact on fertility, but also some specific fertility formulations that definitely make the grade when it comes to helping you get pregnant faster and easier.

But as excited as I am to introduce you to Mother Nature's garden of fertility treatments, I would be remiss if I did not add just a few cautions for you to consider.

First and foremost, know that not every treatment works for every couple - nor does every treatment work equally well for everyone. Much like traditional medications, everyone has an individual response. So, if you try a certain formulation and it is not helpful, don't be afraid to sample another.

At the same time I must also caution you to have patience when it comes to using natural treatments, particularly since most work a little differently than common medications you might be used to taking. Indeed, while we have come to expect that 30 minutes after taking an aspirin our headache is gone, or an hour after taking an allergy medication we are no longer sneezing, generally speaking, that's not the way natural fertility treatments work. Most, in fact, will require from two to four months before you see a result - so be patient!

Finally, I also want you to remain aware that as helpful as these natural treatments can be, they are not the answer for serious fertility problems. And by that I mean, if you have a specific fertility issue that has been diagnosed by your doctor - such as a blocked fallopian tube or an inability to make healthy eggs - then natural treatments alone are not going to totally turn your pregnancy odds around. Certainly they may improve your overall fertility potential - and in some instances may offer a great deal of help. But they cannot, for example, cure a fertility-robbing infection or accomplish what only a surgical procedure can do.

So while I encourage you to give mother nature a try, if you are under age 30 and not pregnant within 12 months, or over age 30 and not pregnant within six months, it's important that you also see a fertility specialist for a baseline check up to ensure that everything is okay. And if, indeed, everything checks out okay, and your fertility is in good shape, you can continue to use the herbs and other natural treatments in this book with the confidence that a pregnancy will happen soon.

> *Herbal supplements not only help encourage a natural pregnancy but they can also give an extra boost to most fertility treatments – but be sure to tell you're doctor about everything you're taking!*

Moreover if your doctor discovers there is a problem – not to worry! There are many fast and easy medical "fixes" available and I'm very certain that whatever is keeping you from getting pregnant can be quickly and easily resolved. What's more, *everything* you will find in this book – particularly the information in this chapter - will not only work in harmony with high tech fertility treatments, in many instances they can enhance the outcome! Just make certain to tell your doctor or fertility specialist about *every* treatment you are taking or using – including prescription drugs, over-the-counter medications, and especially natural products. Remember, if it is strong enough to have an effect, it's important for your doctor to know you are taking it.

So with this in mind, I hope you will read on to discover some of Mother Nature's most useful fertility secrets! Remember, however, that eating a healthy diet, and taking the vitamins and minerals discussed in previous chapters is also important. When used in combination with the herbal supplements featured in this chapter, their power will go even further in helping you optimize both your good health and your chances for a quick and healthy pregnancy!

FERTILITY BOOSTING HERB # 1: CHASTEBERRY (VITEX)

While you may have recently heard a lot about the power of this beautiful flowering plant to boost your fertility, the truth is, chasteberry has been around for hundreds of years! Known by its botanical name Vitex -agnus-castus - L or "Vitex" – it has been used by a variety of different cultures around the world as not only a general reproductive tonic, but a treatment to boost fertility as well. Among the many claims is the ability of Chasteberry to re-balance hormones, and especially to aid in a condition known as "luteal phase defect". This means that a deficiency of the hormone progesterone in the second half of the menstrual cycle can prevent an embryo from reaching the uterus, or successfully attaching to the uterus so it can begin growing. In Germany, where I first learned about the successful use of Chasteberry, doctors routinely "prescribe" this supplement as the first line of defense in the treatment of luteal phase defect.

Most recently chasteberry has been the subject of several new medical studies, some of which have proven its effectiveness under some very strict laboratory conditions. What have we discovered?

- In one recent study of just under 100 women, doctors compared daily treatment with Chasteberry to placebo for three months. The result: In those women who had amenorrhea or luteal phase insufficiency, the use of chasteberry doubled the rate of pregnancy, compared to the group taking the placebo! And while there were also a few additional herbs included in the compound used during the testing period, researchers believed it was the chasteberry that exerted the most prominent effects.

- In another study involving 52 women all diagnosed with luteal phase defects, those who took chasteberry not only saw an increase in progesterone, but also a better balance between estrogen and progesterone. As you read earlier in this book, when hormones are in balance, your reproductive body chemistry works in harmony making it much easier to get pregnant.

- In the most recent research on chasteberry – a double-blind placebo-controlled study of 30 women – 27 out of the 30 showed an increase in mid-cycle progesterone levels, and an increase in the number of pregnancies when compared to women who did not use this herb.

In fact, in most of the studies Chasteberry has been shown to have some remarkable hormone balancing properties. Today, the German E commission –

which is much like the American FDA - approves the use of Chasteberry as a treatment for cycle irregularities as well as the symptoms of PMS.

The most recent studies also suggest this herb may also be helpful in treating the symptoms of PCOS – which you'll learn about in Chapter 17.

How Chasteberry Works

Although technically Chasteberry is thought of as an herb, in reality, its effectiveness traces back to many of the same compounds and properties found in many fruits and vegetables. Among the most potent are compounds known as flavonoids. As you read earlier, these are phytonutrients that can support your health and your fertility in several key ways. The flavonoids found in chasteberry include casticin, kaempferol, orientin, quercetagetin and isovitexin.

But that's just the beginning of what this powerful herbal remedy can offer. Because Chasteberry also contains compounds known as "glycosides" – and here is where the real effect on your reproductive system begins. It is these compounds which are believed to influence the production of several key hormone-related chemicals. These include the peptide prolactin (which is related to the production of your breast milk) the hormone progesterone, and the brain chemicals FSH and LH.

What is somewhat unique to Chasteberry however, is that the effects are intimately tied to dosing in a way that can dramatically alter its effects. Unlike other herbs or even medications where too little results in less effectiveness and too much results in an overdose, with chasteberry, the amount you take is specifically linked to dramatically different results.

And here's an example of what I mean : Low doses of Chasteberry extract, are believed to *inhibit* or reduce the production of FSH or follicle stimulating hormone, the compound that tells your eggs to grow, while higher doses have no effect on FSH. Low doses also cause an increase in LH or luteinizing hormone, the compound which helps signal ovulation and increase progesterone production, while again, higher doses have little or no effect on LH. Researchers have also documented that low doses of chasteberry can cause a decrease in estrogen but an increase in progesterone and prolactin. So, it's easy to see how and why proper dosing and balance are the keys to getting not only good results, but the results you want.

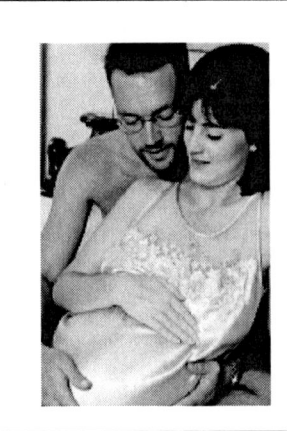

> *If you suffer with even mild symptoms of PMS, if you have been diagnosed with luteal phase insufficiency, or if you simply want to help insure that your hormones remain in good balance, then chasteberry could be the herb that helps you get pregnant!*

How To Use Chasteberry To Help You Get Pregnant

As a fertility aid chasteberry appears to be most helpful to those women who are doing battle with hormone imbalances – specifically a progesterone deficiency. And whether you've been diagnosed as having a hormone imbalance by your doctor, or your tell-tale PMS symptoms are giving you strong clues that something is amiss, in most instances where a menstrual-related hormone imbalance exists, Chasteberry can offer at least some help.

Chasteberry is also used to treat amenorrhea (a lack of menstrual cycle that usually results from a hormone imbalance) and sometimes, for the general treatment of *unexplained infertility*.

Most importantly all these conditions have been shown to respond to Chasteberry with obvious improvement – including increased fertility.

The bottom line: If you suffer from even mild symptoms of PMS, if you have been diagnosed with luteal phase insufficiency, or if you simply want to help insure that your hormones remain in good balance, then chasteberry could be the herbal choice for you!

How much will you need to see an effect? Remember, dosing is important, so how much you take can be dependent on the problem you are trying to solve. That said, to increase fertility research published in the journal of the American Family Physician (AFP) suggests 4 mg per day of a standardized extract. In the United States, this formulation is available as Femaprin from Nature's Way – but other companies provide similar formulations. Just be sure to check the label to ensure you are getting a "standardized" formulation of 4 mg daily.

If you are using the fruit extract as your source, (and the label would note that it is a fruit extract) then the AFP study recommends 20 to 40 mg per day, although higher doses (up to 1,800 mg per day) have been used with no safety issues or change in effectiveness noted. If your extract is fluid, this equals about 40 drops per day; if you are using a tincture then the dosing is 35 to 45 drops, three times daily.

You can use chasteberry in any form either continuously every day, or for just half your cycle, beginning right after your menstrual bleed stops, and continuing through ovulation, and stopping within 24 hours afterwards. You would begin again at the start of the next cycle.

While some women prefer to use this as a single herb preparation, more recently several blended products containing this herb and several others have come on the market as "fertility supplements. " One such is known as "Fertility Blend" , and it has been the subject of a very favorable medical study. If you would like to learn more about Fertility Blend or try any mixed herbal fertility supplement, check out the section on these products later in this chapter.

While Chasteberry appears to be safe and have no specific adverse reactions, as with all natural compounds there is always a chance for side effects or even an occasional allergic reaction. Signs to look for include an increase in headaches, gastrointestinal difficulties, and lower abdominal complaints, and of course any typical signs of allergy including hives, itching, redness or swelling. If these symptoms do appear stop taking Chasteberry immediately and talk to your doctor.

FERTILITY BOOSTING HERB # 2: BLACK COHOSH

I'll never forget the look on the face of one of my fertility patients when I suggested she could increase her chances for conception by taking the herb black cohosh.

"Black cohosh? That's a menopause herb! I want to have a baby, not stop a hot flash! " she said quite exasperated! And the truth is, I could not blame her since it is true that black cohosh has garnered quite a reputation as helping to quell menopause symptoms – including hot flashes.

But as I went on to explain to my patient, the same kinds of hormonal upsets that are responsible for many of the symptoms of menopause, can, in younger women, also cause infertility. Indeed, one reason women approaching menopause have so many symptoms is because they are ovulating much less frequently. This in turn causes a hormone imbalance that ultimately turns their body chemistry upside down.

When a younger woman is having problems getting pregnant, very often she too suffers from a slow down in ovulation similar to that which occurs in midlife. Likewise she may suffer a similar type of hormone imbalance, and may even experience some of the same symptoms of menopause including mood swings and even hot flashes.

So, it's easy to see how an herb that helps quell hormonal upsets related to mid life symptoms, can do an equally good job soothing fertility-related hormonal upsets in younger women.

Moreover, black cohosh has another important property that allows it be so useful for both groups of women : It is known as an "adaptogen". In herbal - speak this means it can literally "adapt" to what your specific body needs are at the moment. So, for example, if your hormones are low and they need a boost, black cohosh can work on those pathways that help increase hormone production. If you are producing too much of one hormone and not enough of another, it can also help normalize levels. In this respect, Black Cohosh is almost the "perfect" fertility herb, - working in a way that helps your body to have more of what you personally need to optimize your reproductive health and, if you are under age 45, optimize your chances of getting pregnant.

How Black Cohosh Works

The herb black cohosh – also known as Actaea racemosa or sometimes as Cimicifuga racemosa – is native to North America. It's first recorded use in the United States was by Native Americans, who used it to treat many types of gynecologic disorders.

Like other plants - including fruits and vegetables – black cohosh contains many different phytonutrients, including healthful, beneficial compounds such as flavonoids and tannins. But the star player, in terms of fertility, appears to be a compound known as "triterpenoid glycosides" which several studies have shown has mild estrogenic effects.

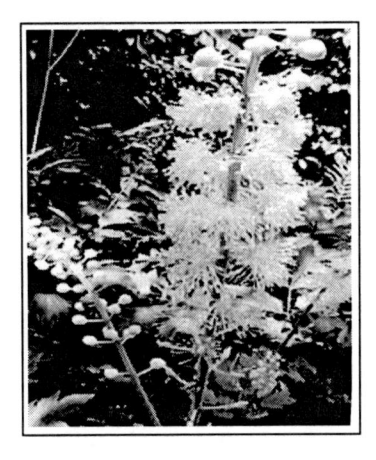

For the most part, these studies have been conducted on women *approaching* menopause – a time when estrogen levels naturally begin to decline. But what's important to remember is that it's not just women in this time of life that can have low estrogen levels. Indeed, this is also a condition that occurs in younger women, and when it does its most often related to ovulation problems. In fact, one reason women approaching menopause develop symptoms is because they are no longer ovulating on any kind of regular basis – and of course, egg production dramatically slows down and eventually stops.

For younger women who suffer from ovulatory problems the same thing can happen: Egg production slows down, so ovulation becomes irregular - and can sometimes even stop altogether. So, it makes sense then that the same herb which helps balance hormone levels affected by dwindling egg production in older women, would help younger women in much the same way.

Moreover, there is also evidence that black cohosh has anti-spasmodic properties which may prevent your newly fertilized egg from being pushed down your fallopian tube too quickly – before the lining of your uterus is thick enough to facilitate a healthy implantation. When this occurs early miscarriage is often the result - so early in fact, that many women do not even realize they are pregnant.

For all these reasons I agree with many natural medicine experts who believe that black cohosh can be a very helpful fertility herb - particularly if you know that you do not ovulate on a regular basis (and you can use the ovulation testing methods in Chapter Three to know for sure) or if you already know you have some specific ovulation or egg-making difficulties.

NOT ALL BLACK COHOSH IS ALIKE!

As helpful as this herb has proven to be, it's important to note that not all black cohosh is alike. Indeed, many experts believe that the success of this treatment is intimately tied to the specific black cohosh formulation you use. The reason? Like all medications, how well it works is dependent on the level of active compounds it contains – in this instance, triterpenoid glycosides.

To date, the vast majority of clinical trials conducted on black cohosh and yielding favorable results have all used a single brand of this herb : Remefemin. In fact, Remefemin has been the subject of over 90 scientific papers and more than 20 clinical trials and it has been tested on over 3,000 women.

Not surprisingly, Remifemin is also the brand of black cohosh that is most often recommended by doctors, and I frequently recommend it as well.

In terms of dosing, the average amount needed to quell menopause symptoms is between 40 mg and 80 mg per day. To use this herb as a fertility enhancer I would recommend that you start with 40 mg daily and take it for at least eight weeks before increasing the dosage.

FERTILITY HERB # 3: DONG QUAI

In the world of Chinese medicine, the herb known as Dong Quai has been a mainstay of good health for hundreds of years. In fact the root of Dong Quai is considered one of the most honored herbs in Chinese medicine, with a history of use that goes back more than 2,000 years.

A member of the celery family, it comes from the plant Angelica sinensis, and has been used to treat a variety of illnesses related to reproductive health. These include menstrual cramps, irregular cycles, and infrequent or absent periods, as well as taming most symptoms of PMS.

But Dong Quai also has a very special place in the herbalists medicine bag, as the herb that can reduce the risk of recurrent miscarriage. Indeed, while it contains several key compounds, among the most important is a natural chemical known as "coumadin" - which, not coincidentally, is the basis for the blood thinning medication by the same name. And it is, in fact, due to its blood thinning properties that many believe Dong Quai helps prevent miscarriage.

Indeed, while any number of factors can cause pregnancy loss, among the most common is the formation of tiny clots in the vessel pathways leading to the placenta – the sac which surrounds your developing baby and through which your baby receives all the nutrients necessary to thrive. When these small clots block the route to the placenta, your baby simply fails to thrive – sometimes right from the very earliest stages of implantation.

Dong Quai is believed to reduce those risks by helping to keep these tiny clots from forming. But as a compound, coumadin also has another beneficial aspect:

It works as both an anti-inflammatory and an anti-spasmodic, particularly in the uterus. For this reason many experts believe it can also increase fertility by helping to reduce the presence of inflammatory compounds that might otherwise damage or even kill sperm before fertilization can occur. Moreover, the antispasmodic effects on the uterus may also reduce the risk of miscarriage, as well as make certain your newly fertilized embryo has a smooth and effortless trip from your fallopian tube to your uterus.

Additionally, Dong Quai also contains a compound known as ferulic acid which is a natural muscle relaxer - one reason why this herbal treatment works to relieve menstrual cramps, which actually occur when the uterus goes into spasms.

Dong Quai also helps tone the muscles in the uterus, so you actually become less prone to cramping as time goes on, which can also work to reduce the risk of miscarriage. Once you do get pregnant, a strong, toned uterus can be a real asset, helping you to have a more comfortable pregnancy and even an easier labor and delivery.

DONG QUAI: MY PERSONAL PRESCRIPTION AND SOME PRECAUTIONS

The usual dosage of Dong Quai for women is three to four grams a day. Supplements of powdered Dong Quai root can be found in capsule form, as well as in tablets, tinctures and extracts. It can also be brewed as a tea.

Since Dong Quai has an extremely low toxicity profile, there is little chance that you can overdose or have a bad reaction.

That said, some side effects have been reported. Among the most common is a sensitivity to sunlight, particularly if you have fair skin.

Dong Quai can also impact blood sugar and should not be used if you have diabetes or insulin resistance - or a related fertility condition such as PCOS.

If you have a very heavy menstrual cycle, or if you bleed excessively from fibroid tumors or polyps you should also not use Dong Quai. You should also stop this herb as soon as you believe you are pregnant.

You must also remain aware that Dong Quai can interact with several common prescription and over-the-counter medications including anti-inflammatory drugs, diuretics and some lithium based drugs used to treat bi polar disorder .

It can also interfere with blood thinning medications such as coumadin or Wafarin, or some medications for high blood pressure.

If you are regularly using any of these drugs make certain to check with your doctor before beginning a regimen of Dong Quai.

Dong Quai & the Chinese Fertility Cocktail

While Dong Quai can certainly be helpful on its own, in Traditional Chinese Medicine (known as TCM) it is almost always prescribed as part of a group of herbs that work synergistically to achieve a desired result.

Indeed, most traditional Chinese doctors prescribe Dong Quai as part of a "fertility cocktail" - a group of herbs that work together to tone your uterus, improve hormone balance, reduce blood clotting and inflammation, and in general improve the health of your reproductive system.

The herbs most often combined with Don Quai include Ligusticum, Rehmanii, and white peony – all of which are thought to work together in a way that promotes a quick and easy pregnancy.

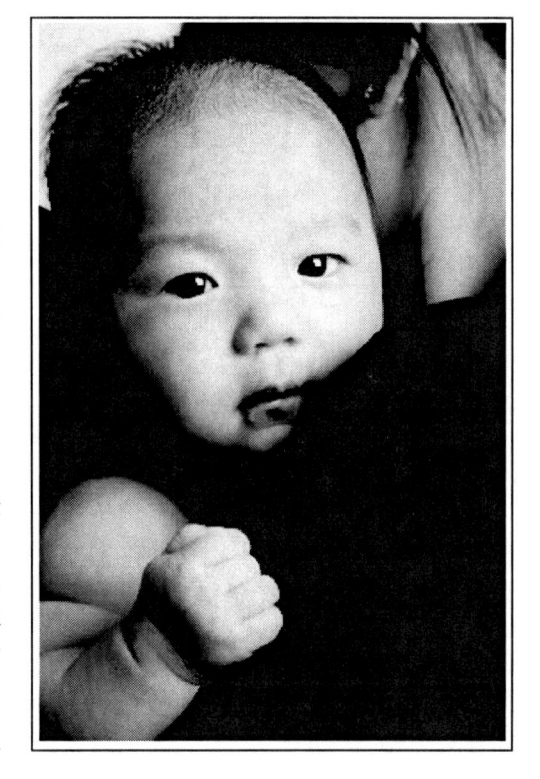

While there are a number of companies offering this or a variation as a fertility supplement, if you are really serious about using Chinese medicine to improve your reproductive health, I would strongly suggest you seek out a Chinese medicine doctor who can customize your treatment based on your specific fertility needs.

While most universities and teaching hospitals can refer you to a Chinese medicine specialist in your area, you can also contact:

- The American Association of Oriental Medicine (http://www.aaom.org/)
- The National Certification Commission for Acupuncture and Oriental Medicine (NCCAOM) http://www.nccaom.org/

In addition to providing you with more information both groups also have a referral service that can help you find a TCM physician in your area.

Additional Herbs To Promote Fertility

In addition to the herbs already discussed, there are a few lesser known compounds that many herbalists believe can impact fertility and help you get pregnant faster. Here is a quick look at what else is available – and how it can help you.

Raspberry Leaf

One of the oldest herbs in recorded history, raspberry leaf has traditionally been used by women as far back as the bible to help reduce the risk of miscarriage and encourage fertility. It's primary mode of action is to relax the uterus, thus helping to prevent contractions that might otherwise expel a newly implanted embryo. Some naturopathic doctors believe that when taken while you are trying to get pregnant, red raspberry leaf can help a newly fertilized egg attach to the uterine lining and to remain attached, again reducing the risk of miscarriage.

In addition, raspberry leaf also has toning effects that not only benefit your uterus, but your entire reproductive system. In addition to encouraging a healthy conception raspberry leaf extract is also prescribed by herbalists for morning sickness, menstrual cramps and heavy menstrual bleeding.

Moreover, if you have been diagnosed with a luteal phase defect, or if you suffer from bouts of PMS – both of which are related to a reduction in the production of the hormone progesterone - raspberry leaf extract can also help. Indeed, in herbal circles this plant is actually known as a "phyto-progesterone" - a plant source of the hormone progesterone.

As a bonus, if you are trying to get pregnant during the hot summer months, Raspberry leaf can also help you avoid dehydration – a problem which can upset the balance of minerals in your body and temporarily impact your fertility. Because this plant works to bring liquids into your cells, it not only protects you from dehydration, it can provide an instant energy boost when you feel thirsty and tired.

Raspberry leaf is available in powdered form and sold as capsules, or in liquid form as a tincture. The usual supplement contains about 400 mg per dose, and most herbalists recommend one to two capsules up to three times daily.

For most women, however, the easiest and most enjoyable way to gain the benefits of red raspberry leaf is by drinking a tea brewed from this herb – which by the way, is really delicious served icy cold on a warm summer's day! Be certain, however, that your tea actually contains raspberry leaf and not just raspberry flavoring or raspberry extract. You need the leaf, not the fruit to get the best results. Several cups per day should be sufficient to get the desire effect.

FALSE UNICORN ROOT

With a long history of use within the Native American Indian community, false unicorn root is best known for its ability to help prevent miscarriage.

The active ingredients are compounds known as saponins, which, as you read earlier, act as precursors in the production of several key reproductive hormones, but particularly estrogen.

Working somewhat like black cohosh, and a little like red clover (see below) false unicorn root is believed to act like a weak form of estrogen to encourage ovulation. In fact many herbalists prescribe False Unicorn Root when a woman fails to ovulate.

But this herb is also considered to be "adaptogenic", allowing it to adjust its activity based on what your body needs at any given time. So, this herb not only reduces the risk of miscarriage, but also offers you better hormone balance overall. This, in turn can impact not only egg production and ovulation but also the ease with which you get pregnant.

If you'd like to try this herb it is usually available as a liquid extract and the normal dosage is 1 teaspoon (or 6 to 8 drops) in a cup of water, two to three times daily. You can also use 1 to 2 grams of the root brewed into a pot of tea and it's safe to drink up to three cups per day. If you take the root tincture on its own, 1 teaspoon 3 times a day is the standard dosing. Be aware however that in some women anywhere from 5 to 15 drops of the extract can cause nausea and vomiting, as can 3 to 4 cups of tea per day. For this reason I always recommend that you start slow with small amounts and gradually build your tolerance level. If you do begin to feel nauseous you'll automatically know your threshold – and how much to cut back to relieve your symptoms.

RED CLOVER

Although Red Clover is often thought of as an herb, in reality, it's a legume that comes from the same family as soybeans – and therein lies some of its power as a fertility treatment.

Although Red Clover has garnered a strong reputation as a hormone-balancing compound able to alleviate menopausal symptoms, much like Black Cohosh these same effects can be equally important if you are a young woman. As you read earlier, when ovulation is irregular, or doesn't occur at all, many of the same types of imbalances seen in older women develop in the childbearing years as well. And this is where Red Clover can help.

What can it do? Like soybeans, red clover derives its power from the phytonutrients known as "isoflavones". As you read in the section on fruits and vegetables, isoflavones have been shown in studies to exert some natural estrogenic effects that may be helpful in overcoming hormonal imbalances linked to some forms of infertility.

So why not just eat soybeans? Because in addition to the two types of isoflavone found in soy - - genistein and daidzein - red clover also contains two more. They are known as biochannin A, and formononetin – both of which are believed to exert an even greater estrogenic effect.

Additionally, like soy and black cohosh, red clover also works as an "adaptogen" So, if your estrogen levels are low red clover will step up to the plate and become estrogen's " understudy" - helping to rebalance your hormone profile. Likewise, when estrogen levels are too high, red clover becomes a "down regulating" compound, that keeps your body from experiencing a hormone overload, once again achieving a more normal balance.

Although red clover is technically classified as a legume, you really can't eat it like you would soybeans. You can however, purchase red clover teas, infusions or various dried products. But if you're really serious about giving this compound a try, I would suggest you immediately look to red clover supplements.

CHOOSE YOUR RED CLOVER WISELY: WHAT TO LOOK FOR

While there are a variety of different types of red clover supplements available, how this plant is harvested, when in its life cycle harvesting occurs, and where the plant is grown can all impact the effectiveness of any supplement – one reason why not all red clover supplements are the same. That said, among the most widely used brand name – and the one that has been the subject of most clinical trials - is Promensil. It is standardized to contain 40 mg of the four key types of isoflavone, plus another weak plant estrogen known as coumasol, a compound similar to what is found in Dong Quai.

Indeed, studies on Promensil were conducted on more than 1,000 women worldwide, and published by doctors from Tufts University, School of Medicine,

NYU School of Medicine, and Oxford University in England and all showed Promensil to be an effective red clover treatment. And while the bulk of the research has been in regard to menopause symptoms, I and many natural medicine experts agree that if you suffer from a hormone imbalance and particularly if you have PCOS, you too can benefit from red clover.

The suggested amount for menopause symptoms is one 40 mg capsule of Promensil daily, with up to two capsules daily for severe symptoms. I recommend that for re-balancing fertility hormones you stay with one 40 mg capsule once daily for at least eight weeks during which time you should monitor your cycle for regularity, and use various natural methods (including basal body temperature and cervical mucus) to also monitor ovulation. I am quite certain you will see some positive changes towards more regularity in both areas - which is a good sign that your fertility is blooming!

A few precautions: Red clover can interfere with the processing of any medication that requires certain liver enzymes for breakdown. As such if you are taking prescription medications or any over the counter drugs on a regular basis, talk to your doctor before using red clover supplements. Also if you are taking any drugs to control blood sugar (particularly if you are using Metformin with or without Clomid for the treatment of PCOS) talk to your doctor before using red clover as it has been known to lower blood sugar. This in turn may alter the effects of some drugs used to treat type 2 diabetes or PCOS.

Also Important: Stop taking red clover as soon as you know you have conceived as it is not recommended for use during pregnancy.

Q: *I have a lot of grass and ragweed allergies. Is it safe to take red clover?*

A: The red clover plant is related to fescue grass, ragweed, and timothy grass, so if you have a severe allergy to any of these pollens, there could be a problem. The best way to know for certain is to see your allergist and be tested for a red clover sensitivity. You should also stop taking red clover the moment you know you are pregnant as it is not recommended for use during this time.

The Buzz Is On:
The Birds, The Bees and Your Fertility

If you're ever been stung by a bee – and particularly if you have had an allergic reaction to that sting - then you probably can't imagine how anything associated with these sometimes nasty insects can be helpful! But in truth many people claim that help is exactly what they get from an assortment of products related to bees – particularly bee pollen, bee propolis and royal bee jelly.

Moreover, just a quick trip around the Internet will show you that all three have been cited as treatments for various problems related to infertility. But, the big question is are the claims real – and more importantly have they been verified in medical studies?

While there have been a handful of very small studies on these substances, because results have varied widely it seems there is simply not enough evidence either pro or con to say for sure that these compounds work – or that they don't.

If, however, you do decide to give bee products a try, here's a quick guide to what they are, how they work, what the studies show about their link to fertility – and most important, some precautions you should heed.

Bee Pollen: What You Need To Know

As bees visit flowers to suck the nectar, they pick up pollen, which sticks to their legs and body. As they fly from plant to plant they spread the pollen – which is actually how flowers are pollinated, so they can bloom each spring. When the bees return to the hive, bee keepers remove the pollen from their legs and body and eventually it's processed, usually into loose granules that are sold much like any other herbal powders.

Currently there are no specific medical studies linking the use of bee pollen supplements to an increase in fertility . That said, anecdotal testimonials abound, particularly on the Internet. So where does the truth lie? Well in my opinion, if there is any power in bee pollen at all, it is likely due to the large variety of nutrients it contains, including polyphenols, enzymes, fatty acids, amino acids, minerals, and vitamins – particularly B vitamins . Perhaps most important is the high antioxidant levels found in bee pollen – with certain types shown to have up to 4 times the antioxidant rating of wild blueberries and twice the level of black raspberries, which are believed to be the fruits rated the highest. As you read in

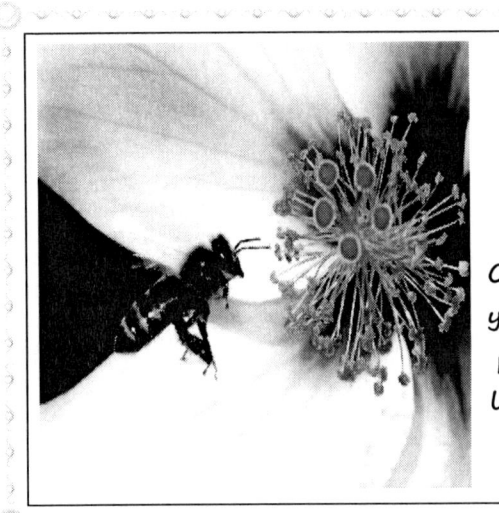

> Bee pollen is loaded with B vitamins and it's a powerful source of antioxidants. And therein may lie it's link to fertility!
> One caution caution however: If you are allergic to tree or flower pollens, then you might be allergic to bee pollen as well — so be cautious when trying it.

the previous chapter, I am a huge believer in the power of nutrients to boost fertility but particularly antioxidants and B vitamins. So, if it fact some women do find it increases their fertility, my guess is that is related to the high nutrient content, particularly the antioxidants.

While most bee pollen products claim that there are no side effects, evidence indicates that if you are allergic to flower or tree pollens, or if you have asthma, bee pollen may worsen your symptoms. In some cases it can bring on serious, even life threatening reactions. In addition, depending on where the bees themselves picked up the pollen, it's also possible it can contain pollutants, including toxic heavy metals like lead, which we know can be harmful to fertility. This can be particularly the case with bee pollen supplements imported from China, where there is very little in the way of growing or packaging regulations. So, this should be another consideration if you are going to use these supplements.

If you do decide to give bee pollen a try follow the dosing on the package insert. It is most often available as loose granules which you can sprinkle on cereal or put in tea or juice. The usual dosage is one tablespoon daily.

Finally, it's also important to note that you can get almost everything that is in B pollen if you eat a healthy diet - particularly fresh fruits and vegetables, and if you take a high potency vitamin/mineral supplement with B complex.

BEE PROPOLIS: WHAT THE BUZZ IS ALL ABOUT!

Although propolis is often mentioned in the same breath as bee pollen, except for the fact that both involve bee activity, they are vastly different substances. Propolis is, in fact, a natural resin that is extracted from trees by various types of honey bees. It is then mixed with bees wax and other secretions made by the bees, and brought back to their hive where it is used as a kind of natural glue to shore up cracks and holes. To make the supplements, the propolis is then taken from the hives and processed into an ointment, a capsule, an extract, or a nasal spray.

Bee propolis first came to medical attention because of its strong anti-microbial activity. It has also long been considered a powerful anti-inflammatory and wound healing agent and was a staple in folk medicine, with use dating back to Biblical times or even earlier.

In more modern times it has been used by natural medicine doctors as an antibacterial, antiviral, anti-ulcer and anti-inflammatory treatment, and many believe it can stimulate the immune system and even work as a local anesthetic. It has also been used as an ointment to treat herpes as well as cervicitis, an infection of the cervix.

In terms of fertility, there is some evidence it may have healing properties on the reproductive system – particularly in women who have mild endometriosis. In one study of some 40 women published in the journal *Fertility & Sterility* in 2003 bee propolis did indeed appear to boost their fertility. In this research project, all 40 women were diagnosed with endometriosis and all had unsuccessfully tried to get pregnant for at least two years. Half the women in the group received 500 mg of bee propolis twice a day for nine months, while the other half received a placebo.

The result: Sixty percent of the women taking the bee propolis became pregnant, while only 20% taking the placebo pill conceived. More importantly, no adverse effects were seen in the women taking the propolis. What's important to realize however, is that sometimes, endometriosis can be difficult do diagnose. As such any subsequent infertility that results may not be properly categorized as being related to this disease. So, in this respect, if you are having problems getting pregnant with no obvious obstacles in the way, then you might have a mild to moderate case of undiagnosed endometriosis – in which case bee propolis might make an important difference in your ability to get pregnant quickly and easily.

In terms of dosage, since Bee Propolis comes in many forms, follow the package insert. But in general, dosing for the powdered form is usually one teaspoon three times a day mixed with food or drink (it does have a somewhat bitter taste). Adult dosing for the extract is 10 to 20 drops two to three times per day.

ROYAL BEE JELLY: IS IT FERTILITY MAGIC?

Although Royal Bee Jelly is often confused with both bee pollen and bee propolis, again, this is a completely separate compound with properties all its own. Moreover, this is the only compound of the three to actually be created by the bee itself in response to a species-specific need. That need is to feed bee larvae, one of which will actually develop into a Queen bee, who then also feasts on royal bee jelly.

The compound itself is formed from secretions that come from the glands of the worker bees, but it is considered to be a highly nourishing nectar – one that eventually helps the queen bee to grow larger, live longer and be more fertile than ordinary worker bees . And therein lies the beginning of the reputation that royal jelly is blessed with " fertility magic".

In terms of its actual composition however, there isn't much magic going on. It's made up of 60 to 70 percent water, 12 to 15 percent protein, 10 to 16 percent sugars, 3 to 6 percent fats, plus a sprinkling of vitamins, salts and amino acids.

That said, throughout the history of natural medicine, royal bee jelly has been credited with successfully treating or preventing a variety of ailments including not only infertility but also arthritis, multiple sclerosis, high cholesterol, liver disease, insomnia, fatigue, ulcers, digestive disorders, skin problems, and some symptoms related to cardiovascular disease. It's also believed to reduce symptoms of menopause, stimulate hair growth, slow the signs of aging, increase immunity to disease, and heal bone fractures.

While there are some small studies which support some of the claims, as a doctor and researcher myself I can tell you that it's always wise to question the effectiveness of any substance – even a drug – that purports to impact such widely diverse ailments, and so many of them. Clearly, some of these conditions are related, but many are not - which in turn makes one question the validity of any of the claims.

However, in regard to fertility I'm happy to report there are a few small , but well designed published studies showing that royal bee jelly has some properties that can be helpful. Among the most important is its ability to act somewhat like

> There are some aspects of Royal Bee Jelly - including it's mild estrogenic effects - that could make it an excellent natural fertility treatment source if you have PCOS - a condition where estrogen levels are low.

estrogen, particularly in regard to controlling the dilation of blood vessels, and controlling blood pressure and cholesterol. It also appears to have some of estrogen's anti-inflammatory properties. All these reasons are what led many health experts to recommend royal bee jelly as a tretment for menopause - a time when estrogen levels naturally decline.

But how exactly does royal bee jelly accomplish all this? In one study published in the *Journal of Complementary and Alternative Medicine* researchers determined that two factors isolated from royal bee jelly – sterols and fatty acids – are largely responsible for most of it's estrogenic effects.

As such, there also seems to be some scientific "common sense" behind using royal bee jelly supplements to encourage fertility in women who appear to have an estrogen deficiency, including those with irregular ovulation and irregular menstrual periods. And if this sounds like it might be the case for you, then it could be worth your while to give royal bee jelly a try.

The common dosage is 50 mg to 100 mg daily – but that can vary due to the potency of the individual supplement. As such you should follow the directions on your specific product to get the best results.

While most adults can easily tolerate even larger doses of royal bee jelly, you should not use it if you are allergic to bees or to honey, or if you have asthma. Adverse reactions can include bronchial spasms, skin irritations and asthma attacks, or in rare cases anaphylactic shock. It is also not recommended for use during pregnancy or while breastfeeding, so if you do conceive, stop your supplements right away.

If you don't know if you are allergic to bees (for example if you've never been stung) you might also want to forgo the use of this supplement. Not only are there other sources of all the vitamins and amino acids found in royal jelly, there are also other food and nutrient sources of the sterols and fatty acids – some of which are featured earlier in this book. You can also find more information on other foods containing these nutrients in my book "Eat, Love, Get Pregnant" or at FertilityDietGuide.com.

ADDITIONAL SUPPLEMENTS TO INCREASE FERTILITY

While vitamins, minerals and herbs make up the largest share of natural fertility boosters, there are, in fact, a number of other supplements that fall outside these three categories that can also help. While some are derived from foods – and actually considered dietary supplements – others are blends of nutrients and herbs that have been shown to work synergistically to enhance fertility and improve your reproductive profile in a number of ways.

What follows are what I believe to be the best of the lot – the supplements that have the most clinical research behind them and have been shown to help the largest number of women. Many are also the supplements I have found to be helpful for my patients.

As with other supplements mentioned in this and previous chapters, remember, however, that results do take time. So, have patience and keep a positive outlook and I'm quite certain you will benefit from at least one of these formulations.

BOOST YOUR FERTILITY WITH OMEGA-3!

As you read in an earlier chapter, Omega-3 fatty acids are a group of nutrients which can have a profound impact on your fertility. The two Omega-3 compounds most useful to fertility are called EPA (Eicosapentaenoic acid) and DHA (docosahexaenoic acid). Found primarily in fish oil, among their many benefits is countering the fertility-robbing effects of insulin resistance. And, if you are diagnosed with PCOS or another ovulatory - related problem, these fatty acids can be particularly helpful to you.

In fact, in one study researchers found that simply adding more Omega-3 fatty acids to the diet worked to kick-start ovulation even in women who were not ovulating at all. There is also evidence to show that the anti-inflammatory effects of Omega-3 fatty acids can also help re-balance hormones and increase blood flow to the uterus, which in turn can help foster a healthy implantation.

Although these compounds are considered "essential" to your health as well as your fertility, your body is unable to make Omega-3 fatty acids on its own.

Indeed, they must be derived from dietary sources. And while I have always believed that natural foods are among the best ways to get all your nutrients, when it comes to Omega-3 , I have found that even women who have a relatively "good" diet, can come up short. For this reason – and because this nutrient is so important to your overall health and your fertility – I also frequently recommend supplementation.

Although there are many types of Omega-3 fatty acid supplements, most experts agree that those which come from cold water fish such as salmon, mackerel, and New Zealand hoki are among the best. That said, it's important to note that not all fish oils – even from these fish - are created equal! This is particularly true when it comes to issues like mercury contamination. Indeed, one reason I have found that so many of my patients were not eating more fish was because of fears and worries over contamination from mercury and other potentially harmful chemicals.

FINDING FISH OIL SUPPLEMENTS THAT ARE SAFE

The good news: There *are* fish oil supplements that are safe – in some instances much safer than eating fish. So, how do you find the ones that will help without doing harm? There are actually two ways to do this.

First, you can visit a web site called ConsumerLabs.com. This is a well run, objective laboratory that analyzes supplements of all kinds (including vitamins, herbs, food supplements, etc) for purity, contamination, formulation integrity, and other important factors. For a very small yearly subscription fee you can have access to all their reports on all types of supplements. I am not connected in any way to Consumer Labs but I frequently recommend them as one of the few organizations where consumers can access "inside" information on products that normally is available only through expensive laboratory testing.

So if you can afford to join the information they provide can be very valuable in terms of finding the healthiest and best supplements of all kinds.

If you'd rather try to go it alone in choosing what to buy, when shopping for Omega-3 supplements look for the words " molecularly distilled" on the label or within the product literature. This is a process that uses high heat to remove all toxins from the fish oil - and in the process also removes that "fishy" aftertaste that can repeat on some people.

While there are some product manufacturers who claim that molecular distillation also removes some of the potency of the fish oil (mostly by changing the original ratio of all the nutrients found naturally in fish) when it comes to fertility I believe molecular distillation can be helpful, particularly since some of the chemicals contaminants found in unprocessed fish oil have been linked to reproductive problems. My personal opinion is that it's better to have a fish oil supplement that is slightly less potent but clean in terms of contaminants that can impact fertility. If need be you can always increase your dosage to get more benefits.

Another option is to seek out supplements that are made from fish that swim in pristine clean waters. These include hoki fish from protected waters off the coast of New Zealand as well as salmon from the pristine clean waters off the coast of Scandinavia. While these fish generally are not subjected to the harmful chemical pollutants found in other parts of the world, some of these supplements can also be very costly, so if you're on a tight budget this might not be an option for you.

POTENCY MATTERS: HOW TO FIND THE BEST OMEGA-3 SUPPLEMENTS

And while you're out shopping, it's important to recognize that it's not just contamination that can make a difference in your Omega-3 supplement - potency also matters. In short, your supplement has to contain enough of the key nutrients EPA and DHA to make a difference.

How much do you need? The most helpful products contain a minimum of 180 mg of EPA and 120 mg of DHA in conjunction with other fatty acids so you get a good balance without sacrificing the therapeutic levels necessary to see results. Products that contain lesser amounts usually make up the difference with fillers and binders - things you don't need and which won't have any effect on your fertility.

Finally, because fish oil tends to oxidize rapidly - and lose potency - preservatives are necessary to keep it fresh and effective. When possible, look for products that use vitamin E or other natural preservatives to keep the oil fresh. In fact, fish oil products preserved with vitamin E offer you the advantage of some extra antioxidant protection with every dose!

Recommended Supplement Prescription: Although supplements vary in both the amount and ratio proportions of EPA and DHA, a common amount found in high quality supplements is 0.18 grams (180 mg) of EPA and 0.12 (120 mg) of DHA

My Fertility Prescription: 800 - 1000 mg or 1 gram of EPA and DHA once daily. This usually translates to one to two capsules daily depending on the strength. According to the FDA you can safely take up to 3,000 mg (or 3 grams) daily with no adverse effects, but I definitely would not go above that amount without talking to your doctor first. In fact, because this supplement can have blood thinning effects, you should definitely check with your doctor before taking any amount.

The Fish Oil Alternative

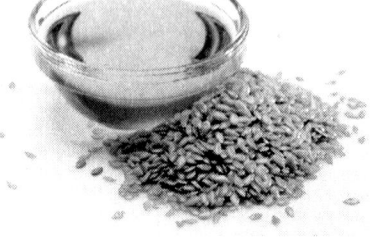

Although fish oil capsules supply the most potent form of Omega-3, for some they can be difficult to take. First, some of the less expensive supplements do have a bit of a fishy odor and some have a fishy aftertaste that many of my patients did not like. If this is a problem for you, try a product such as Core-Omega, which does a great job of hiding the "fishy" taste and smell with fruit flavors and even chocolate. Some flavors however also contain stevia (a sugar alternative), menthol and eggs, so if you have a problem with these ingredients, be sure to check the label before buying or trying.

That said, if you want to avoid fish for any other reason – a food allergy, or a vegetarian commitment – then you can also seek out Omega-3 supplements made from flax seed oil. If this is your choice, then know that you will not be getting either EPA or DHA directly. Instead, these sources provide a compound known as ALA (alpha linolenic acid) which the body converts to omega 3 fatty acids. Although it's not quite as powerful as fish oil, it can be very helpful. .

If you choose this form of supplementation look for products containing at least 1000 mg of flax seed oil with at least 500 mg of alpha linolenic acid, 110 mg of linoleic acid and 110 mg of oleic acid. These numbers – or those close to them – should be on the label.

EVENING OIL OF PRIMROSE: NATURE'S FERTILITY PROMISE

Frequently heralded as one of Mother Nature's "perfect female foods" - Evening Oil of Primrose has been considered both a magical "cure all" and a promising fertility herb by many cultures the world over.

And although most of its claims to fame are steep in folk lore and not science, when it comes to fertility there is some evidence to suggest it may have a mild to moderate impact on inflammatory conditions that might otherwise interfere with pregnancy.

Derived from the Evening Primrose plant, the oil is rich in vitamin E, as well as some essential fatty acids including linolenic acid (the same compound found in flax seed oil) and gamma linolenic acid also known as GLA. And therein may lie the seed of its benefits. How so? GLA is a potent anti-inflammatory compound involved in regulating a number of key reproductive hormones, as well as impacting the healing of endometriosis. So certainly if you have been diagnosed with an inflammatory condition, this supplement might help you.

While in the past Evening Oil of Primrose was routinely suggested as a treatment for PMS – and some women have indeed found help with this compound - at this point reports favoring it's use are largely anecdotal and not science-based. That said, if , in fact, you are among the many women who suffer from PMS , and you are also having difficulty getting pregnant, this supplement may be worth a try. Indeed, if it can help re-balance some of the hormonal activity and symptoms related to PMS, it is likely to have a positive influence on your fertility.

In addition, there also appears to be some evidence - though largely anecdotal - that Evening Oil of Primrose may increase the quality of cervical mucus, including making it more plentiful as well as thinner and more "sperm friendly." While there is no true scientific evidence to show Evening Oil of Primrose alters cervical mucus, there are isolated reports from women who say that it does. So again, if you find that your cervical mucus production is low, or that it is very sticky and thick, you might want to give Evening Oil of Primrose a try. If you do, take this supplement daily beginning right after your period ends, and stopping mid-cycle as soon as you ovulate. This is important since there are some isolated reports that Evening Oil of Primrose may increase uterine contractions. As such, using it during the second half of your cycle might actually work against your fertility. Indeed, if fertilization does take place, contractions might rush your embryo down your fallopian too quickly (before your uterus is fully prepared for implantation) . If your fertilized egg does reach your uterus in the correct amount of time, these same contractions might prevent it from properly adhering to the uterine wall.

You can however, safely use either Omega-3 supplements or flax seed oil supplements during the second half of your cycle to help continue the anti-inflammatory and other positive effects of essential fatty acids.

My Fertility Prescription: I recommend between 1500 mg and 3,000 mg daily – taken in 500 mg doses spread throughout the day. While Evening Oil of Primrose has an excellent safety profile it should not be used during pregnancy, or again, during the second half of the menstrual cycle if you are trying to conceive. It should also not be used prior to surgery, (even fertility procedures) or if you are at risk for seizures. Do not use this supplement if you are taking phenothiazine-related medications, anti platelet drugs, thrombolytics, low-molecular-weight heparins, or anticoagulant drugs. It's also important to point out that The German Commission E has not approved the use of Evening Oil of Primrose for any condition at this time.

DHEA : THE NEW FERTILITY SUPPLEMENT

While the use of some supplements, particularly herbs, goes back hundreds if not thousands of years, others are new to the world of alternative medicine, and some are brand new to the world of fertility. Such is the case for DHEA – short for **Dehydroepiandrosterone** , a precursor compound that the body uses to make steroid hormones, including some that are directly involved in reproduction.

According to New York fertility expert Dr. David Barad, who has conducted studies on DHEA, the link between this compound and conception lies in its ability to help stimulate and support the development of your eggs . It does so by increasing production and metabolism of steroid hormones including estrogens and androgens. It also appears to increase certain other compounds related to egg development, thus providing a kind of overall boost to fertility for some women – particularly those who are over 40 and are having difficulty producing eggs.

Indeed, this was in fact, the age group on whom Dr. Barad's studies were conducted. More specifically, over the course of two years he treated 120 IVF patients over the age of 40 with DHEA supplements. Most had been told by other fertility experts that donor eggs were their only option for getting pregnant. However, after treatment with DHEA, Dr. Barad reports he observed a marked increase in natural egg production and quality in all the women - a remarkable finding which was later reflected in pregnancy rates. Indeed, when compared to women who did not take DHEA supplements the pregnancy rates of those who did were significantly higher. Of the original 120 women in the study, to date, over two dozen were able to get pregnant using traditional IVF procedures and their own eggs.

CAN DHEA INCREASE YOUR FERTILITY?

So, can DHEA help increase your fertility? Although the studies were conducted on women who were involved in IVF treatments and also using fertility medications, my thought is that if you are over age 35 and having problems getting pregnant naturally, it is certainly worth giving DHEA a try.

As to whether or not it can encourage fertility in younger women, we can't say for certain. And certainly if you know you are ovulating regularly, and your egg production is already good, this is probably not the right supplement for you.

That said, if you are over age 35, and/or you are not ovulating regularly or you know you have a problem producing quality eggs, then DHEA may prove helpful.

Be aware, however, that while in small amounts DHEA is essential to egg production, because it is essentially a male hormone, in larger amounts it can cause some unpleasant but not necessarily dangerous side effects. These primarily include oily skin and hair, and some acne. On the plus side, however, some women have reported an increased feeling of well being while on DHEA and some have noted an increase in their sex drive.

My Fertility Prescription: The recommended dosage of DHEA used in the fertility studies is 25 mg, three times a day.

If you are not certain if you are ovulating, or you are under age 35 I would suggest you begin with 25 mg twice a day, and add more if needed. If you are over age 35, then 25 mg three times a day would likely help you.

When purchasing a DHEA supplement, it's important that you seek out a compounding pharmacy, which makes products from scratch. They can insure that you are getting a top quality product with the proper potency.

If you are unable to find a compounding pharmacy in your area, several experts who have done clinical testing on DHEA recommend the website www.DHEA.com, as a source for high quality, pharmaceutical grade supplements.

THE FERTILITY NUTRIENT: CO Q 10

Because it's so often mentioned in the same context as vitamins, many people believe that the nutrient known as CoQ10 is in fact a vitamin. But in truth it's really a compound that is produced naturally by every living cell in the body. It is necessary for the production of another compound known as ATP (adenosine triphosphate) which is actually the "fuel" of all living cells.

Without adequate CoQ10, ATP supply dwindles – and that means cells won't get the nutrients they need to thrive – including those involved in egg production and maturation. So, from this respect, keeping CoQ10 levels high can be a huge health advantage as well as a boost to your fertility.

Additionally, CoQ10 is also a powerful antioxidant. So, much like vitamins A, C, E and others it provides the antioxidant power necessary to stabilize your cells and neutralize fertility-robbing free radicals - which in turn automatically gives your conception efforts a natural boost!

> *Not only can the nutrient CoQ10 help safeguard your fertility, once you are pregnant studies show it can reduce the risk of miscarriage!*

Moreover, CoQ10 can offer you just a bit more in the way of fertility protection by helping reduce your risk of miscarriage. Indeed studies have shown that directly following miscarriage, levels of CoQ10 are exceedingly low - a fact which has led to some serious speculation concerning the role of CoQ10 in preventing miscarriage. While we have no definitive studies showing that this is the case, there is certainly enough scientific suggestion - along with some clear cut evidence on the antioxidant powers of CoQ10 - to recommend it as a fertility supplement.

Also important to note: Because CoQ10 is involved in energy production, studies reveal it also has a somewhat energizing effect on sperm – and you'll learn more about how and why it helps a little later in this book.

When it comes to making sure you and your partner are getting adequate levels of CoQ10, you should consider supplements. Although there are some food sources of this nutrient – with organ meats such as liver having among the highest levels – still, what you generally find in food is minuscule compared to what your body needs to insure against a deficiency. So, for this reason I always recommend supplements as the major source of this nutrient.

My Fertility Prescription: 60 mg – 100 mg capsules, once daily.

Although side effects are rare they can include nausea, diarrhea, and appetite suppression. If you are taking the blood thinner wafarin, or if you have been prescribed heparin for the treatment of recurrent miscarriage, check with your doctor before adding a CoQ10 supplement to your regimen.

FERTILITY BLEND & OTHER SUPPORT SUPPLEMENTS:
WHAT YOU MUST KNOW

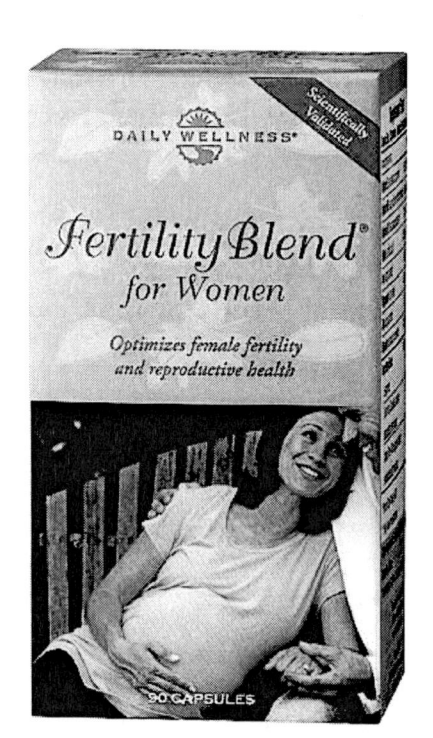

Among the most popular of the "new age" fertility supplements are what I like to call "pregnancy cocktails" - combinations of various herbs and other nutrients in a formula designed specifically to enhance fertility. While most contain nutrients, herbs and compounds similar to what you've already read about in this book, still, many companies claim that their particular way of combining these ingredients contributes to the success of their products.

While this may be true, to the best of my knowledge, only one of these supplements for women has undergone testing within the fertility medicine arena – and I'm happy to say it did appear to have at least some impact on getting pregnant. That supplement is known as *Fertility Blend*.

Currently it is available in two formulas. One is specifically for men, and you'll read about that in my chapter on male fertility. The other is specifically for women, which is the one I want to concentrate on right now. The female formula contains a proprietary blend of amino acids, herbs, vitamins and minerals. These include the herb chasteberry, green tea, vitamin E, selenium, folic acid, vitamins B 6, B 12, iron, zinc and magnesium, and the amino acid L-arginine. The amounts of each ingredient and the specific way they are combined has been shown to have clinically significant results. Indeed in a small but significant double blind study conducted at Stamford University doctors tested Fertility Blend on 93 women aged 24 to 42, all of whom had been unsuccessful in getting pregnant for a minimum of at least 6 months. Each of the women took either the supplement or a placebo, once daily for a minimum of three months.

The Result: When compared with the group taking the placebo, the women taking Fertility Blend appeared to have an increase in progesterone production. Moreover, among those women who initially had the lowest progesterone levels, improvement was the greatest.

The average number of days with an elevated BBT (basal body temperature) during the second half of the menstrual cycle also increased significantly in the Fertility Blend group, which may be especially important if you have been diagnosed with a luteal phase defect - a hormone deficiency that occurs after ovulation.

Finally, for those women who had the shortest menstrual cycle length, Fertility Blend increased cycle length; among those with an abnormally long cycle, the supplement shortened the cycle length. In this regard the herbs acted like an adaptogen - immediately sensing what the body needed to restore fertility.

In all instances, the results suggest that Fertility Blend's main advantage is the ability to achieve a better hormone balance - a factor which, as you already read, can play a major role in encouraging fertility.

But, did any of this translate into a higher pregnancy rate? According to the University of Stanford study, it did.

After six months time 17 of the 53 women taking the Fertility Blend (some 32%) were able to get pregnant, with no negative side effects from supplement use. By comparison, only 4 women (just 10%) of the placebo group conceived

WILL FERTILITY BLEND HELP YOU?

Right about now you may be asking yourself why, if Fertility Blend has such good results, should I even bother taking any of the individual herbs, minerals or

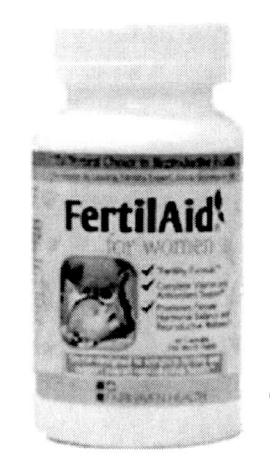

> ## Prenatal Vitamins & Fertility Herbs Combined!
>
> In a unique formulation that combines the protection of pre natal vitamins with the fertility promoting power of herbs, *FertilAid* is yet another option for boosting your fertility. Although it hasn't seen the kind of scientific testing afforded to *Fertility Blend*, still, *FertilAid* was developed by a obstetrician/gynecologist and it does contain many of the key herbal ingredients I have found to be most helpful for female fertility. In addition, *FertilAid* also contains PABA - a compound that one clinical trial reported was particularly effective in boosting female fertilty in just a few months time. Patients who take fertility medications such as Clomid are often recommended to take PABA as it is believed to boost estrogen activity in the body. However, be aware that allergic reactions have been reported in some women who have allergies to para-aminobenzoic acid based compounds. **FertilAid for Women** also offers complete **antioxidant** support plus it's all natural,
> containing no artificial dyes, colors or preservatives. Learn more about it at GreenFertility.com

vitamins discussed in these last few chapters ? Well the truth is, Fertility Blend does contain a great many of the individual nutrients I have recommended thus far. So in this respect I would say that taking this supplement might indeed be a good place to start your experimentation with natural fertility formulations.

That said, it's also important to remember that every woman's body is slightly different – which also means that what it takes to encourage fertility can be slightly different as well. Your individual body *chemistry, weight*, diet, even your overall health are all factors which not only influence your fertility, but also the effectiveness of any treatment you take.

So, for some women the exact blend of nutrients found in a product like Fertility Blend may be spot-on in terms of offering exactly what is needed to maximize fertility.

Other women, however, may find they need more, or less, or perhaps something different altogether in order to maximize *their fertility*. Indeed, while a 32% pregnancy rate is impressive, it's wise to remember that 68 % of the women taking Fertility Blend *did not get pregnant*. This doesn't mean that the formulation failed– or that the women failed. It only means that for these women perhaps a slightly different configuration of natural ingredients was necessary to enhance their individual fertility profile.

And if this turns out to be the case for you, you can confidently use the information I've provided on herbs and supplements to create your own personal "fertility blend". You can do this by adding additional herbs and vitamins to the Fertility Blend product, or by replacing it completely with your own customized formulation of herbs, vitamins and minerals. Either way the end result can be a blend of ingredients that are best suited to enhance your personal fertility profile and help you get pregnant.

Choosing Fertility Supplements: What To Look For

As you no doubt have already seen, in addition to Fertility Blend there are many more pre-packaged fertility supplements on the market – many of which claim they are "Doctor Approved", or that they have been "shown in testing " to work. What's key to remember however, is that unless the company can provide references to published medical studies – claims made by the products may be just that … claims, and nothing more. Does this mean they won't be effective or help you ? It does not mean that. Some of these products may work as well as Fertility Blend, some may work better – and others may not work at all. So how can you tell which ones are worth trying?

In terms of individual results, *you really can't tell until you give them a try*. However, you can narrow your chances of getting a more effective product if you look for the following information associated with the product:

- Standardization: All herbs used in the product should be labeled "standardized" meaning it contains the exact amount of the effective ingredients it says it contains.
- Effective Levels of Nutrients: Using my suggested supplement recommendations as a guide you should read product labels to see if the blended formulations contain enough of the key ingredient to make a difference. If for example I am suggesting 60 mg of a particular herb and

the blend contains just 5 mg, it's doubtful you will get the desired effect.

- Choose products with a minimal number of fillers, binders, artificial ingredients or preservatives.
- When possible look for herbal ingredients harvested from organic crops.
- Avoid products with too many ingredients. If a fertility supplement label starts to look like a recipe for vegetable soup, then it's doubtful that any one ingredient will be represented in a large enough dose to have an impact on your fertility.

SOME FINAL WORDS OF ADVICE

While it's true that the herbs and other nutrients mentioned in this chapter are natural products, it's important to remember that they must be taken in balance, since too much of any one thing could harm you. Indeed, when it comes to enhancing fertility *more is not always better* – so remember not to take everything you hear about all at the same time!

Certainly maintaining a healthy diet, one that is high in fruits, vegetables, fiber and lean proteins, should always be your foundation – along with a high potency vitamin-mineral supplement. From here you can add any of the herbal or other suggested supplements – but do so with some selectivity in mind. You can try a few compounds simultaneously, but don't try to take the whole shopping cart at once! If you watch your body, and more importantly, *listen to your body* – you will begin to know instinctively which of these compounds are helping you to feel better, normalizing your menstrual cycles, encouraging regular ovulation, and ultimately optimizing your personal fertility profile so you can get pregnant fast.

Likewise, if you take a product and either you don't feel well, or you see negative effects on your menstrual cycle or symptoms of PMS, either reduce the dosage or stop taking it altogether. I have always believed that our bodies instinctively know when something is right for us. And if you tune in to your own "natural health frequency" you'll soon learn to decipher your body's signals as well. In fact, some of you may remember one of my earliest books was titled "Listen To Your Body" and I called it that for a reason - because I know that when you do listen to your body you can achieve your personal best in all areas of your life.

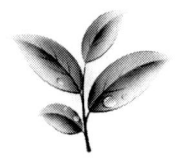

Chapter Twelve

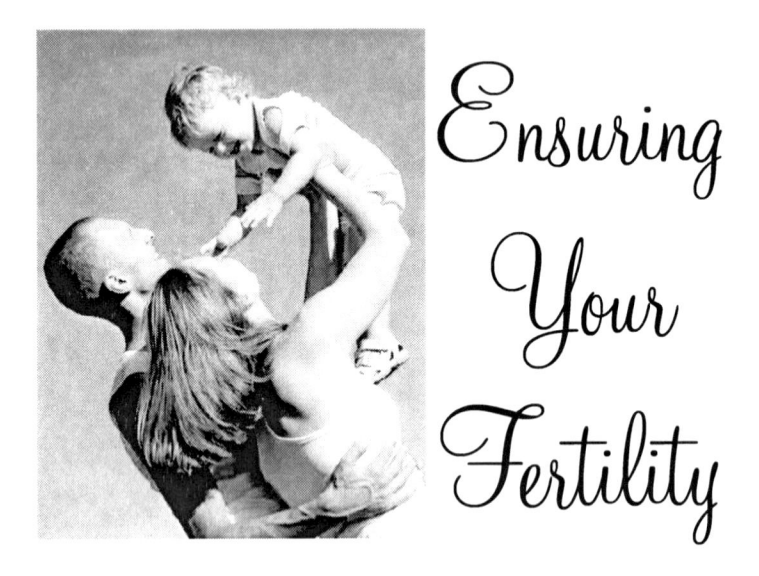

Ensuring Your Fertility

The Small Lifestyle Changes That Make A Big Difference!

When the world first began to turn, the human body was created to live in harmony with nature. Every organ and system in our body – and that includes our reproductive system – was designed to function within that natural state of being. I, and many doctors have always believed that the closer we can get to that *original plan,* the better our body works – and in the end, the more robust our fertility will be.

But I also know that today's world is a far cry from that idyllic Garden of Eden. Of course in many ways it is a much better, much more productive world.

At the same time, however, there are some things about our brave new world that can present our bodies with some unique challenges – at least some of which can impact fertility.

In previous chapters you have learned about some of the lifestyle changes that can make a difference – including diet, nutrition, stress, exercise, and weight control. In this chapter, however, I'd like to take you down a slightly different path – one that involves certain habits and the way in which they can sometimes compromise the ability to get pregnant quickly and easily.

But as important as I know this information will be, I don't want you to become worrisome or fearful. While it may be important to make some changes, I fully understand that change doesn't happen overnight - even when we can clearly see the benefits. So, certainly, work towards making those changes but don't stress yourself to the point of worry or fear. If you take it one step at a time, one habit at a time, I promise you will get there - and your health and your fertility will be reflected in your efforts!

Don't Let Your Fertility Go Up In Smoke!

Since almost the beginning of my medical practice – more than 40 years ago - by far the most common question couples would ask is "What is the best way to increase our chances of getting pregnant." And my answer to them has remained steadfast throughout four decades: "Don't smoke". Indeed, even before we knew all the current health problems related to cigarettes, I always believed there were dangers associated with smoking – particularly when it comes to fertility.

If you're like many of my patients, then I'm sure you're aware of most of the general health dangers linked to smoking – an increased risk of heart disease, high blood pressure and even cancer. But what you may not realize is that smoking is also one of the major threats to fertility. In fact, according to the American Society for Reproductive Medicine, up to 13% of *all* cases of infertility are caused by smoking.

But how exactly do cigarettes affect fertility? To begin with smoking increases the amount of time it takes to conceive. In one study of nearly 15,000 women doctors learned that on average, those who smoked took up to 12 months longer to get pregnant than non-smokers. What's more, the delay was dose related: The more

> **The Good News:**
> While smoking can clearly compromise your fertility & keep you from getting pregnant, just 24 hours after you quit your body begins to rid itself of the harmful toxins & starts to repair your fertility. Just two weeks after you quit smoking your ability to get pregnant dramatically increases!
>
> If you quit smoking today you could get pregnant next month! Wow!

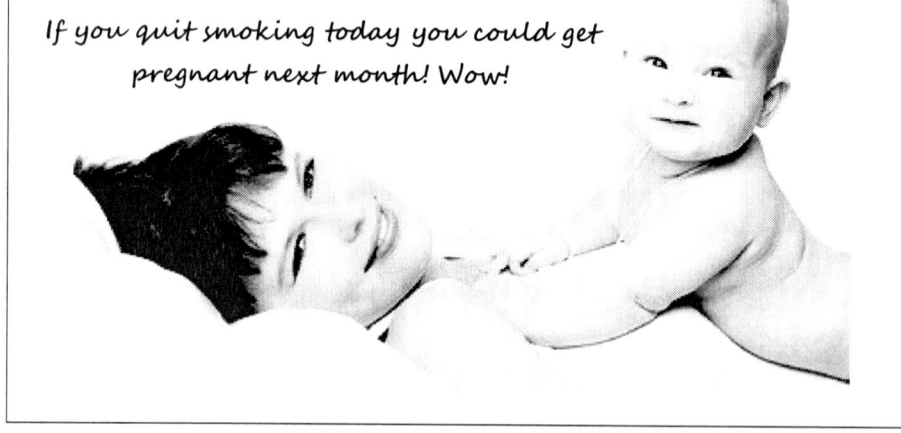

cigarettes a woman smoked, the longer it took her to conceive. For women who smoked 20 cigarettes a day or more, the risk of not getting pregnant after 12 months was 54% greater than it was for non-smokers.

But a delay in conception is not the only problem linked to smoking. For some women cigarettes can be a deciding factor in whether or not they get pregnant at all! Why? According to the American Society For Reproductive Medicine, chemicals found in cigarette smoke have a direct impact on egg follicles, in particular, accelerating their depletion. In simplest terms this means that every time you light up, the toxic chemicals found in tobacco smoke kill some of your egg follicles – the tiny seeds inside your ovary that your body uses to manufacture eggs. In fact studies show that in women who smoke, follicular fluid (the liquid that surrounds each egg and helps it grow and develop) is contaminated with the very same toxins found in cigarette smoke! When this goes on long enough, eventually few, if any egg follicles are left - and that means few or no eggs can be produced.

While this is important for all women, it crucial if you are over 35 and trying to conceive. Why? As you age, your follicle supply naturally dwindles - meaning you make fewer and fewer eggs. Moreover, the eggs you do make are not quite as healthy as they were when you were young.

So, if you add smoking into the equation, the rate of follicle depletion increases dramatically – and with each passing year the chance for getting pregnant plummets equally as dramatically.

Indeed, even if you are undergoing IVF treatments to increase your chances of pregnancy, smoking can still have a detrimental impact. In fact a number of studies have shown that smokers require twice the number of IVF cycles - and much more fertilty medication - to get pregnant than non smokers.

Indeed, smokers also had consistently lower estrogen levels, fewer eggs available for fertilization and a lower rate of fertilization overall, as well as the highest risk of conception failure. In fact, the impact of smoking on fertility can be so great that sometimes even medical reproductive technologies can't overcome all the problems that cigarettes create.

Moreover, if you do happen to get pregnant naturally, smoking increases your risk of both ectopic (tubal) pregnancy and miscarriage , with the level of both chromosomal and DNA damage occurring in direct proportion to the number of cigarettes you smoke.

Also important to note: Even if you don't smoke, but you live or work in a smoke-filled environment, you can be affected as well. Studies show that women with partners who smoke experience the same delay in conception as women who smoke - so getting him to quit is also vital!

In fact, a little later in this book you'll discover how smoking harms male fertility – plus how *he* can suffer if *you're* the smoker in the house!

BOOSTING YOUR FERTILITY: WHAT EVERY WOMAN CAN DO RIGHT NOW!

The good news in all of this is that from almost the moment you stop smoking – or reduce your exposure to second-hand smoke - your body begins an important restorative process that greatly benefits your fertility.

In fact, not only can quitting smoking immediately put the brakes on the potential for damage, within 24 hours after the toxins begin to clear from your body, an important rebuilding process begins. And that can very often translate into an increased ability to get pregnant, sometimes in as little as two weeks.

The effects of reducing exposure to second hand smoke can be even more powerful. Indeed, removing yourself from a smoke-filled environment for as little as one week can have positive effects on your fertility. Stay away from second hand smoke for just a month and you dramatically increase your chances for a successful pregnancy!

If you do smoke and you're having problems quitting, remember that even cutting down can have a positive impact. Because much of the fertility-related damage of smoking is dose-responsive, the less you smoke, the less damage there will be. So, while I strongly urge you to quit smoking, as you head towards that goal remember that cutting down can also help.

Moreover, since nicotine is one of the least toxic of the chemicals found in cigarette smoke, if you're having problems quitting talk to your doctor about nicotine replacement products to help you reach your goal. The safest form of nicotine replacement to use while trying to conceive is the gum. While the nicotine patch has not been shown to cause any major problems when used in pregnant women or women trying to conceive, studies are still inconclusive as to whether or not it might cause a problem.

In terms of the nicotine replacement nasal sprays and inhalers you should try to avoid them while trying to conceive. Both are categorized as Class D drugs – and considered unsafe to use during pregnancy. Since you could easily be pregnant 6, 8 or even 10 weeks and not know it, it's best not to use these products at this time.

The other smoking cessation product believed safe to use while trying to conceive is Zyban (bupropian) . Although this same medication is also marketed as the antidepressant Wellbutrin, the form and dosage used for smoking cessation is somewhat different. As such it is categorized as a Class B drug making it relatively safe to use during pregnancy and safe to use while trying to conceive. That said, it should only be used under a doctor's supervision. In fact, , be sure to check with your doctor before using any of these products and make certain he or she knows you are actively trying to get pregnant.

The best news of all: If you have tried to quit smoking in the past and you have failed, your chances of doing so now are greater! Indeed, studies show that with each attempt to quit smoking, the chances of success increase!

> **Q:** Since trying to conceive, my husband only smokes in front of an open window and exhales through the screen. Are there still any secondhand smoke risks to me? Also, does second hand smoke linger in a car - so that if I use the car after him, will I still get the effects of second hand smoke?
>
> **A:** Blowing the smoke out the window will dramatically decrease the amount you are exposed to in the air - so long as none of the smoke comes back into the apartment. That said, if the cigarette is burning inside the window and he's only blowing the smoke out, then you are probably still getting enough to make a difference in your health. A good barometer: If you can smell the smoke while he is smoking or right afterwards, you're still getting significant exposure. In terms of the car, it's the same issue: If the smell of smoke is strong when you get in, chances are at least some of the chemicals are lingering in the air and the upholstery.
> **The best answer:** He needs to quit smoking for the sake of your fertility as well as his. Smoking is one of the major "sperm killers" around today.

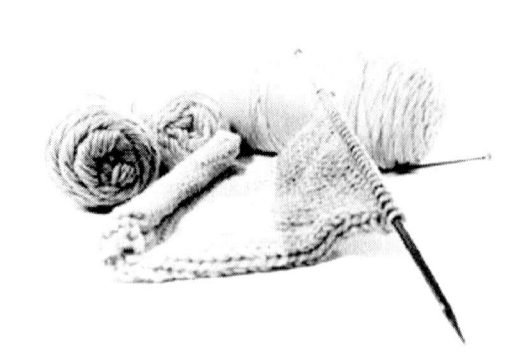

Knit To Quit & Boost Your Fertility!

You may have already noticed that the age-old craft of knitting is enjoying a robust new popularity. While once thought of as an activity for the golden years today, more and more young women are not only learning to knit – but embracing the craft with gusto! One of the reasons is it's body calming effects. Indeed in today's high tech and very stressed out world, knitting has been shown to offer many of the same stress reducing benefits as yoga. In fact, studies show an hour of knitting has the same calming effects on brain chemistry as an hour of meditation! And now, the popular line of yarns known as Lily Sugar & Cream by Bernat are making knitting even more relaxing! The yarn which is all natural cotton, is encapsulated with invisible micro beads scented with essential oils like lavender, vanilla, and chamomile. As you knit the beads release the scent so each stitch you make provides an extra calming aromatherapy effect!

Moreover because of it's ability to calm and soothe the nerves, a number of workshops called "Knit To Quit" are springing up all around the world. Here, knitting is used as a way to help ease the tensions of quitting smoking, while also providing smokers with a physical activity that uses the hands, and in doing so takes the place of some of the physical activity involved in smoking. Because knitting also offers such important meditative effects, it can go a long way in helping to reduce stress - and that can promote your fertility!

So if you knit to quit smoking while also gaining the benefits of a soothing aromatherapy meditative experience, you'll be giving your fertility an even bigger boost

Wine, Cocktails & Infertility: What You Should Know

There's no question that over the past decade, and particularly in the past several years, links between alcohol and health have captured the headlines. From the heart-healthy powers of red wine, to the increase in B vitamins found in beer, to the blood vessel relaxing effects of almost any alcoholic drink, we now know that in moderation, alcohol can have a powerful and healthy effect on the body.

When it comes to your fertility, however, the healthy links are not so clear cut. Indeed, while some studies report alcohol provides fertility benefits, others show it may be harmful. For example, a recent Swedish study of nearly 7,400 women revealed that as little as two drinks per day significantly decreased fertility when compared to women who had just one drink per day.

Conversely, a large self-reporting study of nearly 30,000 Danish women found that those who drank a glass of red wine a day got pregnant faster and easier than women who drank no alcohol!

Rounding out the confusion is an Italian study of nearly 1800 women who found no correlation of any kind between alcohol and fertility!

So, what's a gal to do ? Certainly all alcohol intake should be moderate - less than two drinks per day.

But that said, since we do know that alcohol intake during pregnancy can be extremely harmful to your baby, I prefer to err on the side of caution and recommend against alcohol consumption while trying to conceive. Since it's possible you could be pregnant weeks before you know it, abstaining from alcohol while trying to get pregnant is one way to ensure you will give your baby the absolute best start in life possible!

If you find that eliminating alcohol completely is not an option, red wine is among your best choices, followed by white wine and champagne. If you can avoid hard liquor, that would be a plus.

And be certain to read the chapter on male fertility for some eye-opening facts about how alcohol affects sperm!

COFFEE, TEA & SODA:
HOW CAFFEINE AFFECTS GETTING PREGNANT

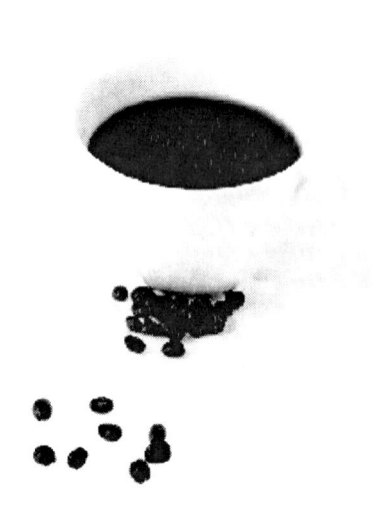

If you just can't start your day without a steaming cup of coffee, if you just can't get through the afternoon without a gulp of cola or the crunch of a chocolate bar, then you already know the power of caffeine. As one of the most potent natural ways to jump start energy levels, caffeine can certainly have some powerful effects.

But these powerful effects aren't just limited to boosting energy. Studies show caffeine can also impact your body in other ways, including affecting estrogen production. Indeed, some studies have shown that when caffeine consumption is high, circulating levels of estrogen increase, sometimes quite dramatically.

Certainly, if you are estrogen deficient, this might not be a bad thing. However, if you have even a slight hormone imbalance (a very common occurrence in women) then caffeine just might throw your reproductive hormones into a tailspin. When it does, your periods may become irregular, your ovulation can go off track, and ultimately you may derail or at least delay your ability to get pregnant. Indeed one study published in the *Journal of Epidemiology* reported women who drank 5 cups of coffee a day or more had greater difficulty conceiving than women who drank less.

Moreover, if you suffer from even mild endometriosis (a menstrual related disorder that is a major cause of infertility) I have found that the caffeine found in just one or two cups of coffee will worsen this condition and in doing so increase your risk of related fertility problems. Finally, studies also show that high levels of caffeine can increase the risk of tubal factor infertility. While the exact cause isn't known, my hunch has always been that the stimulation of the caffeine causes spasms within the fallopian tubes that can push a newly fertilized egg to the womb too quickly – before conditions are right for implantation. And indeed, some studies do show that high levels of caffeine intake early in pregnancy may increase the risk of miscarriage.

The good news however, is that for most women keeping caffeine intake between 300 mg and 500 mg a day (equal to about 3 to 5 cups of coffee) will help ensure that your fertility is not affected. If you can stick to the limit recommended by the March of Dimes – which is the caffeine equal to 2 cups of coffee a day – you'll be doing even more to help encourage a quick and healthy pregnancy.

That said, what you might not realize is how many foods and drinks contain caffeine. While you might be limiting your coffee intake - or maybe not drinking any coffee at all - you could still be taking in too much caffeine, simply because so many different foods contain significant amounts.

For example, many sports drinks as well as high energy drinks are loaded with caffeine, as are many sodas including Coke, Pepsi, and Mountain Dew. Tea and chocolate both contain caffeine as do some over-the-counter medications such as certain headache remedies or menstrual pain products.

Q: *I've heard that the chemicals used to remove caffeine and create decaffeinated coffee are more dangerous than the caffeine found naturally in coffee. Is this true?*

A: It can be true ...depending on the type of process used to remove the caffeine. In the past a series of chemicals were always used to pull caffeine from coffee beans and there was some concern that resides were being left on beans - and that they might have some residual effects.

Today, however, many coffee companies use a chemical-free water process to remove the caffeine, which means the end product is more natural and safer to drink. To know for sure, check the label or website for the coffee you use - it should tell you how the caffeine is removed.

How Much Caffeine Are You Getting?

To help you gauge how much caffeine you are getting each day, I've put together the following list of the amounts found in common foods and drinks. Remember, your maximum daily target is no more **than 500 mg total, and if you can stay below 300 mg you'll definitely give your fertility a boost!** Also be aware that some herbal energy products contain as much as 200 mg of caffeine or more per dose, so do check the bottle before taking.

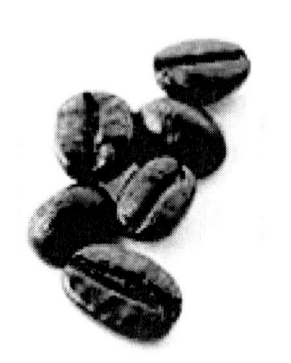

COFFEE:

- Drip (8 oz) = 234 mg
- Percolated (8 oz) = 176 mg
- Regular instant (8 oz) = 85 mg
- Decaffeinated instant (8 oz) = 3 mg
- Espresso (1-2 oz) = 45 to 100 mg
- Starbucks grande (16 oz) = 330 mg

Tea:

- 1 minute brew = 9 to 33 mg
- 3 minute brew = 20 to 46 mg
- Instant = 12 to 28 mg
- Canned ice tea (12 ounces) = 22 to 36 mg
- Snapple Flavored Teas (Reg. or Diet) 31.5
- Nestea Sweet Iced Tea -26.5
- Nestea Unsweetened Iced Tea - 26.0
- Lipton Diet Green Tea with Citrus (16.9 oz)23.0

SOFT DRINKS: (12 OUNCE SERVING)

- Pepsi One - 55.5
- Mountain Dew - 55.0
- Tab - 46.8
- Diet Coke - 45.6
- Shasta Cola - 44.4
- Shasta Diet Cola - 44.4
- RC Cola -- 43.0
- Diet RC - 43
- Diet Sunkist Orange - 41.0
- Sunkist Orange 40.0
- Pepsi-Cola - 37.5
- Diet Pepsi - 36.0
- Coca-Cola Zero - 35.0
- Coca-Cola Classic - 34.0
- Cherry, Lemon or Vanilla Coke - 34.0

- A & W Creme Soda 29
- Dr. Pepper (diet & regular) - 41.0

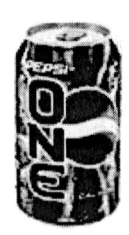

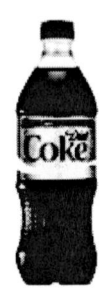

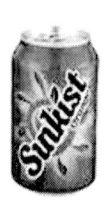

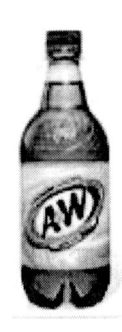

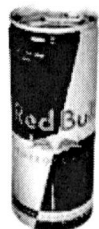

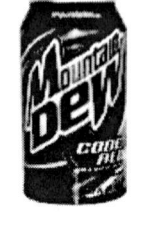

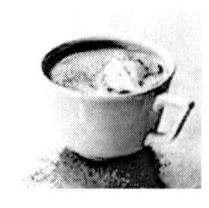

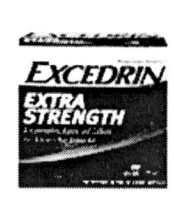

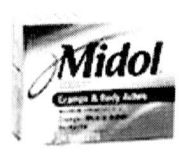

Energy Drinks:

- Red Bull (8.2 oz) - 80.0
- Jolt - 71.2
- Mountain Dew Code Red – 55 mg
- Kick Citrus 54 mg
- Surge : 51 mg
- Mellow Yellow – 52.8 mg
- Red Flash- 40.00

Cocoa and chocolate:

- Cocoa from mix (6 oz) = 10 mg
- Milk chocolate (1 oz) = 6 mg
- Baking chocolate (1 oz) = 35 mg

Over The Counter Medicines:

- Excedrin, extra strength
- Maximum Strength Midol
- Vanquish
- Anacin
- Dexatrim (diet pill)
- No Doz (wake up pill)
- Efed II (energy pill)

Your Medicine Chest:
The Prescription Drugs That Impact Fertility

Generally speaking, when taken correctly most prescribed and over-the-counter medications will not interfere with your ability to get pregnant. This is particularly true when used on a short term basis.

That said, there are a few precautions concerning the way in which some medications can interfere with fertility. While this doesn't occur with a lot of drugs, it can happen with some – which is why it's always a good idea to mention any medications you are taking to your doctor during your pre conception exam. This is especially true if you see more than one doctor and no one physician has all your records.

You can also talk to your local pharmacist, who is an excellent source of information on drug side effects and interactions. If you have all your prescriptions filled in one place, then speak to your pharmacist confidentially and ask them to review your medication list to see if anything you are taking could interfere with your ability to get pregnant – and make sure your partner does the same as well. If you have prescriptions filled by more than one pharmacy, compile a list, along with a list of any over-the-counter drugs you or your partner use on a regular or semi-regular basis. Then, ask your doctor or a trusted pharmacist to review the list with an eye towards protecting and encouraging fertility.

To help get you started looking in the right direction, what follows are the major categories of medications known to impact fertility. Remember however that every woman's body is different, and much of the effects are dose-related. Also remember that not every drug in these categories can cause problems with fertility so it's important that you do not stop taking any medication prescribed or recommended by your doctor until you speak with him or her first. I can't emphasize this enough, particularly for those of you who may have a chronic health concern.

It's also important to note that in many instances your doctor may be able to substitute the drug you are taking now with another that could have less impact on your fertility - which is another important reason to keep at least one physician in the loop concerning your fertility plans.

DRUG CATEGORIES TO DISCUSS WITH YOUR DOCTOR:
-
- Antidepressants
- Pain Relievers
- Thyroid medication
- Antibiotics
- Gastrointestinal aids
- Older blood pressure medications
- Allergy pills
- Cold and cough remedies
- Steroid drugs (such as prednisone)
- Epilepsy Drugs (particularly carbamazepine and valproate).

Remember, not every drug in each of these categories is considered harmful to fertility. As such it's very likely that if one of your medications is a potential problem you doctor can find a suitable substitute. In any event never stop taking a medication prescribed by your doctor until you discuss it with him or her.

No Keeping Secrets!

It's absolute essential to the health of your fertility *and* the health of your baby that your pre-conception exam doctor know about every medication you and your partner are taking, be it prescription drug, an over-the-counter medication or an herbal product.
It's absolutely essential, so don't hide anything!

Pain Medications & Your Fertility:
What You Must Know

Among the medications in most use today are pain relievers, particularly NSAIDs (Non Steroidal Anti Inflammatory Drugs) such as aspirin or ibuprofen, and their "cousins" known as Cox 2 inhibitors. Used to control a variety of aches and pains, from joint stiffness and muscle aches, to menstrual cramps and headaches, they come in varying strengths and are used both long term to control chronic pain as well as short term for quick relief.

When used only occasionally or for a short term, there is almost no chance that your fertility will be compromised – and certainly not on any kind of long term or permanent basis. However, that can change a bit if you are using these medications on any kind of regular basis - and particularly if you are using them for an extended period of time, even at a low dosage.

How Pain Medicines Impact Fertility

Indeed, a number of studies have shown that with continued regular use NSAIDs can interfere with ovulation as well as increase the risk of a condition known as as luteinizing unruptured follicle syndrome (LUF or LUFS). In this condition, your egg follicle fails to "burst" and release an egg which makes getting pregnant impossible.

In fact, in one study published in the journal *Histology and Pathology* in 2006, doctors reported that regular use of even over-the-counter pain NSAIDs (such as aspirin and ibuprofen) for such things as menstrual pain, could be a major contributing factor to infertility in some women – particularly in those who may already be experiencing irregular ovulation or other ovulation-related issues.

Other studies have found that even on a short term basis, ovulation can be effected for up to 7 hours after a NSAID is used. This is particularly important since many women suffer from a condition known as "Mittlesmertz" – or pain on ovulation. As a result, some doctors routinely prescribe NSAIDs drugs – or recommend OTC drugs such as aspirin or ibuprofen – to be taken every few hours beginning a day or two prior to ovulation and continued until ovulation passes.

When you are not trying to conceive, this is a good pain reducing strategy. But if you are trying to get pregnant, the use of these drugs during this pre-ovulatory time frame could definitely delay conception.

The good news: Any fertility problems related to the use of NSAIDs is completely reversible! By simply avoiding the drugs for up to 30 days prior to when you want to get pregnant (and for many women, 14 days can be sufficient) you can guarantee that your system is free and clear of the effects of these medications and that your ovulation won't be affected.

If, however, you have been using these drugs regularly for an extended period of time, it may take several cycles for egg release to get back on track and normal ovulation to resume.

Remember, however, to check with your doctor before stopping any NSAIDs he or she has prescribed for a medical condition.

- **Prescription NSAIDS include** : Diclofenac, Etodolac, Fenoprofen, Flurbiprofen, Ibuprofen, Indomethacin, Meclofenamate, Mefenamic Acid, Meloxicam, Nabumetone, Naproxen, Oxaprozin, Piroxicam, Sulindac, Tolmetin

- **COX-2 inhibitors** include celecoxib.

- **Over The Counter NSAIDs include:** Aspirin, Motrin, Aleve, Advil and some menstrual pain medications.

Q: I get a lot of stomach pain around the time I ovulate. Is it safe to take a pain reliever only during this time - we are trying to get pregnant?

A: Used only occasionally most pain relievers are very safe, even in regard to fertility. That said, if you are having pain during every ovulation, then you should ask your doctor about an ultra sound exam around to be done mid-cycle. This painless, radiation-free test will tell you if there are any cysts or other abnormalities causing the mid-cycle pain. If everything checks out okay, then you are probably experiencing "mittleschmertz" - a type of pain that occurs during ovulation. One of the best natural remedies for this is heat. So in lieu of taking any pain killers try warm compresses of moist heat (try a "Bed Buddy" - it's all natural and you heat it up in 2 minutes in the microwave). You can also try massaging your lower stomach with warm olive oil to help relieve the pain.

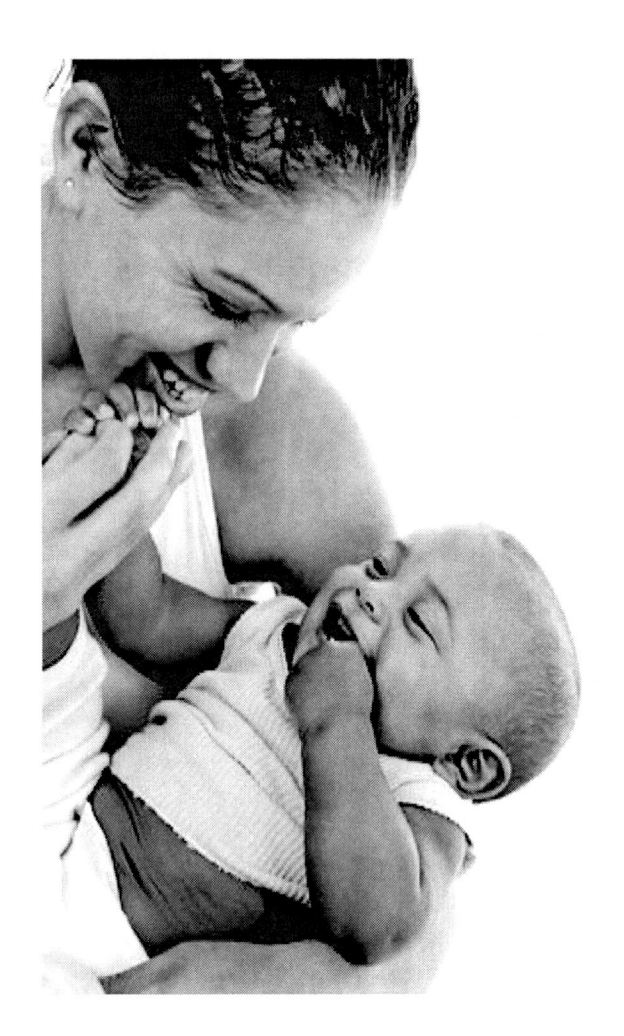

Increase Your Pregnancy Odds!

While there is considerable evidence linking NSAIDs to fertility problems, many doctors believe the problems are essentially dose-related. Indeed there is some evidence to show that low dose NSAIDs, in the form of one baby aspirin daily, is not only safe to use while trying to conceive, but may actually help encourage conception.

In fact, in one study which looked at 149 women enrolled in an IVF program, doctors found that one baby aspirin daily (about 100 mg of NSAID), increased ovarian responsiveness as well as increasing blood flow to the ovaries and uterus.

Not only were the women taking the daily baby aspirin able to make stronger and better eggs, their rate of pregnancy was nearly double that of the women who were not taking this treatment.

In addition, previous studies have shown that taking one baby aspirin a day during the first trimester may help reduce the risk of miscarriage.

If you are actively trying to conceive, talk to your doctor about whether one baby aspirin a day might help encourage a faster conception. I have routinely recommended this for most of my fertility patients and always found it to be a helpful treatment with no adverse outcomes.

ALLERGIES, SEX AND INFERTILITY: SOME IMPORTANT LINKS

If you suffer from the sneezing, coughing, stuffy nose and watery, itchy eyes of seasonal or other environmental allergies then you may already be using one of several allergy medications to control symptoms. And for most people they can offer life changing relief!

At the same time however, if you've noticed that your desire for sex is not quite what it used to be – or if despite how you feel you're trying to conceive and can't get pregnant – then it's important to look to your allergy medicines as one possible source of problems.

Indeed, studies show that in some folks certain allergy medications can have sexual side effects ranging all the way from a decrease in libido in women, to a complete inability to have an erection in men.

Moreover, while there is no direct proof, many doctors now believe that certain allergy medications designed to dry up mucous may impact fertility by also reducing cervical mucous. This not only hampers the ability of sperm to reach egg, but can also lead to a loss libido and/or painful sex - which in turn can cause muscle tensions in the pelvic region capable of impacting conception.

If you or your partner are taking an allergy medication and find that your sex drive is decreasing, or if you personally are experiencing a dry vagina and find that sex is not as pleasurable as it was in the past, speak to your doctor. In many instances there may be another prescription drug available with fewer of these kinds of effects, or there may be something you can add to your treatment regimen to counter the effects on mucous.

> *Certain allergy medications can impact fertility in women by decreasing mucous secretions necessary to carry sperm to egg. If you regularly use any allergy medication talk to your doctor about whether it might be making it harder for you to get pregnant.*

Marijuana, Cocaine & Other Drugs: Some Important Precautions

Studies show that the recreational drug most commonly used by women is marijuana. Unfortunately, of all recreational drugs it's the one most harmful to female fertility. According to a number of studies, marijuana can have a major impact on ovulation, with regular use leading to a disruption of the menstrual cycle and nearly all ovarian activity, making it extremely difficult to get pregnant. When marijuana is combined with alcohol – which it frequently is – the impact on fertility can be even greater, even among young, otherwise healthy women.

But that's not the only problem we see. Indeed, if you should happen to get pregnant while you have marijuana and alcohol in your body, your pregnancy could end in crisis, with the combination of these drugs increasing the risk of miscarriage by over 100%.

In addition, any regular use of cocaine – in any form – can also have a major impact on your fertility. The key mode of damage here is linked to the fallopian tubes, with studies showing that regular cocaine use can cause a type of damage that eventually destroys all chances for a natural conception.

Currently it is estimated that up to 10% of all women of childbearing age use recreational drugs on a regular basis – or they abuse prescription drugs such as tranquillizers or barbiturates. While the reproductive risks of any drug can be based in many factors - including the substance itself and a person's individual metabolism - as a general rule you should consider permanently giving up the use of all recreational drugs as soon as you begin trying to conceive.

Moreover, be aware that the impact on fertility is often dose-related. So, the more drugs you use and the more often you use them, the greater your risks. While it's highly unlikely that a single dose of any drug will cause your fertility harm, regular or habitual use can, indeed be harmful. Moreover, the younger you are when you begin abusing drugs, the more likely it is that any damage you do sustain could become permanent.

The bottom line: If you are trying to conceive , you and your partner should strive to live as "clean" and as healthy a lifestyle as you possibly can - no only for the sake of your health and your fertility but also the health of your baby.

Chapter Fourteen

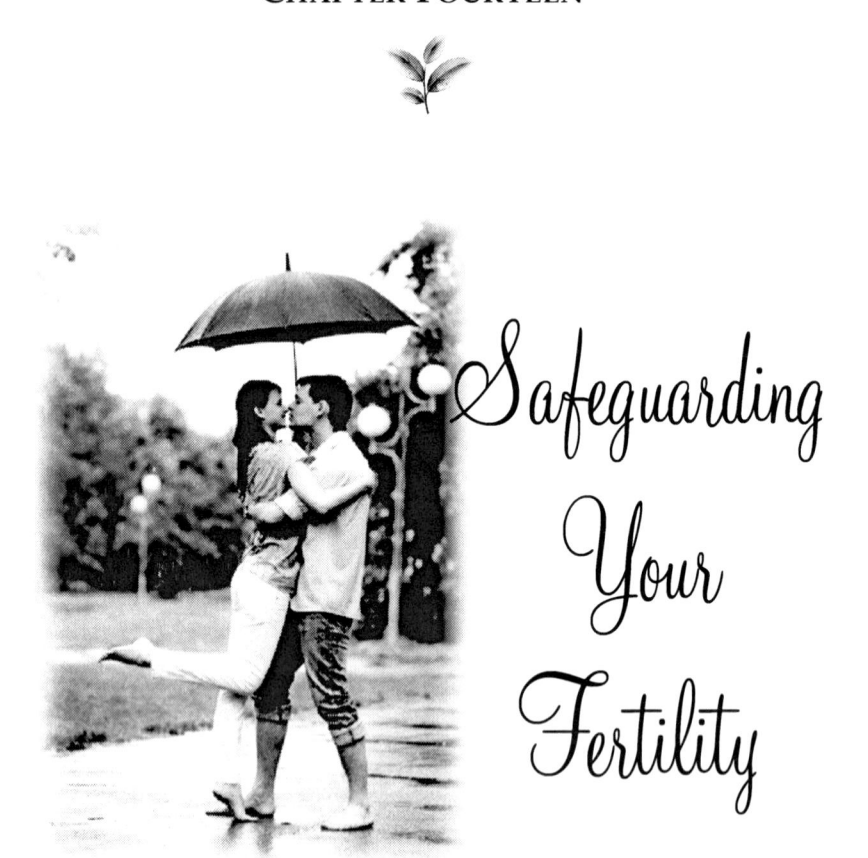

Safeguarding Your Fertility

Make Your World Healthier And Get Pregnant Faster!

There is no question that over the last several decades the number of couples struggling with infertility has increased. While a number of factors may play a role – including more couples delaying childbearing into their 30's and even 40's – this doesn't account for the fact that the fastest growing segment of women with impaired fertility are under age 25. According to the Centers for Disease Control the number of women aged 25 and younger who are struggling with infertility has increased by a stunning 50% in the past decade.

Now certainly, for some of these young women, a poor diet, along with increasing stress levels and weight issues, are the basis for their fertility problems.

But what I, and many fertility experts now believe, is that there is still another factor lurking in the background and robbing a young couples ability and right to have a family - and it's happening in a way that most of us don't even realize.

So what is this mysterious "fertility thief"? It is the environment, and the preponderance of ever-compounding chemical exposures we face every single day.

Indeed, from the soil to the water, from the food supply to the air supply, from the cosmetics on your vanity to the household products under your sink and the fertilizers used to make lawns green and weed-free, every day your body is forced to deal with a staggering number of chemical assaults . To date, there are some 80,000 chemicals registered for use in the United States alone – substances that were never part of the environment for our ancestors.

How Protected Are You?

Now one might think that with all these chemicals in use there have to be some safeguards in place. Well there are …. but only a scant few. Unlike drug manufacturers who must prove their products are safe before they can come to market, by and large there is little in the way of regulation forcing chemical industry manufacturers to do the same. Any testing that *is* done ultimately falls on the backs of federal and state agencies, most of which don't even have the opportunity to test a product until it's on the market and already in the environment. Moreover, due to the sheer number of chemicals in use, testing usually only occurs after significant health risks have been raised – a process that can take years, if not decades.

The result:

- More than 85% of the synthetic chemicals registered for use in the US today have never been assessed for potential health risks.

- Of those that have, a significant number have been shown to be reproductive toxins. In fact, some are so potent that even decades after they have been banned, traces are still showing up in our bodies.

Such is the case with PCBs (polychlorinated biphenyls) which were a staple chemical ingredient in a wide variety of products for years – including many glues and most house paints. Although PCBs were banned from use in the late 1970's – when research found they increased the risk of certain cancers - traces of this chemical still exist to this day in our lakes, rivers and soil. What's more they continue to permeate food and water which is how they ultimately end up in your body. Because PCBs accumulate in fatty tissue, every small exposure compounds every other small exposure and eventually we can be facing a significant health threat.

We see the same kind of continuing threats from the pesticide DDT. Although it's use was banned in the US in the 1970's, residues still remain – and they are still detectable in our bodies, even today.

But it's not just these banned chemicals that are continuing to haunt us. According to the *National Report on Human Exposure to Environmental Chemicals* by the US Centers for Disease Control (CDC), over 90% of Americans have a virtual "stew" of chemical compounds swimming in their bloodstream. In fact, according to one study conducted jointly by the Mount Sinai School of Medicine in New York City and the Environmental Working Group researchers found 167 different contaminants in the blood and urine of study subjects, along with some 200 contaminants in the umbilical cord blood taken from 10 newborn babies!

In addition to residues from pesticides, plastics, and industrial chemicals, compounds also included solvents (including dry cleaning fluids), and waste byproducts of various types of fuel. Indeed studies have found a preponderance of chemicals accumulating in our body including:

- Dioxins (found in some personal care products).

- PBDEs (a popular flame retardant found in everything from your PJs to your living room couch).

- Perfluorinated compounds which make your pots and pans non-stick and your living room furniture stain resistant.

- Phthalates, a chemical found in everything from food packaging to cosmetics and fragrances, vinyl flooring, plastic toys, even medical tubing.

Most recently, studies have focused on the chemical known as bisphenol A, which is found in everything from the cans of food in your kitchen pantry to plastic water bottles, to your baby's feeding bottle.

Now as frightening as all this sounds, it also begs a very important question – namely, do chemical contaminants in our environment, and eventually, in our body, necessarily equate with infertility?

The short answer is that at the moment, we don't have the kind of definitive evidence we would like. But that said, it is safe to say that suspicions are strong – and studies on workplace exposures validate these suspicious.

At the same it also doesn't mean that your personal pregnancy odds will be affected by exposures to even the most dangerous chemicals. Indeed, there are many things you and your partner can do to not only reduce exposures but also to compensate for the exposures you do experience - and in the process optimize not only your fertility but your overall health as well.

A little later in this chapter I'm going to offer some specific things you and your partner can do to protect yourselves from many of the most serious environmental threats. But first I want to take a few more minutes to detail just how the environment can impact your health and your fertility. When you know where your "enemies" lie you can be that much smarter about protecting yourself from harm!

HOW THE ENVIRONMENT AFFECTS YOUR FERTILITY

Depending on the compound environmental chemicals can have a varied number of effects on your body – and in doing so impact your fertility in a number of ways.

Among the most common is for the chemical itself to act like a hormone. When this occurs, the chemical in question binds to the hormone receptor in your body, thus "tricking" your system and initiating a number of "false signals" . This is often the case with chemicals known as "xeno estrogens" found in many pesticides.

Acting much like an estrogen in our body these chemicals can turn natural hormonal signals off and on at will, and in doing so throw your entire reproductive circuitry into a bit of chaos! Indeed, investigations into chemicals found in pesticides, cigarette smoke, fuel, hobby and industrial glues, solvents such as benzene found in dry cleaning fluids, even chemicals used to disinfect the water supply have all been shown to cause immediate changes in the menstrual cycle and ovulation significant enough to delay conception. At their most destructive some of these chemical contaminants may be strong enough to even cause a miscarriage – sometimes occurring at such an early stage a woman does not even know she is pregnant.

In other instances, scientists believe chemical "hits" to a woman's reproductive system are more subtle, occurring over time and causing either a gradual decline in fertility, or, the gradual development of fertility-robbing conditions such as endometriosis. (See Chapter 16 for more information on how this occurs).

BPA and Your Fertility

In a very interesting and enlightening study on just how chemicals can impact our fertility a team of scientists from Case Western Reserve University began studying fertilized mice eggs. In the course of the study they found that some of the eggs were developing with chromosomal damage - similar to that which causes both early miscarriage and Downs Syndrome in humans.

After months of being mystified over what was causing the problems, they finally traced it to a chemical residue found in a common detergent used to clean the plastic components of the mice cages. What they found specifically was that after being cleaned the plastic was releasing a chemical known as bisphenol A (BPA), a known endocrine disrupting compound.

Before long, the mystery was solved. Mice exposed to the BPA were the ones whose eggs were becoming damaged. But if you're thinking it's just mice in a cage who are at risk for BPA exposures, guess again. BPA is a form of synthetic estrogen that is a significant component in polycarbonate plastic – and that means it's present in many products each of us uses in the course of our daily lives.

Moreover, because it acts much like estrogen in the body, it's impact can be widespread, causing hormonal imbalances leading to infertility in women, as well as estrogen overloads that have recently been linked to impotence and sexual dysfunction in men (see Chapter 15). In the worst case scenario, over exposure to estrogen stimulation – even synthetic estrogens – can increase the risk of breast and endometrial cancer in women and prostate cancer in men.

WHERE IS THE BPA HIDING?

While BPA it has long been a "chemical of controversy" among many consumer health groups, that controversy made recent headlines when BPA was found in high levels in some baby bottles and in canned infant formula. Now that's bad - but it's not the only place you'll find this chemical. As a component of "hard" plastic, BPA is found in literally thousands of consumer products used in food preparation or serving - including kitchen utensils, food storage containers, plastic mugs (especially travel mugs), and inside the linings of some food and beverage cans. And it is, in fact, this food connection that is the cause for alarm. Why?

Studies show the BPA in these containers and utensils can leach into food, and eventually, our bodies. Moreover, certain related factors, including heat, acid, age, micro waving and the use of certain harsh detergents can increase the likelihood of this happening, according to Frederick vom Saal, a biology professor and BPA researcher at the University of Missouri.

The latest concern: In a study commissioned by the Environmental Working Group and carried out by scientists at the University of Missouri , BPA was also found on many cash register receipts – like the kind you get from the grocery store, pharmacy, or even your favorite restaurant, bank or ATM. Indeed, the new report examined 36 different receipts collected in seven US states from such places as Safeway, Whole Foods, CVS, Walmart, Chevron, McDonalds, the US Postal Service and cafeterias in the House of Representatives and the US Senate, and various bank ATM receipts. They also collected receipts from Starbucks, Kentucky Fried Chicken and McDonalds located in Japan.

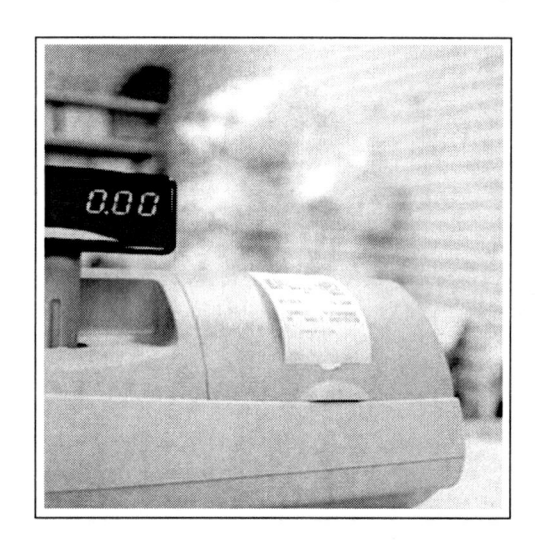

The result: Of the 36 receipts, all but 7 contained BPA. Moreover, sixteen of the receipts – almost half- contained levels of BPA averaging 1.9 percent and as high as 2.8 percent (of the total weight of the receipt). According to the report, one receipt for the purchase of a McDonald's Happy Meal in Clinton, Connecticut contained a whopping 13 mg of BPA. The EWG says that equals the BPA found in 126 cans of Chef Boyardee Overstuffed Beef Ravioli in Hearty Tomato & Meat Sauce - which is one of the highest concentrations of all canned foods tested!

According to the EWG report receipts from Safeway contained 3 of the 6 highest overall levels of BPA, with receipts from the Washington, DC Safeway store containing an astounding 41 mg of BPA per receipt.

Overall the study reports that 40% of the collected receipts contained high concentrations of BPA while others contained about 1/100th of that amount. Indeed, Target stores in three states and three Walmarts issued receipts that were nearly 100% BPA –free.

But if you think you can win this round of Chemical Jeopardy by patronizing only those store chains that came up relatively clean, guess again.

Indeed, one of two Whole Foods stores tested had totally BPA-free receipts, while the other was issuing receipts coated with substantial amounts of BPA! Yes, the truth is, levels can vary from store to store, even within a franchise.

> Of the stores receipts tested for BPA chemical residues, those issued by Target stores in three states, and three Wal-mart stores were nearly 100% BPA free, while one of two Whole Foods stores tested were BPA free . And that means it's entirely possible for all receipts to be BPA-free - and you can make it happen!

The question of course remains whether or not the BPA found on these paper goods will necessarily end up in your body. To find out for sure, the EWG scientists did a "damp wipe" of four receipts to see how much could be removed simply from handling them.

THE RESULT: As much as 3.8 percent of BPA could be easily wiped off. So if your hands are even the least bit sweaty – or possibly damp from just washing them –

touching these receipts allows you to pick up up at least some of this chemical contaminant. Just handling the receipts, say experts, can increase the risk of both inhalation and skin contact contamination. While casual exposures certainly won't harm you, the concern is that, over time, these exposures build in your body to the point where they are having a hormonal influence.

In fact, one federal study found that 90 percent of Americans have traces of BPA in their urine due to continued and constant use of products containing these chemicals.

But perhaps the worst scenario of all is not the result of handling paper we know contains BPA, but what happens when those papers are recycled – and end up in products we have no clue could contain these chemicals, such as toilet tissue or feminine hygiene products?

Indeed, a number of years ago reports surfaced at a European environmental conference showing that BPA from recycled thermal paper was making it's way into recycled paper products, including toilet tissue.

Since the vaginal mucosa are among the most porous tissues in the body – it virtually sucks up every chemical it comes in contact with – there's no telling how much contamination could get into your body by using something as benign as toilet paper or a sanitary napkin!

REDUCING BPA EXPOSURE: WHAT YOU CAN DO

With new research linking the synthetic estrogen bisphenol A (BPA) to increased sexual dysfunction and some forms of infertility in men (see Chapter 15) and previous studies suggesting a link to birth defects in babies and infertility in women – many couples are looking to reduce exposure.

But with BPA found in literally thousands of consumer products, avoiding it can be a bit of a task. The good news: Even cutting down on exposures can help. And to this end there are some small but significant changes you can make that will not only benefit your fertility but your overall health.

12 Easy Ways To Cut BPA Exposures In Your Life!

1. Check The Bottom Of Plastic Drink Bottles – If you're buying water or juice in plastic bottles, look for the clear "hard" plastic type with the "recycle" triangle symbol stamped with the number 1, 2, 4 or 5 on the bottom. This indicates the product is a less reactive form of plastic. Steer clear of bottles with a number "3, 6 or 7" stamped in the triangle – they are considered more reactive forms of plastic and many contain BPA. When you can, buy sodas and other drinks in either glass bottles or waxed paper cartons.

2. Replace Canned Fruits and Veggies with Fresh or Frozen – In one study conducted by the Environmental Working Group (EWG) researchers tested 97 cans of food ranging from soda and tuna to fruits, veggies and more and found that 1 in every 10 cans contained enough BPA to exceed government safety levels for chemical contamination by some 200%. By comparison, frozen fruits and veggies contain no BPA and may retain more of the nutrients that are good for your fertility in many other ways.

3. Make Your Own Chicken Soup – and Toss Out The Cans! Doing so could not only help foster your fertility, but also your good health. Indeed, in the EWG studies of canned foods those containing the highest levels of BPA included canned chicken soup. Other canned soups varied by brand and content.

4. Eat Tomato Products Out Of Glass Jars - This includes not only sauces and pesto, but also salsas and particularly ravioli or other pasta products. The reason? The EWG study found that canned goods containing tomatoes also ranked high on the list of products containing significant amounts of BPA. With so many sauces now available in glass jars this is an easy switch that could make a huge difference in your health and your fertility.

5. Switch Out Canned Beverages for Glass Bottles - Because the levels found in beverage cans can vary dramatically depending on the lining, if the manufacturer doesn't tell you their product is BPA-free, then switch to a glass bottled product – they are always BPA-Free.

6. DON'T STORE FOOD IN PLASTIC CONTAINERS – When possible, put your leftovers in glass bowls – and save glass jars, wash them well and use them to store foods as well. Just make sure to wash the lids by hand using a mild detergent – they can often contain BPA in the cap liners.

7. SWITCH OUT A PLASTIC TRAVEL MUG FOR A STAINLESS STEEL BOTTLE OR GLASS LINED THERMOS. These will keep beverages hot or cold without BPA exposure.

MORE BPA-FREE TIPS: If you must use plastic containers take these extra precautions to reduce exposure.

- Never pour a warm beverage, soup, citrus or tomato product into a plastic container. The heat and the acid can exacerbate the leaching of BPA from the container into your food.

- Use only ceramic or glass to microwave foods. The microwaves will break down the BPA in plastic and cause it to leach into your food.

- Wash all plastic containers by hand using a mild detergent. Harsh detergents and the ultra hot water in dishwashers can break down the plastic allowing more BPA will leach into the foods placed in those containers.

- Toss out any plastic containers that are cracked, "hazy", sticky, or just look "old". As plastic products age they may release more BPA.

- Look for plastic products containing recycling numbers 1, 2, 4 or 5 – they are less reactive forms of plastic and are less likely to cause chemical leaching. Avoid products marked 3, 6 or 7.

Additionally, keep all receipts in a small plastic bag inside your wallet and when possible wash your hands after handling them - especially before eating anything with your hands. If you forget now and again, don't panic - occasional exposures aren't going to harm you. But when you can cut down on overall exposures.

To avoid BPA contamination in paper products that haven't been tested – such as toilet tissue or feminine hygiene products - whenever possible choose organic items, or at the least, items which are not made from recycled paper. At least in this instance, it's better to *not* be so environmentally correct!

In fact, you can actually help the environment – and help protect everyone's fertility – if you toss out those grocery and thermal paper receipts with the regular trash and DO NOT recycle them. While I generally believe that recycling is great for the environment and good for the earth, when it comes to further BPA contamination I say it's better to toss than recycle.

WHEN HELPFUL CHEMICALS DO BAD THINGS

As anyone whose ever purchased a couch, a pillow or even a pair of pajamas can tell you, today many of our fabrics are treated with flame retardants – chemicals which help reduce the risk of burning if and when a fire should occur. And in fact, fabrics which are treated with flame retardants have been credited with saving many lives.

But that said, what helps us in one way may harm us in another. Indeed, in January, 2010 a study published in the journal *Environmental Health Perspectives* showed that a specific flame retardant chemical known as PBDEs, or polybrominated diphenyl ethers – commonly used to protect clothing, foam furniture, carpets and some electronic and plastic goods - appeared to make getting pregnant more difficult.

More specifically the study found that for each 10-fold increase in the blood concentration of four PBDE chemicals, women experienced a 30 percent decrease in the odds of getting pregnant each month. Ultimately the women whose blood contained the highest levels of PBDE took the longest to get pregnant.

What is perhaps most alarming is that other studies have reported PBDEs are widely found in house dust with some 97% of US residents having detectable levels in their blood – an amount that is 20 times what is found in those who are living in European countries. In California, where laws concerning the use of flame retardants are extremely strict, exposures of PBDEs are among the highest anywhere in the world.

While doctors aren't sure how PBDE affects fertility it appears as if these chemicals – of which there are some 209 varieties - reduce thyroid hormones, and alter levels of sex hormones, both of which disrupt the normal menstrual pattern .

So, what you can you do? First, if you are purchasing clothing or furniture treated with a flame retardant, find out which one - and if you have a choice, chose those that are PBDE-free. Next, if you already own products that are treated with this

> ### Are Your PJ's Causing Fertility Problems?
>
> A new study has found that the flame retardant chemicals frequently used to treat women's pajamas could decrease the chance of getting pregnant by a significant margin! For each 10-fold increase in the blood concentration of four chemicals found in the PJs, women experienced a 30 percent decrease in the odds of getting pregnant each month!

compound, make certain that you keep plenty of fresh air circulating in your home. This will help reduce the amount of direct exposure you receive. Lastly, use an electronic air purifier or ionizer in your home. This will reduce the amount of house dust in the air, so it automatically reduces the amount of toxins you will be breathing.

HAND SANITIZERS & YOUR FERTILITY

If you're like most folks you've probably got at least one bottle of hand sanitizer in your handbag - and maybe a bathroom or kitchen sink filled with antibacterial soaps and detergents.

Indeed, between the proliferation of new germs that seem to be swarming our earth, and the tainted foods that keep landing on our grocery store shelves it's hard not to give in to the proliferation of new ways to stay germ free.

But if you're a couple trying to conceive you need to pay special attention to some new concerns about one of the most common anti-bacterial ingredients around. It's called triclosan - and it recently became the focus of a new FDA and Environmental Protection Agency (EPA) review for safety concerns.

What kind of concerns? According to the Environmental Working Group's database of hazardous chemicals, studies on triclosan found links to cancer, allergies, immuno- toxicities, irritation of the skin, eyes and lungs.

But what's most important for those of you trying to get pregnant is that triclosan is also connected to a host of developmental and reproductive toxicity issues - mainly because it is believed to be a "hormone disruptor. Much like the xeno estrogens I discussed earlier, these are chemicals that, once absorbed by the body act much like a real hormone - including binding to hormone receptors in our body. As I explained earlier, this "tricks" our system into believing the real hormone is present, and in doing so initiates a number of "false signals" that in turn cause other hormonal and chemical activities to occur.

* In one study recently conducted by researchers at the University of California at Davis, triclosan - and it's chemical cousin triclocarban - were found to disrupt reproductive hormone activity and interfere with a type of cell signaling that occurs in the brain and other cells.

* In another study published in the journal *Endocrinology*, Dr. Bill Lasley a professor of Obstetrics and Gynecology concluded that unlike other classic endocrine disruptors which bind to cell receptors, triclocarban actually impacts that way our natural sex hormones act. This in turn appears to depress the natural production of both estrogen and androgens (male sex hormones) and in the process disrupt our fertility in myriad ways.

Indeed, when a hormone disrupter messes with your reproductive hormones, it can throw your entire reproductive biochemistry into a tailspin.

* Women can experience changes in the menstrual cycle and ovulation dramatic enough to delay or even prevent conception.

* Some exposures are strong enough to cause infertility or even miscarriage - sometimes occurring at such an early stage you might not even know you are pregnant.

* When men are exposed, sperm count may be affected, along with sperm motility and maturity.

In fact, researching just a little deeper we find that **triclosan** is actually a pesticide closely related to dioxin - a known chemical health threat, endocrine disruptor, and carcinogen. According to the FDA, triclosan "could be" and is "suspected to be " contaminated with dioxins - a chemical known to have devastating effects on fertility.

BUYER BEWARE: IS TRICLOSAN HIDING IN YOUR HOME?

While the majority of the triclosan you see is found in products like hand sanitizers and antibacterial soaps, you may be surprised to discover how many products actually contain these chemicals - and don't include it on the label.

You can, in fact, find triclosan in not only many cosmetics, but also in soaps, dishwashing detergents, toothpastes, shampoos, skin creams and moisturizers, shaving gels, kids toys, workout clothes, and socks, to name a few! (See full product list at GreenFertility.com). And because of this, it's also found its way into our environment.

According to Rep. Edward J. Markey (D-Mass.), who has been pushing federal regulators to take stronger action to restrict the use of triclosan and other chemicals, " It's in our drinking water, it's in our rivers and as a result, it's in our bodies. . . . I don't think a lot of additional data has to be collected in order to make the simple decisions about children's toys and soaps that people use. It clearly is something that creates a danger," he recently told *The Washington Post.*

Indeed, the exposure to triclosan is now so great that the US Centers for Disease Control and Prevention report that residues are showing up in the urine of 75% of Americans.

Fortunately, it appears as if the US government, along with those of many other nations, may soon be acting on the recommendations of those who believe there may be dangers lurking in hand sanitizers.

Currently, The European Union classifies triclosan as dangerous to the environment while both the Canadian and Japanese governments have banned its use in cosmetics. In the United States, both the FDA and the EPA have agreed to take a second, much harder look at triclosan, including whether or not it could be causing reproductive harm.

But as anyone who has ever waited for a government report can tell you, answers are not likely to affect what's on supermarket shelves any time soon.

KINDER, GENTLER, ANTI BACTERIALS: THEY'RE HERE NOW!

So what's a couple trying to conceive to do in the meantime? First, remember that studies also show that vigorous hand washing for 20 seconds or more with regular old soap and hot water will go a long way in wiping out most germs destined to do us in.

But if you're looking for an extra edge of protection, there are kinder, safer natural antibacterial products available! Among the best choices are products manufactured by CleanWell - an entire company devoted to killing germs on contact, *with no harmful chemicals!*

Indeed, CleanWell products rely on a combination of the natural herbal antibacterial known as thyme, in conjunction with a series of essential oils to to provide the same (or better) protection as triclosan, without the inherent dangers.

Moreover, these same oils have been shown in independent laboratory studies to kill the "bad" bacteria (including MRSA, salmonella and E-coli) without destroying the "good" bacteria on skin that is designed to keep us healthy.

According to Dr. Larry Weiss, the medical director of CleanWell, "The good bacteria on our hands and skin helps us stay healthy by protecting against bad germs we're exposed to through contact; that's why it's important to choose soaps and hand sanitizers that help your body maintain a healthy balance of bacteria."

But CleanWell is not alone on the store shelves. Companies such as DEFENSE manufacture an all natural antibacterial soap that uses a combination of tea tree oil and oil of Eucalyptus to fight bacteria associated with MRSA, ringworm, staph, impetigo, herpes, jock itch and athletes foot.

California Baby offers a natural antibacterial wash for both children and adults that relies on lemon, tea tree oil and the herb ravensara for natural antibacterial properties along with a recommendation to "vigorously " wash your hands for

20 seconds or more for the best protection.

And that's just the beginning of what you will find. Indeed, if take some time to visit stores featuring natural or organic products you'll find a nice selection of natural products that can help protect you from germs without compromising your fertility. Most companies also make their products available online so a little Googling can't hurt either!

While it's clear we can't completely avoid triclosan and other chemicals that can impact our fertility, the more we can reduce our exposures through better product choices, the less likely we are to experience problems.

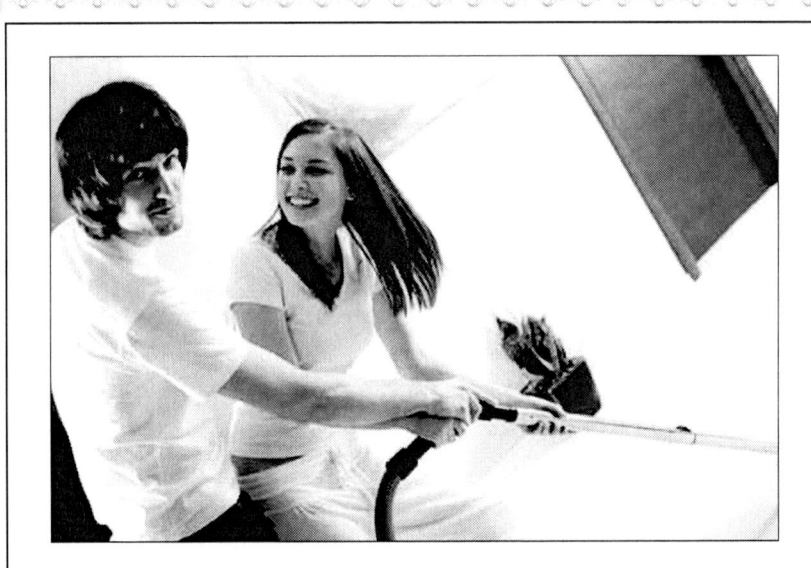

Switching to all-natural household cleaners such as those made by Seventh Generation, Bon Ami or Method and using natural anti-bacterial products made by companies like CleanWell can dramatically decrease your chemical exposures - and help your fertility to prosper! Be sure to visit GreenFertility.com for some great product substitutions!

PROTECTION FROM FERTILITY ROBBING CHEMICALS: WHAT YOU CAN DO

While experts have identified dozens of chemicals with the potential to harm fertility, what follows are some of the basic categories these products fall into. Identified by the Stanford University School of Medicine Collaborative on Health and Environment, they represent those groups of products with the most convincing evidence in terms of impacting both male and female fertility.

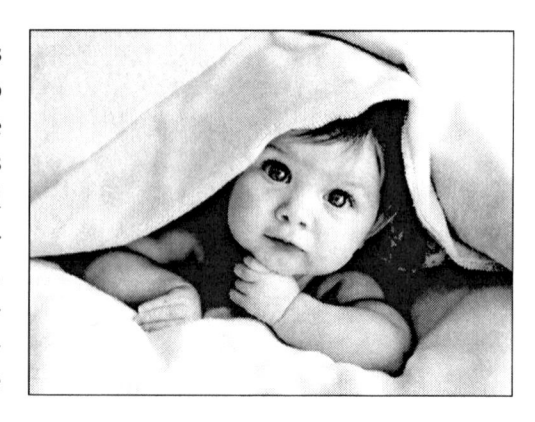

Clearly, it is virtually impossible to eliminate all chemical exposures and still live a somewhat normal life. And you really don't need to do that to protect your fertility. In fact, a little later in this chapter I'll give you some important tips on what you and your partner can do to stay healthy - without having to move into that plastic bubble!

But before I do I felt it was important for you to at least know where some of the potential harm is coming from. In this way you can begin to assess your own personal risk level, and know exactly where you have to take the most urgent steps to protect yourself from harm.

While some of the contaminants listed are easy to identify (some are even listed on product labels) others are a bit harder to ferret out, so when possible, look to the broad category – such as plastic bottles, or stain resistant fabric.

If you're not certain if a product contains an offending chemical, send a note to the product manufacturer and ask. Most companies now have websites and email addresses where you can usually get a pretty speedy response.

What's most important however, is not to let this list scare you! While the information may seem dramatically ominous, remember it's only a guide. What's more, it's important to remember that not every couple exposed to these chemicals will suffer infertility - so please don't be frightened! But for those who are more sensitive to environmental cues, or for those who are already struggling to get pregnant, you may well find some answers in eliminating or reducing some of these factors from your life.

Fertility Robbing Chemicals
At A Glance: What To Look Out For

Contaminant: Bisphenol A (BPA)
Found in: Polycarbonate plastic, resins, bottles, lining of canned goods
Effects on Female Fertility: Oocyte (egg) chromosome abnormalities, recurrent miscarriage
Effects on Male Fertility: Decreased semen quality

Contaminant: Chlorinated hydrocarbons
Found in: Dioxins/furans, PCBs, some pesticides (organochlorines), and wood preservative (pentachlorophenol)
Effects on Female Fertility: Menstrual irregularities, hormonal changes, reduced fertility, Endometriosis, fetal loss
Effects on Male Fertility: Decrease semen quality, hormonal changes

Contaminant: Drinking Water Treatments/ Disinfection by-products
Found in: Drinking water
Effects on Female Fertility: Fetal loss, menstrual irregularities
Effects on Male Fertility: None reported

Contaminant: Ethylene oxide
Found in: Chemical sterilizer used in dental and medical practices
Effects on Female Fertility: Fetal loss, miscarriage
Effects on Male Fertility: Decreased semen quality, partner miscarriage

Contaminant: Glycol ethers
Found in: Home Dec & Hobby products like paint, varnish, thinners, printing inks,
Effects on Female Fertility: Fetal loss, reduced fertility.
Effects on Male Fertility: Decreased semen quality

Contaminant: Heavy Metals
Found in: Products made from lead, mercury, manganese, cadmium (including some costume jewelry).
Effects on Female Fertility: Fetal fertility, menstrual irregularities
Effects on Male Fertility: Abnormal sperm, reduced fertility

CONTAMINANT: Pesticides
FOUND IN: Many classes of insecticides, fungicides, herbicides, rodenticides, and fumigants
EFFECTS ON FEMALE FERTILITY: Menstrual irregularities, reduced fertility, fetal loss
EFFECTS ON MALE FERTILITY: Decreased semen quality, reduce fertility, miscarriage in female partner, sperm chromosome abnormalities, hormonal changes

CONTAMINANT: Phthalates
FOUND IN: A plasticizer added to soften plastics like PVC; also found in cosmetics, hair care products, toys, pharmaceuticals, some medical devices
EFFECTS ON FEMALE FERTILITY: Fetal loss, ovulatory irregularities, reduced fertility
EFFECTS ON MALE FERTILITY: Decreased semen quality

CONTAMINANT: Solvents
FOUND IN : Products containing benzene, toluene, xylene, styrene, 1-bromopropane, 2- bromopropane, perchloroethylene, trichloroethylene, and others (Look for it in glues, adhesives, dry cleaning products including home dry cleaning, gasoline.
EFFECTS ON FEMALE FERTILITY: Reduced fertility, fetal loss, hormonal changes, menstrual irregularities
EFFECTS ON MALE FERTILITY: Decreased semen quality, reduced fertility, miscarriage in female partner, hormonal changes

CONTAMINANT: Cigarette smoke
FOUND IN: All brands of cigarettes; second hand smoke.
EFFECTS ON FEMALE FERTILITY: Reduced fertility, miscarriage, early menopause, hormonal changes, reduced fertility.
EFFECTS ON MALE FERTILITY: Reduced fertility, decreased semen quality, hormonal changes

CONTAMINANT: Perfluorinated compounds (PFOS, PFOA)
FOUND IN: Home Care Products such as stain resistant fabrics, water replants, coating in cooking pans, floor polish, some insecticides, bathroom cleaners, some upholstery shampoos, room deodorizers
EFFECTS ON FEMALE FERTILITY: Hormonal Changes;
EFFECTS ON MALE FERTILITY : Hormonal Changes

CONTAMINANT: Radiation
FOUND IN : Medical x-rays, airport scanners, some department store scanners
EFFECTS ON FEMALE AND MALE FERTILITY : Overexposure can result in mutagenic effects on the reproductive organs, including damage to the testes in men and ovaries in women, sometimes causing complete infertility.

Let The Sun Shine In!

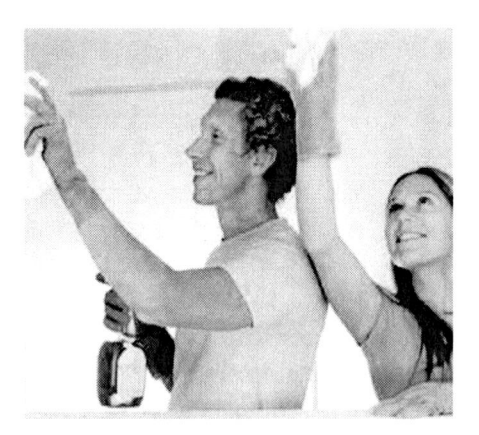

*You can reduce the impact of many potentially toxic home decorating chemicals, as well as home cleaning products by simply keeping the windows open while you work!
The more fresh air that circulates inside your home, the more the toxins will be diluted. And that means they will become much less harmful to you!*

Personal Care Products And Your Fertility

If you are like most women, then you no doubt use a variety of personal care products made of paper, including sanitary napkins, tampons, and panty liners. And there is no question that each of these items provide a convenient and hygienic way to care for your body.

Unfortunately, however, there is also downside to their use. In the process of manufacturing some of these paper products a chemical byproduct known as "dioxin" is formed. The problem is that residues of dioxin can remain on the products themselves. While dioxins are also present in our soil, water and even the air we breathe, what makes their presence on personal care products so disturbing is that these items come in direct contact with vaginal mucosa - one of the most porous areas of the body. In fact, the tissue that lines your vagina is almost like a natural sponge, soaking up pretty much anything that it comes in contact with. So, when a tampon contaminated with dioxin is placed inside your vagina - or a sanitary pad or panty liner is in close proximity – the likelihood of contamination increases, with a direct route to your uterus.

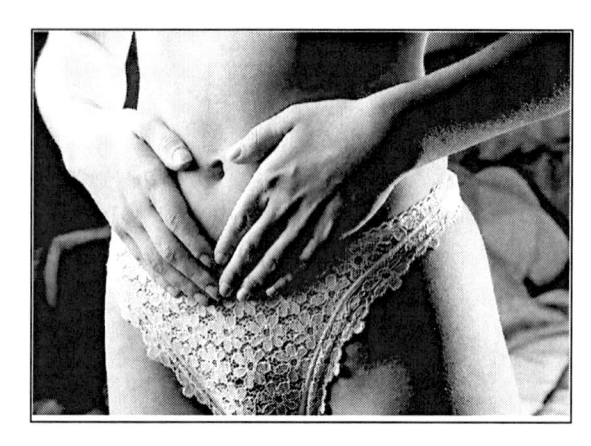

While manufacturers of these products vehemently deny any such related dangers, in reality, the only safety testing that has occurred, was done by the manufacturers themselves. Any independent studies that have been conducted have, indeed, raised questions about safety, with some researchers now solidly convinced these products can cause a problem for some women. Currently legislators in several states including Representative Carolyn Maloney in New York State, have introduced bills calling for more unbiased safety studies on these products.

Until that happens, however, there are things you can do. First, if you can avoid wearing panty liners, do so. If you have to, change your panties twice a day. Next, only wear tampons for your days with the heaviest flows, then switch to a pad. Also wear pads when you are home relaxing, and don't need the extra protection of a tampon. When possible, seek out both tampons and pads made from organic cotton and manufactured without dioxin. You can Google the term "dioxin-free sanitary products" for companies that offer these items.

In addition, you should always avoid douching, particularly with commercial douching products, and especially during the time you are trying to conceive. Research shows that douching can reduce fertility by as much as 30% following each cleansing. For women 18 to 24, studies show the rate of conception can be reduced by as much as 50%. Interestingly, a study published in the *American Journal of Public Health* found that conception rates were equally affected by both commercial douches and homemade vinegar and water solutions. Indeed, even douching with plain water had some detrimental effects on fertility.

The good news: Your vagina is a self-cleaning organism! As long as you shower regularly and use good bathroom hygiene, your vagina doesn't need internal cleansing. If you do notice an odor or a discharge of any color (including yellow, green, grey, or thick cloudy white) then do not douche, but instead see your gynecologist.

Q: *If I don't use a vaginal deodorant every day I develop a terrible odor - and it gets much worse around the time of my period. My husband says he can smell me coming 20 feet away! Will using these products harm my fertility?*

A: While occasional use of vaginal deodorants and fragrances won't necessarily harm you, in general it's a good idea to avoid as many chemical V zone exposures as you can. Using products such as baby powder made with cornstarch, or other natural fragrances can reduce chemical exposures and still help control natural odors. That said, if you have a persistent odor that does not disappear with good hygiene practices, you need to see your doctor. It's possible you have an infection that is causing the bad odor - and it may be keeping you from getting pregnant too.

GETTING PREGNANT IN THE DIGITAL AGE: WHAT YOU NEED TO KNOW

In the not so distant past there was lots of speculation about links between computer use and female infertility – and even more so, miscarriage. At the time the link was thought to be related to radiation leaking from the back of computer terminals and from some monitors.

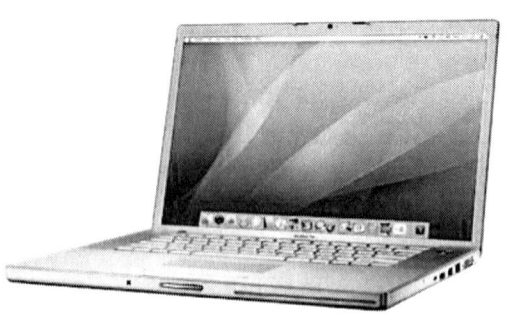

While a number of studies gave us pause for concern, to date there is still no conclusive evidence that computers harm a woman's fertility. This is particularly true with the computers in use today, most of which no longer use the type of components that originally aroused suspicion.

But that said, I and a number of fertility experts remain cautious about not only the extensive use of computers, but also excessive use of many personal electronic devices such as smart phones , MP4 players, even personal video players. Why are we still concerned?

All of these devices – including computers - generate what is known as electro-magnetic fields. This is a type of energy that is produced by any electrically charged object. While almost everything in our environment lies within an electro-magnetic field – including our power lines, our home wiring, and nearly every modern appliance in our world – many believe that the items which are in close proximity to our body, particularly for long periods of time, create the greatest amount of exposure and ultimately the most cause for concern.

But how does this exposure lead to harm? Studies show that continued exposure to any electro magnetic fields can result in headaches, dizziness, depression, anxiety, even the inability to focus clearly. Dr. David Carpenter, former Dean at the School of Public Health, State University of New York has said that it is likely up to 30% of all childhood cancers come from exposure to EMFs. There is also some evidence that some of these emissions can impact sperm production in men – a topic I discuss more fully in the upcoming chapter on male fertility.

But how do electro magnetic fields translate into caution for female fertility? Since at least some of the effects are linked to changes in brain chemistry - particularly that which is involved in depression and anxiety – many believe they can also impact the brain chemistry involved in reproduction, particularly that which controls ovulation. There is, in fact, some evidence to suggest that women who are over exposed to electro magnetic fields may not only have difficulty getting pregnant, but also experience an increased risk of miscarriage.

So, does this mean you should not use a computer, your cell phone or your MP3 player while trying to get pregnant? No it doesn't mean that at all.

What it does mean is that you should take some simple precautions to reduce the *cumulative* amount of exposure you receive.

- If you use a laptop computer, make sure there is something between the bottom of the computer and your lap- don't place it directly over your reproductive organs.
-
- If you are using a desktop computer, try to position the unit so that you are not facing the back, where most of the frequencies are generated.
-
- When using a cell phone, hang up if the reception isn't clear and re-place your call from an area where you can hear better. Indeed, studies show that when reception is more difficult most cell phones automatically amp up their frequency power - which means your exposure is greater.

- Never sleep with your cell phone next to your head (or under your pillow), or fall asleep with the earphones from your MP3 player still on your head, or your lap top computer on your bed.
-
- Purchase products such as Zerofon or Zerocom - tiny ceramic devices you attach to your phone or computer to absorb radiation before it gets to you! Visit GreenFertility.com for more information.

Indeed, if you use common sense in reducing some exposures you can still use all these devices without fear or worry. In fact, by following just a few simple guidelines you and your partner can not only protect your fertility right now, but also insure better health in the future!

Boost Your Fertility:
10 Things Every Couple Can Do Right Now!

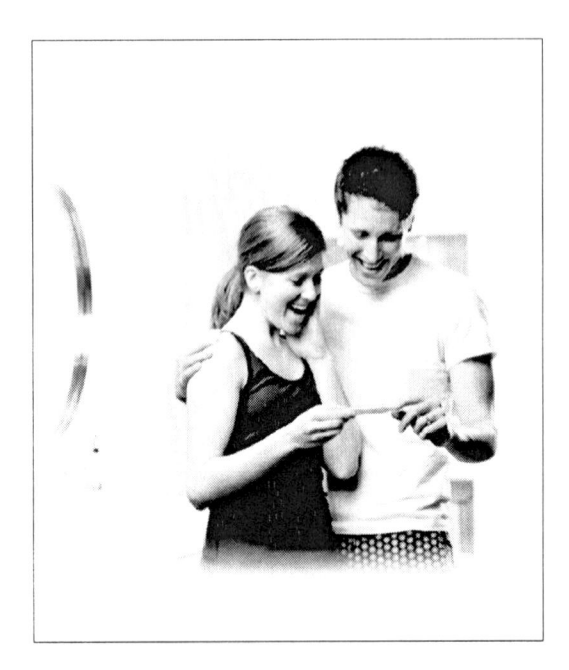

Certainly it's true that our world is filled with many different types of threats, some clearly more harmful than others. But it's also true that avoiding all of them is pretty much impossible – and even cutting down exposures can be difficult.

But that said, there are a few things you can do that will help decrease your exposure as well as bolster your protection against the exposures you do experience.

Together, this can form a powerful one-two punch that goes a long way in protecting your fertility from harm. In many instances protection involves nothing more than a good old fashioned dose of common sense – and if you look around your world I'm certain you'll find many ways to cut down on many questionable environmental concerns.

In fact for many of you, all it will take is a little bit of awareness of the world in which you live to know instinctively what to do to keep yourself safe from harm. And in this regard I say always go with your intuition!

If something in your immediate environment smells bad, looks bad or feels bad, there's a good chance it is bad, so do what you can to make whatever changes are necessary to correct the situation. More often than not, your instincts will show you the way!

But to help get you thinking in the right direction here are my personal Top Ten ways to make your world a healthier, more fertile place to be!

1. **GO ORGANIC -** We often think of the term "organic" in relation to food. But what I'm referring to here is more of an organic lifestyle, in the sense of letting nature rule your environment whenever possible. This means seeking out home supplies like paints and home dec products that are organically based, while opting for lawn care and garden products that are as close to natural as possible. In fact, anything with which you are in constant close contact should, whenever possible, be as natural as possible.

2. **DECORATE NATURALLY!** While I know it's much less expensive to decorate your home or office with products made from "engineered wood", it's important to note that most are manufactured using quite a toxic brew of chemicals including arsenic and formaldehyde. Moreover, many of these nasty chemicals can continue to "off gas" for up to 7 years or more. So, the more "fake wood" products in your home, the more contaminated your air will be – and the more chemical exposures you will have. If you can stick to furniture made from natural wood – even if it means purchasing some items second hand. In the long run they will be safer and healthier for you and for your children.

3. **CLEAN NATURALLY!** Since a great many of the most toxic chemicals are found in cleaning products, simply cutting down on the number of items you use will go a long way in reducing harmful exposures. When possible choose all natural products for household chores, particularly those items you use daily, such as dishwashing detergents, degreasers or floor cleaners.

4. **GO GREEN -** No, I don't just mean buy environmentally safe products – although that's a good idea too! I mean GO GREEN, in terms of house plants! Plants are nature's original air cleaners and they can make an enormous difference in the quality of the air inside your home or office. By reducing the impact of chemical emissions and giving you more oxygen to breathe, placing plants in every room of your house is great way to enhance your fertility and your health naturally!

5. **GO STAINLESS!** When it's time to buy those new pots and pans, skip the coated ones and opt for all natural stainless steel cookware. It's not only a healthier way to cook your food, it can dramatically reduce your exposure to at least one group of chemicals known to impact health and possibly fertility.

6. **DRY CLEAN LESS – AND AIR EVERYTHING OUT!** Is your closet a toxic waste dump of chemicals? It might be if your racks are loaded with dry cleaned clothing still in those plastic bags. When possible have clothing hand laundered and not dry cleaned – and if that's not possible, never put freshly cleaned clothing directly in your closet. Always remove the plastic bags and if possible air out the clothes in a garage or on a porch for at least 30 minutes before putting them in your closet. Because we're so used to many of these odors we sometimes don't even notice when the air in our bedroom is approaching a toxic level.

7. **LET THE SUNSHINE IN!** Winter fuel bills are high, and summer air conditioning bills even higher – a fact that leads most of us to seal up our doors and windows so that nary a drop of outside air comes in. But the truth is studies show that indoor air pollution is a far greater health threat than anything you'll breathe outdoors! As such it's important to regularly ventilate your home, exchanging stale indoor air for fresh air whenever possible. Fresh air will also help dissipate any harmful chemicals that do accumulate from household chemical use, and help reduce the risk of mold and mildew.

8. **CLEAR THE DECKS!** Keep your sleeping area clear of electronic devices. That means don't keep the cell phone charger right next to your bed – or fall asleep with your blue tooth headset on – no matter how important a call you're expecting! Your sleeping quarters should be free of all electronic clutter - which will not only protect your fertility, but maybe even help you get a better night's rest!

9. **SPEAK UP!** If your work environment is pretty much out of your control, but you see or smell or feel something you believe might be a threat to your health or your fertility, speak up! Talk to co-workers and tell your boss – and if need be, contact your local office of NIOSH - the National Institute for Occupational Health and Safety. Here you will find a wealth of information about workplace safety regulations and your right to a clean and safe work environment.

10. **VITAMINS, VITAMINS, VITAMINS!** One of the best ways to counter the effects of any environmental assault is to keep your body as healthy as possible. And that means not only eating healthy, nutritious meals, but also making sure you get a ready supply of vitamins and nutrients. Indeed, one of the ways to protect your body and your fertility from any type of toxic threat is to arm it with the "soldiers" necessary to protect you! And those soldiers include the antioxidant vitamins including A, C, E, and B complex, as well as vitamin D.

I can promise that if you can put even 5 of these 10 suggestions in place in your life, you will not only improve your fertility profile but also your overall health!

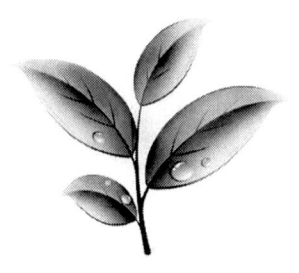

Chapter Fifteen

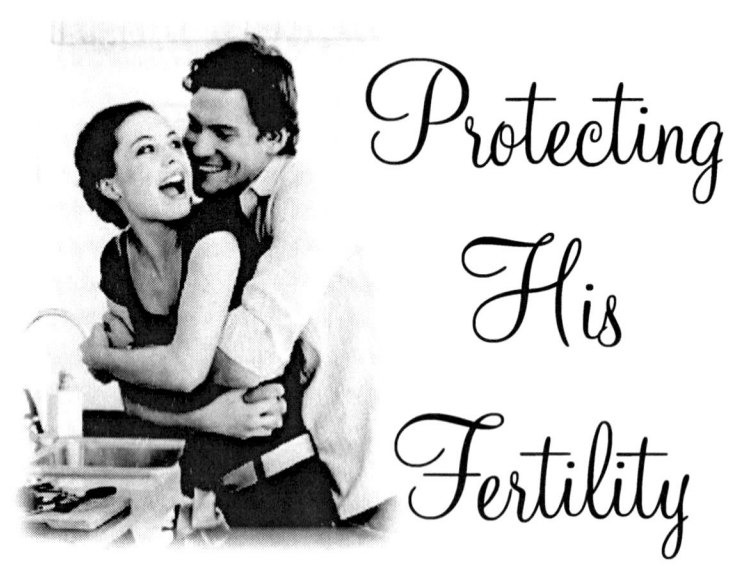

Protecting His Fertility
What Every Couple Needs To Know!

It wasn't so very long ago that the term "infertility" was applied strictly to women. Because a baby was conceived inside a woman's body, not being able to get pregnant seemed like a strictly female problem. Moreover, most men thought of their own fertility as virtually "indestructible." Unlike women for whom the ability to have a baby naturally declines with age, men believed they had no such "biological clock" to contend with.

Today we know how wrong this entire line of thinking is. Indeed, the American Society for Reproductive Medicine reports that today, up to 50% of all cases of infertility are caused by factors in a man's body.

As to the notion that nothing can harm male fertility? The shocking truth is that not only is a man's fertility much more fragile – and more limited - than we ever thought possible, there are a host of lifestyle factors that can rob even fertile young men of their ability to conceive a child.

In fact, in my experience, for the vast majority of couples who have a problem getting pregnant, it is factors in *both partners* that come together to block baby making success. Many times the problems can be so slight – what we call "sub clinical" – that they don't even show up on a test. Yet, when you combine slightly reduced female fertility with slightly reduced male fertility, the result is a couple who can't get pregnant!

You've already learned about the many things you can do to help turn your reproductive odds around. But equally as important are the steps your partner takes to protect and enhance his fertility. Certainly, many of the same dietary, nutritional and lifestyle factors that can help you improve your baby making potential, will also improve your partner's fertility as well. But that said, there are also some unique and specific steps your partner can take to not only improve his fertility profile, but also ensure his virility for decades to come. These steps include not only specific dietary and nutritional recommendations just for men, but also some lifestyle changes that are specific to male fertility.

And that's exactly what you are going to find in this chapter – the specific diet and lifestyle factors shown to boost and support male fertility. I strongly urge you to share this chapter with your partner and to help him understand just how important it is that he takes steps beginning right now to protect his fertility. In doing so, however, I must offer just a few words of advice: Don't be surprised if your partner's initial reaction is total resistance! Indeed, even more men than women fall prey to the rumours and half truths about the "indestructible male fertility. " Moreover, many men confuse "fertility" with "virility" and feel that by challenging their ability to make a baby you are also challenging their ability to be a good partner and lover.

But the truth is, even the most virile, sexually active men can have fertility problems. And it's important your partner understands that he can be a sexy, virile, fabulous lover – while still having weak or defective sperm. So if he resists the idea that he may have a fertility problem – or even refuses to admit that he needs to take care of his fertility – be patient with him. It has been my experience that eventually most men come to realize just how awesome being a father truly is – and in doing so also come to realize the importance of doing everything they can to ensure and protect their ability to conceive. So if at first your partner does resist some of the ideas in this chapter, give him a little time and some understanding – and be sure to let him know that in the end protecting his fertility is just another way of protecting and ensuring his good health for life!

Understanding Male Fertility: What You Both Need To Know

When it comes to making a baby, it all begins with the "mighty" sperm – a microscopically tiny " DNA rocket" that makes it's way to your egg, gets inside, and combines with your DNA to create a baby. While sperm are "ejaculated" from a man's body via his penis, they are actually manufactured in his testicles.

The process begins with a cell known as a "spermatogonium". Following stimulation from a variety of hormones – including some of the same brain chemicals necessary to stimulate egg production in you - sperm cells begin to divide. As they do they form what are called "spermatocytes."

More hormonal stimulation leads to further development , until we have what are called "spermatids" – tiny, immature "baby sperm" that are the male equivalent of developing egg follicles. As spermatids begin to mature they develop the classic "sperm tail" and slowly acquire the ability to move – a feat that is actually accomplished by the beating of the tail.

Once a sperm can move freely, it spends about 12 days passing through a section of his reproductive system known as the "epididymis" – a 21 foot coiled tube that sits inside the sac that holds the testicles. It is here, and ultimately in a small depot-like sac known as the "ampullae", that the final maturation process takes place, including the refining of some key enzymes located in the head of the sperm. Acting much like a kind of biochemical radar it is these enzymes that guide his sperm to your egg and, once there, allow it to attach and get inside.

How Sperm Gets To You

Before any of this can happen, however, sperm must get from your partner's body to your body. And as you no doubt know, sex is the activity that makes this happen! But how exactly does it all work?

As your partner becomes sexually aroused, and his penis becomes erect, it sends a signal to an area of his reproductive system known as the "vas deferens". These are two long tube-like structures which extend out from the area where sperm is stored.

Once they get the "go ahead" message from the penis, the vas deferens tubes begin a series of rapid muscular contractions. This, in turn, begins to pump the sperm from its holding depot through the vas deferens tubing. As it travels along, the sperm passes by what is known as the "seminal vesicle" – another depot-like structure that contains a fructose solution. As sperm pass by, the fructose solution is secreted to help propel the sperm forward toward the prostate gland, where it picks up even more fluid.

Combined, these liquids are known as semen – that gray-white semi liquid secretion that you see and feel when your partner has an orgasm and ejaculates. In fact, the moment an orgasm begins it creates a muscular contraction so powerful it forces the sperm shot-gun style down the shaft of his penis, out the tip, and into your body. Each milliliter of ejaculated semen contains literally thousands of sperm.

Although a new supply of sperm is made every day, what is being ejaculated today wasn't made today. That's because it takes approximately 72 days for each sperm to develop, mature and be ready for ejaculation. And the fact that it does take this long is really key to understanding male fertility. Why?

Because anywhere within that 72 day time period – and during any of the steps that occur during each phase of this time frame - any number of things can interfere with the production of healthy sperm.

When they do a variety of problems can result including:
- A reduced amount of sperm
- Reduced sperm quality - with more deformed or weak sperm
- Reduced sperm motility – meaning a lack of swimming energy and a lack of navigation skills necessary to reach an egg.

When any of these problems develop, either alone or together, it often means reduce fertility for him, and problems getting pregnant for you.

The Male Reproductive System

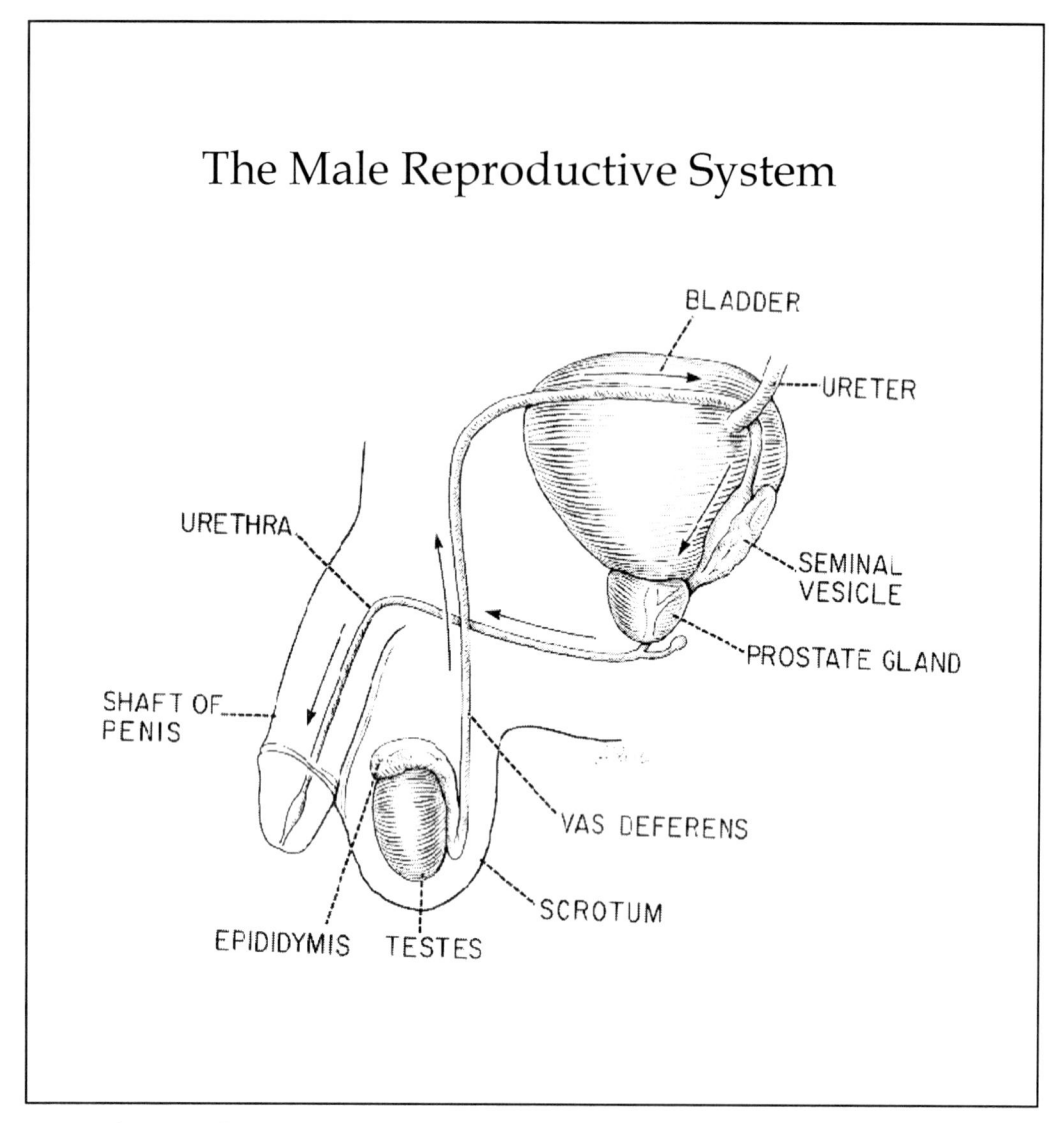

(Diagram labeled: BLADDER, URETER, SEMINAL VESICLE, PROSTATE GLAND, VAS DEFERENS, SCROTUM, TESTES, EPIDIDYMIS, SHAFT OF PENIS, URETHRA)

HOW SPERM GETS TO YOU: Sperm is manufactured in the testes (testicles) and then spends about 12 days passing through the epididymus a 21 foot coiled tube that sits inside the scrotal sac. It then passes through the vas deferens, a long, tube-like structure that winds up through the abdomen, past the prostate gland and eventually connects to the urethra, a long hollow tube inside the shaft of the penis. Sexual stimulation leading to orgasm pumps the sperm and the fluid through the penis and into a woman's body.

What Harms Sperm - And How To Prevent It

In some instances certainly physiologic problems can be behind some or all of the sperm problems a man experiences. For example, a defect in the testicles themselves, or sometimes in the epididymis, can prevent sperm from maturing properly. A blockage within the tubal transport system can keep mature sperm from leaving a man's body, or an over or under production of certain hormones can keep sperm from ever being made.

While these conditions usually exist only in a relatively small number of men, when this is the case there are a number of important exciting and new male fertility treatments that can help. In my book *Getting Pregnant: What You Need To Know Right Now*, I detail what all of those treatments are and how they can help.

That said, in my experience, for the vast majority of couples grappling with infertility - particularly "unexplained infertility" - the most dominant issues affecting sperm are related to lifestyle factors.

Indeed, studies show that a man's lifestyle, including his diet, nutritional profile and personal habits such as alcohol use, smoking and drug use can have overwhelming effects on his fertility. Couple this with environmental exposures both at home and on the job, as well as weight problems and a boatload of stress, and you have the classic "recipe" for fertility chaos.

But what's important to realize is that when lifestyle factors are behind a man's fertility problems, the factors are largely under his control!

Moreover, by following just a few simple guidelines and making a few small changes, your partner can not only prevent many fertility related problems from occurring, but also correct many of those which may already be underway.

In fact, in one very important study of some 800 men, Australian researcher Dr. Anne Clarke found that by simply adding a few nutritional supplements to their diet and making a few lifestyle changes, more than 40% of men who were considered infertile were able to father a child. Moreover, a full 11% of these men were able to do so naturally – without any medical or laboratory assistance!

So, if you and your partner are having problems conceiving – or even if you just want to ensure a faster conception and a healthier baby - I am quite certain that making just a few lifestyle changes will turn your reproductive odds around! In fact, if you follow the lifestyle changes I have suggested in earlier chapters, and your partner heeds those in this chapter, then I can promise you that getting pregnant will definitely be faster and easier.

Five Super Sperm Assassins
& How To Defeat Them!

There is no question that some of the harmful factors in today's world appear to aiming directly for sperm! In fact, I like to call them the "Sperm Assassins" - but don't let the term scare you! Because while they can clearly harm or even kill a man's baby making potential, the good news is they are all factors under his control! In fact, your partner can reverse the effects of even the most potent sperm assassins with just a few simple lifestyle changes! What follows are the five factors I believe are most harmful to sperm – and the important ways your partner can protect his fertility from harm!

Sperm Assassin # 1: Smoking

There's no longer any question that smoking is bad for your overall health. And usually, what is bad for general health is also bad for fertility.

But when it comes to cigarettes, there are some specific fertility related concerns. In fact, an analysis of 27 different studies showed that cigarettes not only reduce sperm production by some 25%, but that smoking also decreases sperm motility (the ability to swim) as well as their ability to function normally.

In one of those studies conducted by researchers at The University of Buffalo, sperm from smokers was shown to have a much harder time sticking to an egg – a major step necessary for achieving fertilization.

The same study also found that men who were heavy tobacco users experienced a significant overall drop in fertility. Research conducted elsewhere revealed smoking can impact hormonal activity necessary for healthy sperm production

But these are not the only fertility problems linked to smoking. There is also evidence it can damage the DNA inside each sperm. So, even if a pregnancy does occur, a smoker risks passing on that defective DNA to his child – a situation that can result in any number of serious birth defects, including an increased risk of disease later in the child's life.

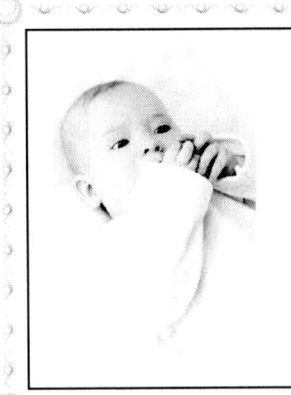

> **THE BEST WAY TO INSURE A FAST CONCEPTION: STOP SMOKING!**
> Twenty-seven different fertility studies have shown cigarettes not only reduce sperm production by 25%, smoking also decreases the ability of sperm to swim and to function normally.
> **The good news:** Even cutting down helps since the more cigarettes a man smokes the more likely he is to suffer from fertility problems.

In fact, studies show that the impact of smoking on male fertility can be so significant it even reduces the effectiveness of a medically assisted pregnancy. This includes procedures such as IVF (in vitro fertilization) and even ICSI (intracytoplasmic sperm injection), a procedure which inserts a single sperm directly inside an egg!

If your partner smokes, quitting is the absolute best option - and doing so often reverses negative effects on sperm within as little as 3 months. Moreover, since new sperm is being made very day, abstaining for even a few weeks prior to attempting conception can be helpful.

In fact, I often advise couples who are having trouble conceiving to stop smoking before turning to expensive fertility treatments for help. Why?

First, being smoke-free improves the success rate of pretty much every fertility treatment. But in many instances the on effects of quitting smoking can be so powerful, you may not even need the fertility treatments at all!

I am very happy to report that a number of my patients who did nothing different in their lives *except* quit smoking were able to get pregnant naturally – sometimes even after years of being infertile. As such I hope you agree that it's certainly worth giving it a try!

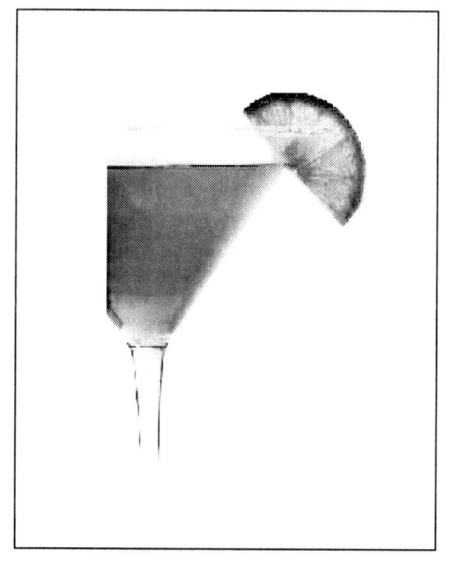

Sperm Assassin # 2: Alcohol

So, I've just told you that you have to stop smoking ….and now I'm telling you stop drinking alcohol too? If you're like many of my fertility patients you're probably thinking I've taken all the fun out of making a baby!

But in reality there is some startling evidence linking male fertility problems to alcohol consumption – and good evidence to show that reducing alcohol intake can dramatically increase baby making success!

Among the most immediate effects is a decrease in sperm count which occurs within 24 hours after becoming intoxicated. Indeed, studies show that sperm count can drop as much as 50% within a day after consuming enough alcohol to be considered " drunk". In one study pregnancy success was reduced by about 50% within 24 hours after the male partner became intoxicated.

But that's just the beginning. When consumed on a regular basis, and often to excess, alcohol affects the entire system of endocrine glands and hormones necessary for healthy sperm production. This includes not only the brain hormones which direct sperm production, but also testosterone, the male hormone made in the testicles and key to sperm maturation and development. Testosterone, by the way, is also key to the male sex drive, which is one reason why men who drink a lot often lose their desire for sex and/or their ability to have an erection.

Moreover, there is some evidence to show that when the body metabolizes alcohol it produces what are known as "oxidants" – molecules that contribute to cell damage, and may play a role in alcohol-induced tissue damage in the testicles. If your partner's diet is also lacking key nutrients (and you'll learn more about what they are in just a few minutes) the oxidants become the dominant cells, creating a condition known as "oxidative stress". This produces even more "oxidants" which in turn causes more cell damage – ultimately causing sperm production to falter even more.

Beer, Wine and Nuts: Can They harm His Fertility

While any form of alcohol can have a detrimental impact on sperm, new studies from The Medical Research Council in Cambridge, England found that both beer and red wine may be especially harmful to sperm – and that the harm can be further increased by adding a handful of the peanuts so frequently served at bars.

Indeed, researchers found that both red wine and brown ale, along with peanuts, were loaded with phytoestrogens – the same plant estrogens that can help a woman increase her fertility. In men, however, phytoestrogens have the opposite effect, reducing sperm count and sometimes overpowering testosterone, the male hormone necessary for sperm production. As such, they are advising any man interested in fathering a child to reduce their intake of both beer and red wine.

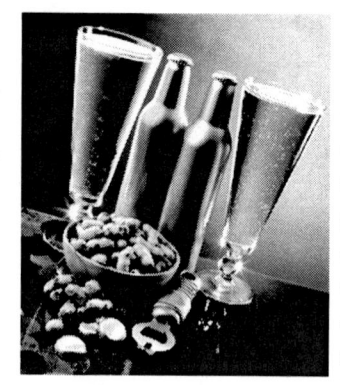

Protection From harm: The Good News

The good news is that reducing alcohol intake dramatically reverses many of these problems, and even helps rejuvenate testosterone production. In fact, research indicates that avoiding alcohol for just 3 months can dramatically increase sperm count – to the point where some men can go from infertile to fertile!

As such, if your partner has been tested and his sperm count was found to be borderline low or even very low, I recommend he abstain from all alcohol for two to three months, and then be retested. You may both be surprised to discover that his fertility problems have self-corrected!

If, at the same time, your partner also improves his diet and stocks up on fertility nutrients (and you'll find out more about what he should eat in just a few moments) he will not only stop most problems related to sperm production, but maybe even reverse some of the damage to his reproductive system caused by the alcohol.

In the event that testosterone levels are still not up to par, early research suggests prescription bio-identical testosterone supplements might rejuvenate sperm production. Be certain that he speaks to his doctor about this, however, and only take legitimate medically prescribed testosterone supplements, and only after adequate blood testing to insure a true deficiency exists.

SPERM ASSASSIN # 3: HOT TESTICLES!

Be it from hot tubs, a hot bath, or jeans that are just too tight, anything that can cause a man's testicles to overheat can potentially rob his fertility. The reason? Sperm is heat sensitive, so, when the temperature inside his testes rise too high, sperm production slows down, or sometimes, can stop completely.

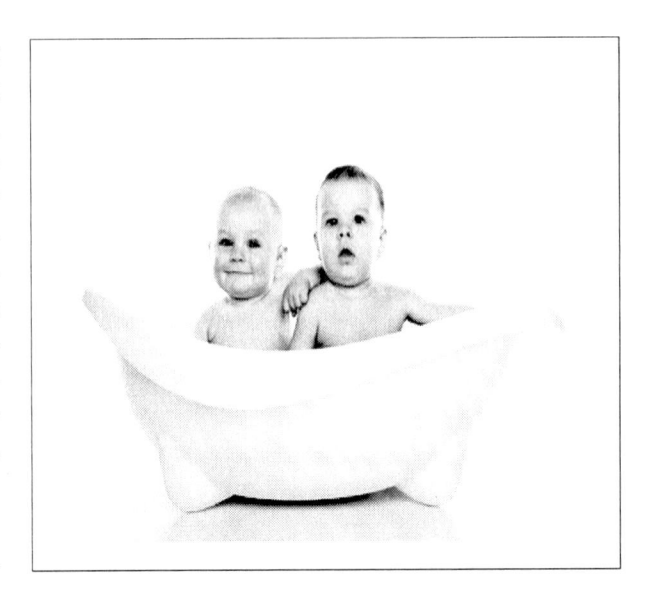

Moreover there is also evidence that prolonged exposure to high heat can effect the epididymis, the part of the male reproductive system that helps sperm mature – and where they learn to swim. When the epididymis becomes even temporarily damaged, it can impact a man's immediate ability to conceive a child. A defective epididymis can also increase the risk of miscarriage or birth defects by increasing the number of defective sperm available for conception.

Although the most common causes of "hot testicles" are traditional heat sources – such as hot tubs, saunas, hot baths, electric blankets, or even laptop computers (see more on this later) - there is also some evidence that certain fitness activities can cause similar heat related issues.

The fitness workouts most likely to increase heat in the testicles include rowing machines, simulated cross country ski machines, treadmills, duration aerobics, jogging or bike riding. That said, all of these activities can be made "sperm safe" if your partner simply wears cool, loose-fitting clothing when working out. In fact, what he wears while doing any exercise can significantly contribute to testicle heat build-up. The workout fabrics to avoid include tight, spandex shorts, synthetic fibers that don't breathe, tight fitting jeans with spandex (worn during or right after working out) or tight spandex or nylon bikini underwear.

WEIGHT & HOT TESTICLES

Also important to note: If your partner is overweight, particularly if he's holding a lot of that weight in the belly area and below, then he may be literally "smothering" his testicles with heat nearly every day. While losing excess weight, particularly belly fat, can be extremely healthy for every man, for some it can make the difference between being infertile and fertile! Once the layers of fat are removed from the belly and below, the testicles are naturally cooler – and that means sperm production can increase.

So what is the ideal temperature for sperm production to flourish? Studies have shown that keeping the scrotum between 94-96 degrees F - which is a couple of degrees cooler than normal body temperature – is really the best. In fact, it seems Mother Nature was quite clever in putting a man's testicles outside his body (instead of inside like a woman's ovaries) which naturally enables them to remain cool and thus encourage better sperm production.

COOL EM' DOWN!

What can also help: Wearing cooler clothes, and staying away from tight underwear – and when possible forgoing pants altogether when he is relaxing at home. If, in fact, if your partner just loves his tight jeans – and he'd rather cut off his arm then wear a pair of baggy boxers – then encourage him to spend leisure time at home in a bathrobe wearing no pants. This will help to compensate for whatever heat build up has occurred during the day.

Also be aware that wearing boxers for a day or two before conception isn't going to make a difference. Again, because the sperm he is ejaculating today were actually made 11 to 12 weeks prior, any heat-related consequences occurring in the few days prior to attempting conception isn't going to make any difference.

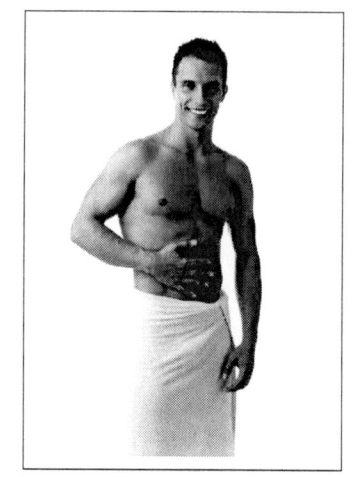

At the same time, however, if he is willing to begin making changes two to three months prior to when you want to get pregnant, then reducing heat exposures can definitely help maximize his sperm count when conception time rolls around.

SPERM ASSASSIN # 4: CELL PHONES & COMPUTERS

There is no question that the rate of male fertility problems is on the rise. In several countries around the world the number of men diagnosed with poor sperm health is staggeringly high – and increasing at regular intervals.

While there are likely a wide variety of reasons behind the increase, many suspect there is also a "high tech" link to male infertility. The main culprits, say experts, are lap top computers and cell phones.

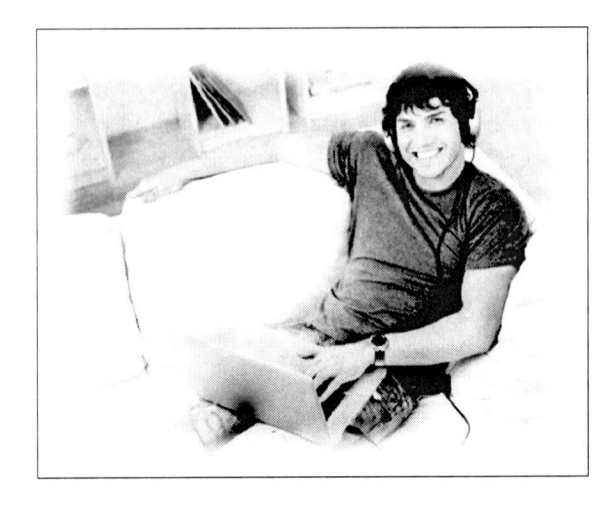

How can they harm his fertility? In the case of the laptops, it's all about the heat! As you just read, the optimum temperature for sperm production is between 94 and 96 degrees F. And if you've ever felt or measured the heat generated from the underside of a notebook computer then you know those temps can soar far above this level. What's more, when the heat continues to generate – focused directly on the testicles - temperatures can continue to rise. How much?

In one study conducted at Stony Brook University in New York researchers found that laptop use can raise the temperature of a man's scrotum by several degrees – which can be equally as damaging as a soak in a hot tub or an hour in a sauna. What's more, the newest laptops – with faster processors – are generating even more heat, particularly during graphics-heavy applications and especially while gaming. All this makes overheating problems even more likely.

Also contributing to the new heat issues are the tiny netbooks now so popular. Although they run slower, because they are smaller, heat generally builds up quicker and is harder to dissipate. They get hotter faster, and so does his lap!

THE SOLUTION: Always make certain your partner has at least some type of shielding between his lap and the bottom of the computer. Almost any type of cooling device will help including gel pads and podiums like the ones made by Targus. But do be careful with any cooling device featuring fans which draw heat away from the computer and focus it towards the lap. Most important, make sure he gives "the boys" some air from time to time by removing the lap top, and/or getting up to walk around , thus allowing some of the heat to dissipate.

The second high –tech link to fertility are cell phones – particularly in regard to where on his body he carries his phone. According to one study published recently in the journal *Fertility and Sterility*, men who carry their cell phones either in their jeans pocket or clipped to their belt - while using a headset to talk - risk damaging their sperm.

How? When in "talk" mode, cell phones emit radio frequency electromagnetic waves. Studies show over exposure to these waves generates free radicals - molecules that damage sperm or reduce production. This may even be more critical when the waves are directed right at the scrotum and testicles.

THE SOLUTION: Make sure he turns his phone off when he's not placing a call, since it delivers the most radio frequency waves in "talk" mode. He should also be aware that when a connection is bad, phones amp up their frequencies in order to keep the call going – and that generates an extra dose of electromagnetic current. When the connection starts to wane, the best idea is to hang up the phone and place the call again from another location where the connection is better.

BOXERS VS. BRIEFS – THE LEGEND CONTINUES!

When it comes to hot testicles, the "hot debate" often centers around boxers vs. briefs . More specifically, the question always arises as to whether or not wearing loose boxer shorts can help encourage sperm production, while "tightie whities" might slow it down. For the most part, the theory is based on rumor – and in fact, a study published in the *Journal of Urology* found that men who wore briefs were not any more likely to have fertility problems then men who wore boxers. But that said, I've always believed that if you do engage in activities that cause heat to build in the testicles, and particularly if you use a lap top computer –on your lap –then wearing tight knit brief underwear could contribute to the problem. If you wear boxers whatever heat is generated will more easily dissipate, and that can only help sperm count to thrive!

Sperm Assassin # 5 – Social Drug Use

Currently it's estimated that up to 10 percent of all men who are actively trying to conceive a baby use some form of illicit social drugs, or abuse prescription medications. And while the degree of reproductive problems depend largely on the substance that is used as well as how much and how often it is used, still, the potential for damage is clearly there anytime these substances come into play.

Among the two social drugs most harmful to male fertility are marijuana and cocaine.

Indeed studies show that regular use of marijuana not only reduces sperm count and semen production, but also impacts the shape and form of sperm that is produced. Moreover, if your partner uses marijuana just prior to attempting conception, sperm can actually get a little bit "stoned" – meaning they can't quite follow a straight path through your reproductive system to your egg. Instead they just swim in circles not really knowing where to go! But if, in fact, they do manage to get to your egg, studies conducted at the University of Buffalo in New York found that compounds in marijuana inhibit the release of enzymes found in the head of the sperm, and are necessary to penetrate an egg. So, even if his sperm bumps smack into your egg, it won't matter - because no fertilization can occur unless that sperm gets inside.

While there is some evidence that stopping habitual use of marijuana will help reverse problems in some men, it does take a while. Since the active component of marijuana – a compound known as THC – is stored in fat cells, de-toxing the body isn't fast or easy. That said, the sooner he quits, the more likely it will be that his sperm count will rise and his fertility will be restored.

When it comes to cocaine use, sperm can also suffer. Men who use cocaine on a regular basis are found to have reduced sperm counts, reduced sperm motility and an increased number of abnormal sperm. Moreover, if your partner has this drug in his body at the time of conception, your baby can experience some dramatic health risks. Indeed, molecules of this drug can attach to the tails of sperm and literally "ride" right into an egg – so the drug and it's effects are present in your baby from the moment of conception. And that, in turn can result in a number of serious developmental problems. In one study published in the *Journal of the American Medical Association* (JAMA) researchers found that the

> ## Stoned Sperm? It Can Happen!
>
> **Q:** *My sister's husband smokes a lot of pot - and her doctor told her that his sperm is too "stoned" for her to get pregnant. Is this true - and can sperm really get "stoned"?*
>
> **A:** As silly as it may sound, the truth is that "yes" sperm can get "stoned" from the resides of marijuana found in the bloodstream after "pot" is smoked. In fact, within minutes after smoking marijuana sperm waiting to be ejaculated can become so "stoned" they can't swim straight - often going in circles and not able to make their way through the reproductive canal in order for pregnancy to occur. Besides all the health implications of smoking pot, if you sister wants to get pregnant her husband must stop using drugs.

embryos conceived by men who regularly used cocaine were much more likely to suffer serious developmental problems. The number of children born with birth defects increases in couples where one or both partners habitually use cocaine.

Other narcotics such as heroin and amphetamines have also been linked to a disruption of hormone production necessary to manufacture healthy sperm.

Also important to note: There is considerable evidence to show anabolic steroids (the kind used by athletes to increase muscle mass) not only reduce sperm count, but also interfere with overall sperm production. Indeed, over the past decade we have learned much about these drugs, which include male hormones such as testosterone, as well as human growth hormone (HGH). When used correctly, under a doctor's supervision, and only when a true deficiency exists, these medications can be a boost to male fertility. But when used without the benefit of medical supervision, and particularly when a deficiency does not exist, disastrous results can occur. This includes testicle atrophy (meaning testicles shrink in size and begin to deteriorate), a dramatic drop in sperm count, and sometimes, complete sterility. In addition, men who use these drugs for body building purposes can also suffer an increased risk of heart problems, and experience both deep depression and excessive rage, sometimes even psychosis.

THE MEDICATIONS THAT CAN IMPACT SPERM

Although it's always a good idea for both you and your partner to approach conception with your bodies free and clear of all drugs, I know this isn't always easy, or possible. Indeed, there are some instances where prescription or over-the-counter medications are necessary – and without them overall health can really suffer. And if you or your partner are currently using medications prescribed by your physician, don't be afraid to take them!

That said, there are some medications that definitely impact male fertility. While your partner should never stop any treatment unless his doctor directs him to do so, it's important to know which drugs have the potential to cause problems. As such, if your partner is regularly using any of the following medications it's important that he speaks to his doctor about your parenting plans. Very often there are other drugs less likely to cause problems that can be safely substituted for the medications he is now taking. But remember, no one should ever stop taking any medication without their doctor's okay!

- Blood pressure medications including Thiazide diuretics, spironolactone, aldactone, beta blockers, calcium channel blockers, alpha blockers.

- Mental Health Drugs – such as anti psychotics, tricyclic antidepressants, MAO Inhibitors, Phenothiazines, lithium.

- Antibiotics including nitrofurantoin, erythromycin, tetracycline, gentamycin.

- Methotrexate – used to treat psoriasis and cancer

- Cimetidine - used to treat heartburn

- Salicylazosulfapyridine – used to treat irritable bowel syndrome

- Phenytoin – Used in the treatment of seizures

- Sulphasalazine – Used in the treatment of ulcerative colitis

- Colchicine – Used in the treatment of gout

Sperm Assassin # 6: Environmental Assaults

If there was ever a good reason to "go green", planning a family is among the best! Why? Because nearly every day we learn just a little bit more about the tremendous impact that environmental chemical exposures can have on our reproductive health. As you read earlier, female fertility can be dramatically affected by these exposures. But in truth, many of the same chemicals that can harm female fertility can be just as devastating to male fertility. Add to this important new evidence on how certain exposures are specifically harmful to sperm and it's easy to see how any couple can fall prey to a toxic brew of chemicals that ultimately robs them of their ability to become parents.

But how exactly do these chemicals cause us harm? Most often it occurs via "hormone disruption". In fact the chemicals which are thought to cause us the most harm are called "endocrine disrupters – named so because once ingested by the body they begin to act much like a hormone, disrupting the natural sequence of bio-chemical events. How does this occur?

First, they bind to hormone receptors in the body thus "tricking" all systems into believing the real hormones are present. This, in turn, initiates a number of "false signals" that ultimately cause other hormones and chemicals to either speed up or slow down production. This is often the case with some particulalry nasty hormone disrupters known as "xeno estrogens" – compounds which mimic the activity of estrogen and in doing so throw the reproductive systems of both men and women into a complete tailspin.

You already learned in a previous chapter how xeno estrogens can impact female fertility. But male fertility can be just as vulnerable – or sometimes even more vulnerable to harm. In most instances, the greatest impact occurs on sperm count – causing either a dramatic drop in the total number of sperm manufactured, or an increase in the number of defective sperm being made. This means that either conception will not occur, or if it does, the risk of miscarriage or birth defects is high.

Now clearly, the most dangerous level of exposure occurs in men whose occupations allow them greater than normal contact with these substances. For example, men who regularly work with organic chemical solvents such as glues, formaldehyde or lead, or those exposed to higher than normal levels of pesticides or radiation are at greater risk than a man who has only occasional or casual exposure. In my book *Getting Pregnant: What You Need To Know Now* I detail the occupations that represent the greatest threats to both male and female fertility.

But that said, while occupational exposures may present the highest level of risk, certainly even small exposures can, over time, also contribute to fertility problems. This is particularly true since many of the most harmful environmental toxins accumulate in fat cells – which means residues remain in our body for years, even decades after a single exposure.

Certainly I don't want to instill fear in either you or your partner. But I do think it's important that you both know which of the most common chemical contaminants are most likely to cause harm to sperm. I do believe that knowledge is power – and when you know what can harm you, you also know what you should avoid. Moreover, even if exposures can't be completely avoided – and many cannot - knowing that you are at risk will allow you to take some protective steps, including increasing your nutritional stores and eating a better diet.

So what are the chemical exposures most likely to harm male fertility? According to a number of studies the following substances are the most likely to act as hormonal or endocrine disrupters and over time impact male fertility.

Potential Sperm Killers	**Commonly Found In:**
Alkylphenols -	Industrial & domestic detergents
Dioxins	Paper products including computer paper, paper towels & napkins, toilet tissue
Organochlorine pesticides including Lindane and DDT	Lawn care products, weed killers, insect or rodent control products.
Phthalates	Fragrances, deodorants, shower gels, soaps, personal care products
Phytoestrogens	Soy, red clover, peanuts, red wine, beer
Synthetic estrogens	Widely used in the livestock & poultry industries.

Canned Ravioli, Beer and Bottled Water: A Common Link To Male Impotency & Infertility

If a group of Chinese researchers are right, you may want to keep your partner from snacking on canned ravioli and beer. The reason: You just might see the after-effects in the bedroom - and *not in a good way*.

Indeed, in research published recently in the journal *Human Reproduction* it was noted that bisphenol A or BPA - a synthetic estrogen found in thousands of consumer products including plastic beverage bottles, the linings of food and beverage cans, even many paper products (see Chapter 12) – may, in fact, be responsible for a wide range of sexual dysfunction problems in men, including erectile dysfunction and possibly infertility.

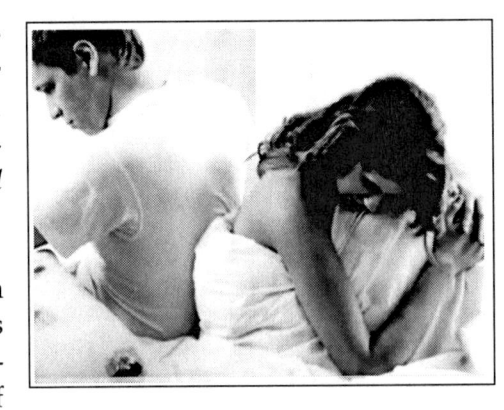

Head researcher De-Kun Li recently told the Washington Post " Critics dismissed all the animal studies saying "Show us the human studies'; now we have a human study and this just can't be dismissed," he said.

The five year study followed 634 male works from four Chinese factories where exposure to BPA was significant. Researchers then compared the incidence of sexual dysfunction among these men with a control group who did not have workplace exposure to BPA.

The result: The men who were exposed to the BPA were four times more likely to suffer from erectile dysfunction and seven times more likely to have difficulty with ejaculation. Moreover, it didn't take long periods of exposure for the sexual problems to kick in. Indeed, men who worked in the factories only a matter of months appeared to be as affected as those who spent years being exposed to the chemical.

In other research it has been shown that men who have either erectile dysfunction or ejaculation problems also experience a higher rate of infertility – and now some researchers are wondering if the two problems aren't "chemically" connected.

Indeed, at this point we don't know if the infertility is simply a result of not being able to transport sperm into their partner's body, or if the BPA is playing an additional role in the infertility as well. Indeed, since animal studies have shown BPS can cause infertility on it's own, it's certainly a possiblity in humans.

Adding more fuel to the BPA fire: A brand new Italian study conducted by researchers at Peninsula Medical School and the University of Exeter. Here researchers found that men who had the highest levels of BPA in their urine also had measurable differences in their blood hormone levels when compared to me who had less BPA in their system.

"BPA has been classed as a 'hormone disruptor' for many years, but until now most of the evidence has come from laboratory or animals studies," says lead researcher Professor Tamara Galloway. "Here we have shown for the first time that higher exposure to BPA is associated with changes in circulating hormone concentrations in normal, healthy adult men."

HOW MUCH BPA IS TOO MUCH BPA?

Clearly, the research shows that the men in the Chinese studies were routinely exposed to levels of BPA 50 times higher than the average North American man. And to this end, the American Chemical Society – which represents many manufacturers who use BPA in products - says the new study holds little concern for most Americans.

Indeed, Steven G. Hentges of the ACC recently told the press " Although this study represents interesting information it has little relevance to average consumers who are exposed to trace levels of BPA," he said.

Unfortunately, however, the "low dose" logic may not apply in this scenario. While traditional toxicology screens equate high doses of chemical contaminants with increased harm, specific tests on BPA indicate lower doses may be even more toxic simply because they " slip by" the body's natural defense system unchecked. In fact, in one study, low dose BPA exposure increased the risk of prostate cancer by 70% over high dose exposure, in lab animals. Moreover, some experts contend that with so many products containing BPA, low level exposure may actually be chronic and continual, making it virtually impossible to calculate how much each man is getting – or how widespread that exposure might be among men already experiencing the symptoms represented in the study.

Obviously some men are exposed more than others, and we do know that genetics also play a role But that said, the association raises a red flag I believe we cannot and should not ignore – and its definitely something that couples who are grappling with infertility should not ignore.

Because food and drink containers are such a large source of BPA, at least some of responsibility for regulating this chemicals falls with the US Food and Drug Administration, which has been widely criticized for not regulating it's use in the United States. Indeed, even their own scientific advisory committee voiced discontent over the fact that the FDA appears to ignoring more than 100 studies linking BPA to adverse health effects in animals and humans, including infertility, weight, behavioral changes, early -onset puberty, cancer and diabetes.

While the agency has reportedly pledged to re-examine the issue, to date, the FDA has maintained that BPA is safe. At the same time, the Canadian government has drafted legislation to prohibit the importation, sale and advertising of polycarbonate baby bottles that contain bisphenol A (BPA), and it has allocated 1.7 million dollars to further research the health effects of this chemical particularly in relation to food containers.

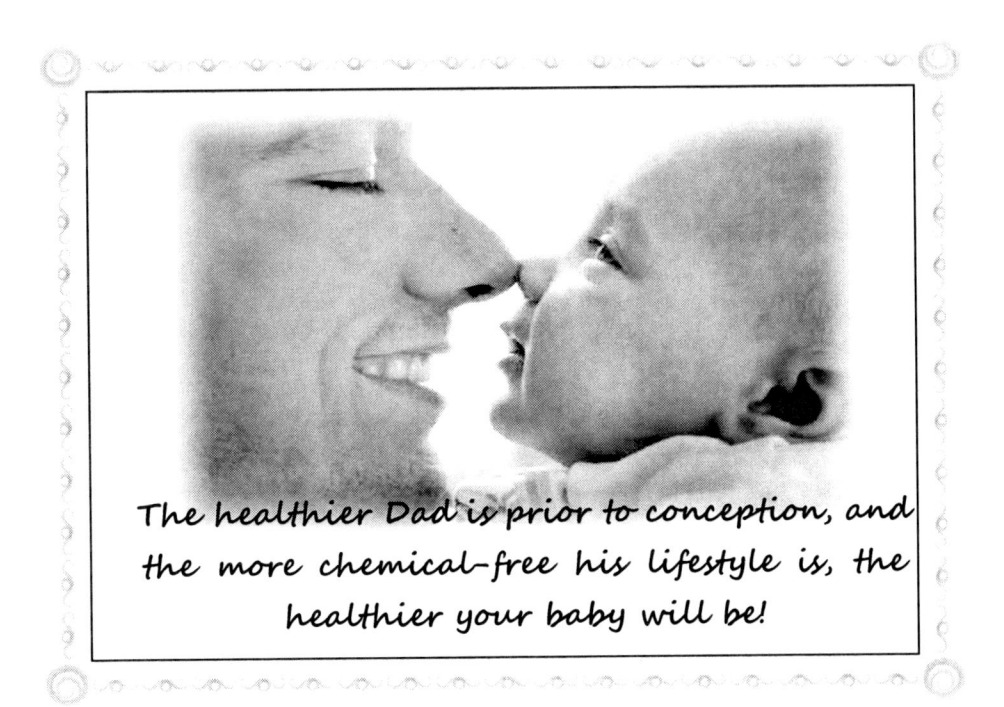

The healthier Dad is prior to conception, and the more chemical-free his lifestyle is, the healthier your baby will be!

MAKE YOUR HOME A SPERM-SAFE ZONE!

While avoiding potentially toxic chemicals isn't always possible, when it comes to your own home turf, you do have a choice. This is why I have always recommended that my patients use "green" products in their home and yard as much as possible. These are items that don't include many of the more harmful chemicals, or if they do, they are present in much lesser amounts.

Products to concentrate on include household cleaners, room deodorizers, insect repellants, rug shampoos, bathroom cleaners, household glue (like the kind used to lay carpet or put up paneling), laundry soaps and other home maintenance products, as well as lawn and garden care.

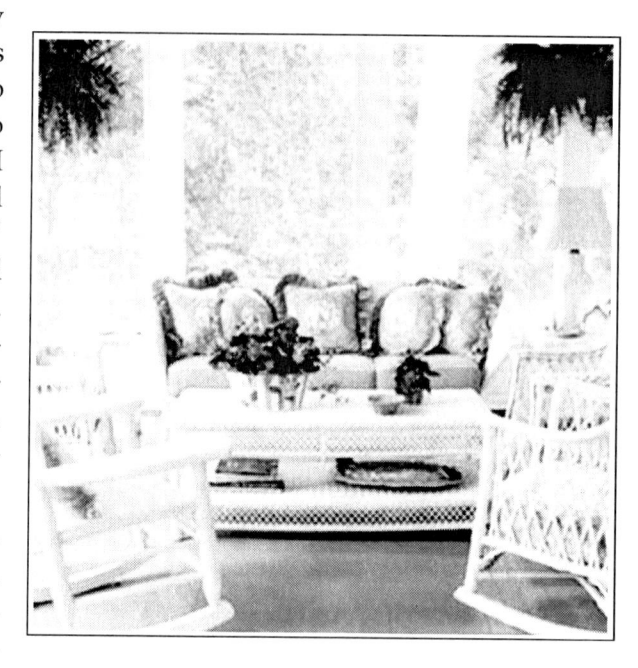

Moreover, you should also pay attention to the contents of many home decorating and even hobby products, since some may contain sperm-offensive toxins. According to studies conducted at the University of North Carolina at Chapel Hill, chemicals and solvents commonly found in many house paints, paint thinners, and paint strippers lead to defects in sperm that increase the risk of abnormalities in the children they conceive.

Fortunately, today there are many safer alternatives to the products we use every day. This includes safer, healthier paints – such as Benjamin Moore's AURA (which carry a "Green Promise" that ingredients meet or surpass chemical safety standards) - as well as natural home care products such as those made by Bon Ami, CleanWell, Method, and Mrs. Meyers.

As such I strongly urge you to use my Green Fertility Shopping List found at www.GreenFertility.com

Protecting His Fertility : Where To Begin

While some of the factors which impact male fertility are clearly under your partner's control, there are others which, due to circumstances simply can't be avoided. In fact, just living in today's high tech- chemical-laden world is a challenge to everyone's health and fertility!

The good news is that every man can take steps to overcome at least some of these challenges and in the process insure not just his fertility, but his sexual vitality and overall health as well. And one of the best ways to do this is via a pre-conception exam.

In much the same way that I recommend you have a "fertility check-up" before attempting conception, I also recommend that your partner have one as well. In many instances his regular internist may be able to perform much of what is needed, however if you have had a problem getting pregnant for while, or if he is over age 45, then I strongly recommend he visit a male urologist - a type of physician who specializes in the male reproductive system.

The Male Fertility Checkup: What It Must Include

Regardless of the type of doctor he sees, his fertility exam should include the following steps:

1. Health History Check - Much like your exam, the male fertility check should begin with a through reproductive history . This should include:

- **Sexual Health History:** Here the doctor is looking for any indications of sexual malfunction including inability to have an erection, loss of sexual desire, inability to maintain an erection, premature or no ejaculation, pain during intercourse or any sexual activity. Any or all of these symptoms may be indications of an underlying problem that can be related to several fertility-robbing diseases and conditions.

- **Sexually Transmitted Disease Check** - This should include any indication of previous sexually transmitted diseases, including when they occurred and the treatment received. It should also include any indication of chronic infections such as Herpes, and the date of the last breakout. This is also an important time to bring to the doctor's attention any suspicious "symptoms" including redness, rashes, itching, bumps or blisters, even if they disappeared on their own.

- **FATHERHOOD HISTORY -** Your partner should mention if he has ever fathered a child, if the child was born, and any indications of problems such as miscarriage, repeated miscarriage, or congenital abnormalities involving any pregnancy with any partner.

-

- **FAMILY HISTORY** - This should focus on any family history of birth defects, genetic abnormalities, inherited diseases, prostate disease or infertility.

2. THE TESTICLE CHECK : Here the doctor is looking for any indication of lumps, tenderness, discoloration, swelling, rigidity of the testicles inside the scrotal sac.

3. THE PENIS CHECK - What matters most here is any sign of discoloration, growths, lesions, blisters, warts or abnormal discharge. The doctor should gently squeeze the tip of the penis for the presence of abnormal discharge. If there is the discharge will be tested for bacteria or viruses and if found, an antibiotic will be prescribed.)

4. THE RECTAL EXAM - This is essential if your partner has a family history of prostate disease or if he has symptoms of prostate related problems, such as difficulty urinating.

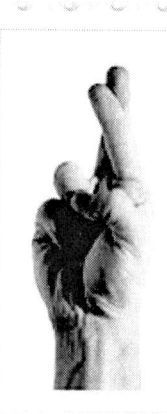

Honesty The Best Male Fertility Policy!

While most men avoid going to the doctor, studies show that those who do aren't always truthful about their symptoms. But when it comes to fertility, honesty is the best policy - so urge your partner to answer his doctor's questions truthfully & not to hold anything back in the way of symptoms or problems.

Protecting And Enhancing Fertility: What Every Man Can Do Right Now!

As many sperm-hating dangers as there appear to be in the world, the good news is there are also many things your partner can do to arm and protect his fertility as well as his virility now, and for years to come. And in doing so increase not just his fertility but your ability to get pregnant!

To help him make the right choices - and choose the right defenses - what follows are the factors I have found most helpful for my patients - foods, minerals, supplements and a few lifestyle changes that I know can make a difference in his fertility profile. I urge you to share this information with him and for the two of you to work together towards achieving that healthy and fertile lifestyle!

So where does it begin ? There's no better place to start than right at the kitchen table – with what research has shown are a number of sperm-happy foods!

Feed His Sperm: Six Super Sperm-Happy Meals Your Man Will Love!

It's not exactly like feeding those guppies in your coy pond, but it is a fact that sperm need good nutrition! This is doubly true in a world where so many of our lifestyle factors deplete essential nutrients.

And certainly, many of the same foods that foster female fertility also promote male fertility. This is particularly true when it comes to fruits and vegetables most of which provide us with an abundance of antioxidants and other nutrients that can boost not only your fertility but your overall health as well. But that said there are also a few key foods that are extra special for men – those high in nutrients proven to have a powerful effect on the production of healthy sperm and the upkeep of a healthy male reproductive system overall.

So what should a man eat to promote better fertility? Here are 6 scrumptious ways to boost his fertility with the foods that can keep sperm happy and healthy! Plus visit us online at GreenFertility.com for the recipes to these and other fertility boosting meals!

SPERM FOOD # 1:
PIZZA WITH GARLIC!

It may not be your idea of the most romantic meal, but studies have shown that this dish contains two of the most important nutrients essential to male fertility: Lycopene and selenium. The lycopene is found in tomatoes, with cooked tomatoes having even more than the fresh whole fruit – and it's one of the most important "sperm foods" your partner can eat.

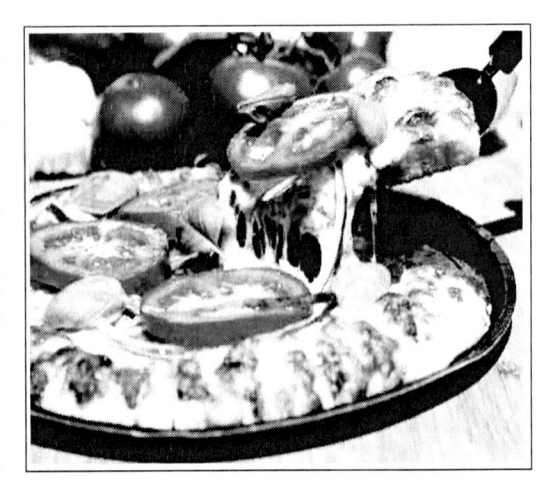

Indeed, in one study conducted on men with low sperm count, researchers at the All India Institute of Medical Sciences in New Delhi found that twice daily supplements of lycopene had a dramatic improvement on sperm.

More specifically, 70% of the men experienced an increase in sperm concentration, while 58% had an actual increase in sperm count - all within 9 months increasing their intake of lycopene.

Moreover, 36% of the men who were unable to previously father a child were able to do so thanks to lycopene! And certainly, supplements of this nutrient are an important option - which you'll learn more about in a few minutes. But I also believe that getting your lycopene from foods is equally important - simply because you also get a boat load of other helpful nutrients at the same time! In addition to tomatoes, lycopene is also found in watermelon, grapes and some shellfish.

To further enhance the effects of the lycopene, garlic is a great garnish! Packed with the mineral selenium – which is a key factor in the production of healthy sperm – garlic also has been shown to help repair damage to DNA.

And this in turn may help protect sperm from some of the environmental toxins that can cause cell damage.

SPERM FOOD # 2:
HOT CHILI WITH BEEF AND BEANS

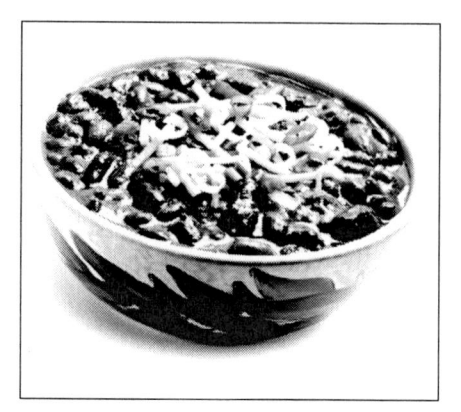

I don't know too many men who can walk away from a steaming bowl of chili - possibly because we are genetically programmed to know what's good for our fertility! And in fact, this is one sperm-happy meal that can make a real difference! What's the secret? Lean red beef is packed with zinc, a critical mineral for male sexual function, and necessary for the metabolism of testosterone, sperm production, motility, and sperm count.

Zinc is also essential for reducing estrogen in male reproductive tissues, which can be extremely important when men are exposed to environmental "xeno estrogens". Moreover, deficiencies of zinc are actually quite common – and the more sex a man has, the more likely he is to be deficient. Why? Each time a man ejaculates he lose 5% of his zinc concentration. Plus, did you know that every drink containing alcohol zaps zinc from his body? It does, along with coffee, tea and very high fiber foods, which also inhibit zinc absorption.

The beans component of a good chili are high in protein and fiber, both important for male fertility, as well as being packed with folic acid – which we now know is not only a key nutrient for female fertility but also male fertility. Indeed, in studies conducted at the University of California, Berkeley and published in the journal *Human Reproduction* researchers found that man who had the highest dietary intake of folic acid also had the lowest level of defective or abnormal sperm. In fact men who had the highest dietary intake of folate – 772 to 1,150 mcg daily – had a up to a 30% lower frequency of several types of sperm abnormalities directly related to birth defects and miscarriage. Moreover, another study recently published in *Human Reproduction* found that men who ate a diet high in lean red beef, potatoes and beans, had a higher pregnancy success rate when participating in fertility treatments such as IVF or ICSI. Almost any type of bean is good for men with the exception of soybeans which should be avoided due to their possible estrogenic effects.

SPERM FOOD # 3:
SALMON BURGERS ON WHOLE GRAIN BREAD
WITH ONIONS, AND A SIDE OF COLE SLAW

This combination of foods is so downright healthy for sperm it's almost magical! And the magic can be found in the abundance of Omega-3 fatty acids, folic acid and selenium – three of the most powerful super sperm foods.

But why are these foods – and specifically these nutrients – so important? Omega-3 fatty acids are found in high concentrations in the tail of healthy sperm. Indeed, in one study recently published in the *Journal of Lipids* doctors found that an ample supply of Omega-3 fatty acids could actually reverse some forms of male infertility related to sperm abnormalities.

Moreover, when levels of Omega-3 drop, there may be a decrease in the number of healthy sperm available for fertilization. Moreover, when it short supply Omega-3 is replaced inside the tail of the sperm with cholesterol, which slows down sperm maturity and affects sperm motility, both of which can lead to infertility.

Fortunately the type of Omega-3 fatty acids on which sperm thrive can be found in great abundance in cold water fish, particularly salmon – so eating fish burgers two to three times per week can offer your partner a real fertility boost. (Also remember that earlier I told you how Omega-3 fatty acids are also important to female fertility – so be sure that you and your partner share these fish meals together!).

When it comes to flavoring the salmon, your partner should definitely load up on onions. Like garlic they contain lots of selenium, necessary for strong sperm production. The side of cole slaw gives him the benefit of not only antioxidant protection – which can keep sperm healthy - but also provides him with a healthy dose of the phytonutrient Diindolylmethane, or DIM. How can this help? DIM has the power to block certain types of estrogenic stimulation which he might otherwise get from environmental exposures, particularly toxins known as endocrine disrupters. Plus, when you add in the folic acid benefits of whole grain bread you have a meal that is a sure male fertility winner!

Sperm Food # 4:
Organic Lean Roast Beef and Mashed Potatoes

If your guy is an old fashioned "meat and potatoes" man, then you're in luck – because while he's satisfying his appetite he's giving a boost to his sperm!

In one important multi center study conducted in the Netherlands, doctors reported that men who followed the traditional "Dutch " diet – consisting of lots of lean beef, potatoes and whole grains - appeared to have better semen quality and a higher concentration of healthier sperm, then men who ate other types of foods.

While some previous studies have shown men who eat a lot of red meat have lower sperm counts, many believe this is ostensibly due to the influence of natural and synthetic estrogens used to stimulate cattle growth.

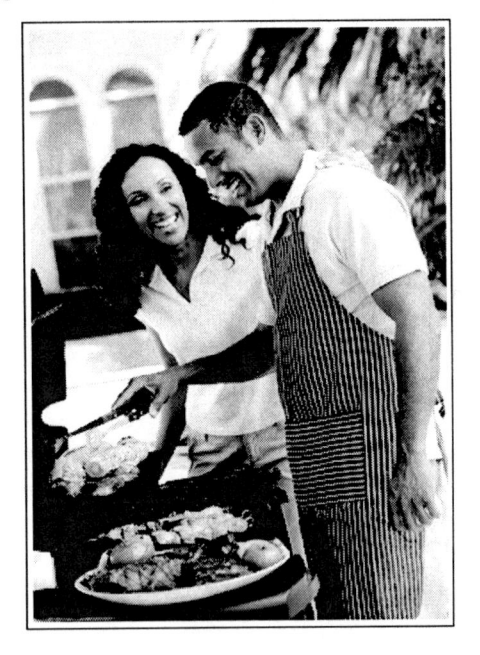

As such the newest studies suggest that moderate consumption of red meat from organically raised cattle not subject to hormone stimulation, will have a favorable impact on sperm.

In general I always recommend to my patients that whenever possible they should eat organically raised beef and poultry, or at least purchase brands that do not give their livestock hormone-laced feed.

As to the potato portion of the "meat and potatoes" meal, the key element here is lots of folic acid, as well as Vitamin C , which as you read earlier, can help keep sperm healthy and cut down on the number of defective sperm manufactured by the body.

Sperm Food # 5: Whole Grain Mac & Cheese & A Cup of Tomato Soup

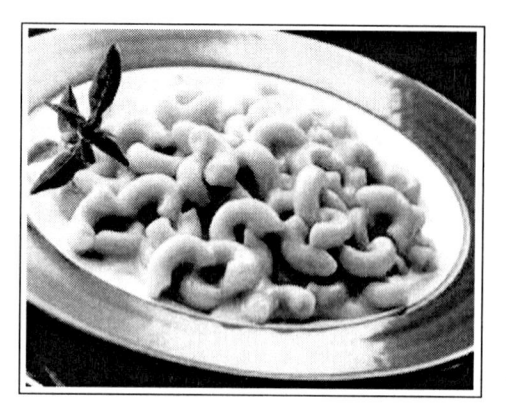

There is perhaps nothing more satisfying on a cold winter day than a steamy bowl of tomato soup and a heaping portion of Mac & Cheese. If the macaroni is whole wheat pasta and the cheese is low fat, this meal will offer your partner one hefty fertility boost!

The whole grains provide both fiber and folate, plus a healthy dose of vitamin B6, which, together with zinc is essential for the production of healthy sperm.

Meanwhile the cheese will offer him a good serving of calcium, another sperm-friendly nutrient. In fact, studies show calcium may be able to reverse completely some forms of male infertility.

In one study published recently in the *Journal of Nutrition* researchers from the University of Wisconsin at Madison found that when male rats with impaired fertility were given either calcium supplements or vitamin D supplements, their mating potential was restored equally as quickly.

While in the past it was believed that Vitamin D supplements were the link to improved male fertility many now believe it may actually be Vitamin D's ability to properly metabolize calcium that offers the real boost.

To give your Mac and Cheese an extra boost, add in a serving of fortified low-fat milk when melting the cheese. This will not only increase the calcium levels but also add in some extra vitamin D.

And of course the tomato soup will add another boost via it's high lycopene content. As you read earlier, cooked tomatoes are even more packed with this nutrient than raw tomatoes, so a steamy cup of tomato soup is like a refreshing gulp of goodness for his sperm!

Sperm Food # 6: Fruit Salad

While it may not be the heartiest of typical "male" meal choices, I can promise that getting your partner to chow down on a heaping bowl of fresh fruit salad will do more for his fertility than he can imagine!

Fruits to concentrate on include blueberries, strawberries, watermelon, peaches, mangoes, cantaloupe and pomegranate. Each one of these fruits is a symphony of antioxidants and vitamins including Vitamin A, C, and E, as well as phytonutrients known as carotenoids. This nutrient is found in great concentration in a man's testes and believed to be intrinsic for healthy sperm production. In addition, the antioxidant vitamins found in these fruits have been shown in studies to protect against the free radical damage caused by environmental assaults - toxins and chemical exposures that can lead to male infertility. If he also adds a dollop of yogurt or even a serving of low fat vanilla ice cream, he'll get the added boost of calcium and vitamin D, for a super fertility snack or dessert.

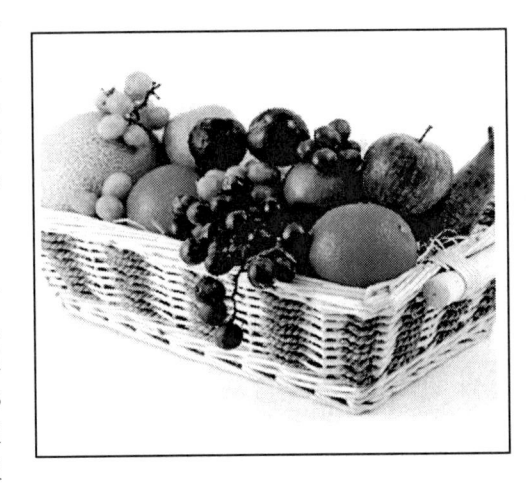

> Q: My husband is trying to lose weight and is using meal replacement supplements. Will this harm his fertility?
>
> A: While meal supplements won't harm your husband on a short term basis, over time they can cause nutrient deficiencies that can harm his sperm. This is particularly true if the supplement does not contain adequate vitamins, minerals and fiber. You should encourage him to lose weight via a nutritionally balanced diet that is simply lower in calories - it's best for sperm and best for his overall health.

Weight And Male Fertility: How Much Is Too Much?

While it may be important to help your partner "feed his sperm" that doesn't mean he shouldn't also remain conscious of maintaining a healthy weight – not only to protect his overall health, but specifically to protect his fertility.

How can this help? As I mentioned to you earlier, one of the fertility perils of being overweight is that excess fat can hold in body heat. And when it does so in the vicinity of the testicles, there can be some real sperm production consequences.

But that's not the only reason men looking to become fathers should control their weight. In one study conducted by the US National Institutes of Health researchers discovered that being just 20 pounds overweight increases a man's risk of being infertile by about 10%. The research, published in the journal *Epidemiology* in 2006 used questionnaires filled out by some 1500 farmers and their wives. The women completed health questions that included their reproductive history while the men reported their weight and height.

The analysis of the data was restricted to those couples who had been trying to conceive in the previous 4 years, and where the woman was under age 40. When the data was compiled the researchers discovered that a man's BMI or body mass index, was an independent risk factor for infertility.

Indeed, after adjusting the results for other factors linked to male fertility – such as smoking, alcohol intake, and chemical exposures - as well as factors in the woman that could have contributed to conception problems, the doctors *still found* overwhelming evidence that a man's weight matters. And the more he weighs, the greater his risk of infertility, *no matter his age*.

More recent studies have shown that men who are obese have lower semen quality in general, as well as hormonal issues that might contribute to fertility problems.

"This study provides data on some additional health problems associated with obesity," said David A. Schwartz, M.D., director of the National Institute of Environmental Health Sciences. "Preventing obesity can help improve men's overall health, perhaps even their reproductive health."

Indeed, the study conclusions make sense - particularly since we already know that being overweight influences the production of hormones.

More specifically, when a man is overweight, a greater portion of his testosterone gets converted into estrogen – and that affects both sperm production and the quality of the sperm that is produced.

THE GOOD NEWS: When a man loses weight and gets his BMI as close to normal as possible, it provides a natural boost to sperm production and *increases fertility*.

COKE, COFFEE AND MALE FERTILITY

If you're trying to get pregnant, your partner might want to cut down on the number of 18 ounce big gulps of cola he consumes every day. Why? The latest studies show that when consumed to excess, high caffeine sodas can have a detrimental impact on male fertility.

More specifically, research on more than 2,500 Danish men found that those who consumed more than 800 mg of caffeine daily - or about 14 liter bottles of cola a week - had both lower sperm counts and lower overall sperm concentrations then men who consumed more moderate levels of caffeine.

The findings, published in the *American Journal of Epidemiology* did not suggest whether the caffeine in coffee or tea had the same effect, and scientists say that other components of the soft drinks, including high fructose corn syrup may be a contributing factor.

But remember, he doesn't have to cut out caffeinated beverages altogether. There is some research to suggest that in moderate amounts caffeine may actually help improve sperm motility.

THE BEST ADVICE: Up to 3 cups of coffee or tea per day, and two 12 ounce cans of caffeinated soda per day should be safe to consume. However, if his sperm count is already low, I would recommend no more than 1 cup of coffee or one caffeinated soda daily.

The Super Nutrients For Male Fertility

In addition to the powerful fertility boost your partner can get from food, there are also certain specific nutrients – vitamins as well as herbs – that studies show increase sperm production as well as improving sperm maturation and motility.

While most young, healthy men will get all they need from eating a balanced diet and taking a daily multi vitamin, if you are having problems conceiving, then your partner may also benefit from taking some additional supplements above and beyond what a standard multi-vitamin pill provides.

So, what does he need to maximize his fertility? The following nutrients and herbs have been shown in a number of studies to support male fertility as well as overall health.

As is the case with your body, it is impossible to separate out healthy fertility from overall good health. They work together and when you "feed" one, you "feed" both!

The Top Nutrients That Sperm Love!

1. **Amino Acids L-Arginine and L-Carnetine.**
   Necessary for both egg and sperm production, amino acids are the building blocks of life that can literally help sperm to develop and mature. One particular amino acid known as L-arginine has been known to be particularly powerful for increasing male fertility.

   In studies on L-Carnetine men who used supplements for just 4 months increased their sperm count by over 30%. Other studies found L-Carnetine was more effective than testosterone in overcoming erectile dysfunction.

Recommended Dosage: L-Carnitine: Start with 250 to 500 milligrams once daily and gradually build to three times daily for a total of 1000 to 1,500 mg daily for 3 to 4 months.
L-Arginine - The average dose is 500 mg but it's safe to use up to 1 gram or 1,000 mg per day. However, your partner should not use these supplements if he has a history of the herpes virus, as this may increase the risk of a break out.

2. **VITAMIN A**
    Simply put, a man's body can't produce testosterone if he is short on vitamin A, making this a "must have" nutrient for him. In fact, without sufficient Vitamin A his overall sperm count will plummet, while the number of abnormal sperm he produces will rise. Vitamin A is also important because as a "carotinoid" phytonutrient it makes up 1/3 of the volume of each sperm. As an antioxidant, Vitamin A protects sperm from free radical damage. And finally, this is also an essential nutrient for the health of the seminiferous tubules, the area of a man's reproduction system which helps sperm to mature.

    Recommended Dosage: Up to 10,000 IUs daily, taken with foods that contain some fat or oil for best absorption.

3. **VITAMIN B6 (PYRIDOXINE)**
    This is yet another essential nutrient for the production of testosterone as well as being a necessary component for sperm production. A deficiency of B6 has been shown in animal studies to result in infertility.

    Recommended Dosage: Up to 500 mg daily. However this vitamin should always be taken in conjunction with a minimum of 100 mg of B Complex, which is a combination of all the key B vitamins. For best absorption, always take B6 with the mineral zinc (see below).

4. **VITAMIN B12**
    When levels of this vitamin are low there is not just a reduction in sperm count, but those sperm which are produced are generally poor "swimmers". Deficiencies also mean an increased number of abnormal sperm. This nutrient is crucial even if sperm count is low-normal.

    Recommended Dosage: 3 - 4 mg daily

5. **FOLATE (FOLIC ACID)**
    A key nutrient in the production of sperm, deficiencies of this B vitamin can also affect sperm motility and lead to a higher rate of abnormal sperm. It's best taken with vitamin C, which increases absorption.

    Recommended Dosage: Up to 1000 mcg daily

6. **VITAMIN C**

   Not only has a deficiency of Vitamin C in men been linked to a higher incidence of birth defects, that deficiency also decreases sperm count and motility. When a deficiency is severe enough, sperm actually "clump" together making it impossible to fertilize an egg. Vitamin C is also a powerful antioxidant that protects against many forms of environmental damage. So, the higher the level of exposures, the greater the need to supplement with this nutrient. Moreover in one study published in the *Annals of the New York Academy of Science*, doctors found that after one week of daily doses of 1,000 mg of vitamin C, sperm counts rose by some 140%.

   Recommended Dosage: Up to 1,500 mg per day.

7. **VITAMIN D**

   For many years doctors believed vitamin D was only important for female fertility. Today however, a number of studies have shown it also plays a key role in male fertility. In fact, in one study of nearly 800 men with fertility problems presented before the Fertility Society of Australia, Dr. Anne Clarke reported more than one-third were severely deficient in vitamin D.

   Recommended Dosage : 2,000 – 4,000 mg daily in winter, 1,500 -3,000 mg daily in summer. (Note: The recommended dosage continues to increase as more research comes in).

8. **VITAMIN E**

   Without adequate amounts of vitamin E, studies show a male simply cannot reproduce. Not only do testicles begin to degenerate, but their ability to manufacture sperm comes to a complete halt. At the same time, when vitamin E is plentiful, it can help sperm penetrate an egg – which means supplements may be particularly helpful to those couples who suffer from "unexplained infertility", of which one cause can be difficulty in sperm penetration.

   Recommended Dosage: Up to 800 IUs daily

9. **SELENIUM**

   This mineral is so key to male fertility that long term deficiencies can result in complete infertility.

   Why is this mineral so important? It helps the body produce enough normally shaped sperm to ensure conception. It also plays a key role in maintaining the health of the epididymis, the area of the male reproductive system where sperm matures and is held before final release.

   And finally, it also functions as a protective antioxidant. In one study published in the *Archives of Andrology* researchers found that the antioxidants vitamin E and selenium improved the ability of sperm to swim - a skill necessary to reach the egg.

   Recommended Dosage: 75 mcg per day

10. **ZINC**

    Considered to be the predominant "male nutrient", the mineral zinc is critical for male sexual function, affecting everything from the metabolism of testosterone, to the growth of the testicles, to sperm production, motility and count.

    Zinc also helps suppress excess estrogen in the male body, so it can be very helpful for those men exposed to environmental estrogens.

    Moreover, most men are zinc-deficient. Why?

    Each time a man ejaculates he loses about 5 mg of zinc. So if you and your partner have a very active sex life, then it's easy to see how quickly he can become deficient in this essential fertility mineral. Moreover, since alcohol, coffee and high fiber foods can also deplete zinc, a deficiency can occur even quicker.

    One study published in the journal *Fertility and Sterility* reported that men with fertility problems who took a daily dose of 66 mg of zinc in combination with 5 mg of folic acid for just 6 months, increased their sperm count by some 74 percent.

    Recommended Dosage : Up to 100 mg daily

11. Coenzyme Q10

Present in large amounts in seminal fluid, research indicates this nutrient energizes sperm, increasing the ability to swim through a woman's reproductive system and reach her egg. There is also research showing fertilization rates rise when CoQ10 supplements are given to men undergoing the male fertility procedure known as ICSI.

Recommended Dosage: 200 mg per day

12. Glutathione

This is a molecule that is made in the body from three major amino acids: L-glutamic acid, L-cysteine and glycine. Together they not only offer a powerful antioxidant punch, but glutathione is necessary for the formation of a protein that enables sperm to swim.

Recommended Dosage : 500 mg per day on an empty stomach

Give His Fertility An Extra Fertility Boost With Essential Fatty Acids!

You've already read about the importance of omega 3 fatty acids in *your* diet. But it's also important that your partner maintain a balance between omega 3 and omega 6 as well since these two essential fatty acids work together to help regulate hormones related to sperm production. Unfortunately most diets are abundant in omega 6 (it's found in so many foods!) while omega 3 is frequently in short supply. Since sperm actually contain high concentrations of omega 3's, and require these nutrients to function, it's essential that these fatty acids remain in good supply. The best way to insure that is by taking supplements!
Recommend Dosage: 2000 mg per day of omega 3

Ancient Chinese & Modern Herbs For Male Fertility

While there are a variety of herbs that have long been associated with male fertility, there is little in the way of medical studies showing they work. Of course this doesn't mean they don't – it just means that we don't yet have the scientific proof to back up what can sometimes be generations or even centuries of successful use.

That said, there are a few herbs that have been tested and found to have some important effects, and I've included four of the most popular ones in the section that follows.

When it comes to dosages, my best suggestion is to purchase a credible product from a well known company, and then follow directions on how much to use. Also remember that when it comes to herbal products, more is not always better – in fact sometimes taking too much of a substance can cause an effect opposite of what you are trying to achieve. So your partner should not deviate too far from the recommended amounts on each product.

Also, it's best to try each of these supplements separately before attempting to combine them – and certainly they should never be taken all at once. By testing out each herb separately for 8 to 12 weeks, it's much easier to judge which is the most personally effective.

Four Key Herbs For Male Fertility

- **PANAX GINSENG** - For centuries this has been known as the " male tonic", used by generations of Chinese medicine practitioners as a way to improve overall male health. Now studies show it may have a direct impact on testosterone, increasing levels of this hormone as well as increasing sperm count. Siberian ginseng (*Eleutherococcus senticosus*) has also been shown to be similarly helpful.

- **ASTRAGALUS** (*Astragalus membranaceus*) - According to a study published in the journal *Alternative Medicine Review*, researchers tested the extracts of 18 major Chinese medicinal plants for their ability to increase sperm motility. Of the the 18, only Astragalus was shown to make a significant difference. While this was an in vitro test wherein the extracts were directly added to the sperm, still , many believe that when taken internally as an herbal extract, the effects on sperm will be similar.

- **SAW PALMETTO** (*Serenoa repens*) – This herb first came to prominence as a treatment for benign prostate disease. Now, however, it is quickly gaining a reputation as an overall tonic for the male reproductive system and may have some positive effects on healthy sperm production.

- **MACA ROOT-** This powerful plant contains a full complement of amino acids, complex carbohydrates, vitamins B1, B2, C, E and the minerals calcium, phosphorous, zinc, magnesium and iron. As such, it has been used by many South American cultures for generations, as a way to increase the production of testosterone, encourage the production of healthy sperm, and generally tone up the male reproductive system – even to the point of increasing libido in some men.

FERTILITY SUPPLEMENTS FOR MEN

As you read in a previous chapter, an off-the-shelf product known as "Fertility Blend" for women is one of the few herbal supplements with some good science behind its use.

Now the same company is also offering *Fertility Blend for Men* - a similar product that blends ancient Chinese medicine with modern western technology to help improve male fertility - with some good results.

While the male version is not supported by the same "gold standard" double blind studies conducted on the female version, the formulation is based on ingredients that have been proven in independent studies to be very effective in boosting male fertility including L-carnitine, Vitamins C and E, green tea and selenium . Another antioxidant known as ferulic acid is found in Dong Quai and it's also present in Fertility Blend as well as zinc, and vitamins B6, B12 and folate.

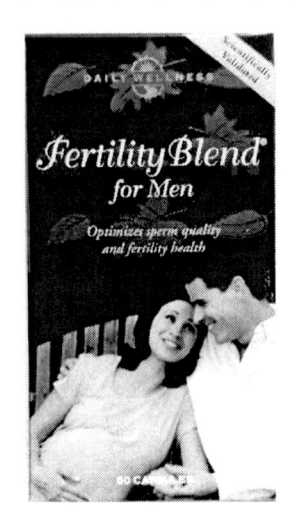

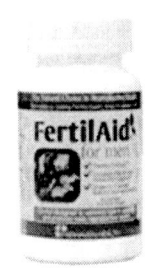

Another option is *FertilAid for Men*. Results from a recent small but important independent clinical study on *FertilAid for Men* indicates significant improvements in sperm health, with marked increases in the total number of motile sperm of 20% or more. The main ingredients in *FertilAid for Men* include L-Carnitine, vitamins C & E, selenium and grape seed extract, zinc, beta carotene and maca root - all natural ingredients that research has shown can make a difference.

In fact, if your partner does not want to take individual herbs and you just can't get him to swallow a vitamin pill, both of these products offer an important combination of herbs and nutrients designed to boost his sperm count and protect his fertility. Other products in the FertilAid line include *CountBoost* and *Motility Boost* -which feature slightly different nutrient configurations. Learn more about all these products at GreenFertility.com

Stress & Sperm & Getting Pregnant: What You Both Must Know

One of the fertility facts that often surprises so many of my patients is discovering just how "delicate" a man's reproductive system can be! Unlike the "macho" indestructible persona that most men assign to their fertility, the truth is that oftentimes something as simple as a cold or a virus can knock a man's sperm count out for days! In fact, everything from the ability to have an erection, to the ability to ejaculate, to the most basic of all sperm making functions, can be affected by some everyday factors we might never associate with fertility.

But if I had to focus on just one of these lifestyle factor that affects men more than any other I would have to say "stress" is at the top of the list. Indeed, when a man is under prolonged stress, or even low levels of ongoing tension, his reproductive system takes a huge hit. What happens?

First, we now know that prolonged stress can affect the functioning of the hypothalamus gland – the area of the brain that helps produce both FH and LH in men and women. In men, however, when production of these brain hormones go down, testosterone production also suffers. And when it does, sperm count can plummet. Moreover, low testosterone not only decreases a man's desire for sex, but also can lead to erectile dysfunction. In short, many men who are extremely stressed can have difficulty obtaining and maintaining an erection – which clearly impacts fertility.

Interestingly, new research has also begun to emerge showing that stress can increase the negative impact of other factors – including exposures to environmental chemicals. In one study published in the journal *Endocrinology* in 2009, researchers from Edinburgh, Scotland suggested that living with a fair amount of daily stress can increase the rate at which chemical exposures can cause adverse health effects.

In short, men who are under significant stress may be impacted by fertility robbing environmental factors sooner and to a greater extent then men who are less stressed.

And when it comes to specific stresses among the most significant for men is that which is associated with loss – be it job loss, loss of a loved one, or even business or financial loss. All can lead to the kind of stress that can reduce sperm count by 10% or more. If a man is already under stress when the loss occurs, or if he is stressed about conception problems or fertility treatments, the impact on sperm can be even greater.

Ultimately this leads to a kind of "round robin" effect where the stress leads to fertility problems which lead to more stress, which impact fertility to an even greater degree.

BLOW OFF STEAM – GET PREGNANT FASTER!

No matter how stressed out your partner may be, taking steps to reduce his tension can have many positive effects on his fertility. In fact, studies show that when men with fertility problems make a conscious effort to reduce their stress levels – or at the very least, make the effort to "blow off steam" and keep stress levels from building - it can reverse even a very low sperm count!

Certainly, stress reduction is a highly personal experience . And what works for one doesn't always work for all. But many of my patients have told me that their partners seem most relaxed when they exercise more. And as long as he doesn't over do it, this may be a great way to blow off steam and increase his overall health.

But that said, don't let your partner overlook the power of *"passive" exercise* as a wonderful way to reduce stress and increase his fertility. Activities can include yoga, meditation and Tai Chi, all of which can not only help reduce stress but in some instances also offer some fertility benefits of their own. In fact, the two of you can work together to reduce stress utilizing any of the relaxation exercises detailed in the section on exercise and female fertility.

Moreover, if you and your partner have been trying to conceive for a while, there is some clinical evidence to show that both your fertility and his might benefit from some counseling specifically geared towards helping infertile couples cope.

Indeed, clinical researchers have found that professional counseling as well as participation in support groups led by professionals can not only reduce the stress associated with conception problems, but in doing increase fertility.

In fact many fertility clinics now routinely offer this kind of group support for their patients. But even if you and your partner are not seeing a fertility expert, many of these centers may still provide a reference to stress reduction groups in your area, so don't be afraid to call and ask.

Of course the one thing you don't want to encourage your partner to do is use alcohol or medications in an attempt to relax. While an occasional glass of wine isn't going to do any harm, with continued use alcohol and drugs can have some devastating effects on fertility. When combined with the damage already caused by stress, the effects can be even greater.

GETTING PREGNANT: SOME FINAL WORDS

When it comes to getting pregnant, there is no question that it's a "couples" effort. But what many couples don't realize is that protecting fertility, and when necessary doing what you can to boost and insure fertility, should also be a team effort shared between you and your partner.

While the steps each of you may need to take can be somewhat different, in many instances, maximizing both male and female fertility often comes down to avoiding or including many of the same factors – be it foods, nutrients or lifestyle habits and practices.

And in many ways and for many reasons, this is a good thing. Why?

I have always believed that when a couple works together towards a shared goal they not only achieve that goal faster and easier, but the support they give each other along the way can work to not only cement their relationship, but in many ways have beneficial health effects that in the end can help bolster their combined fertility – making the sum much greater than either individual part.

At the same time I have seen all too many couples grappling with infertility, or even just trying to get pregnant - turn on each other and begin to pull apart . This an issue that not only increases their individual stress levels, but in doing so moves them farther away from their parenting goals and dreams. For this reason I want to urge each of you to share the information in this entire book with your partner – not just this chapter on male fertility. I also want to encourage you to work together, as team, towards your parenting goals.

Too often I have seen the stress of infertility drive couples apart, causing them to blame each other for what goes wrong and filling their lives with negative energy. Before long, they stop communicating with each other, and finally, they can stop talking altogether, and instead keep their feelings bottled up and their resentments deep inside.

And I can't tell you just how destructive this can be to not only your mental health, but your overall physical health and especially, your fertility.

At the same time, if you keep the lines of communication open, if you talk to one another (and not "at" each other), if you continue to view having a baby as a joint effort in which you both share equal responsibility, you will not only have an easier time getting pregnant, but the two of you will grow much closer together in the process.

Most importantly do not blame yourselves or each other for what might be less than optimal conception conditions. Instead, take that energy and turn it into positive fruitful support for each other. Continue to do as much as you can together – from sharing "fertile" meals, to exercising and relaxing together, to continuing to share your hopes, your dreams and yes your fears. If small changes in diet and lifestyle are necessary, support and encourage one another to make those changes and become a force for positive change in each other's lives.

When you do I can promise you that this wonderful shared journey you are on will be brighter, happier, more memorable and most of all more "fertile".

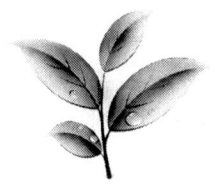

CHAPTER SIXTEEN

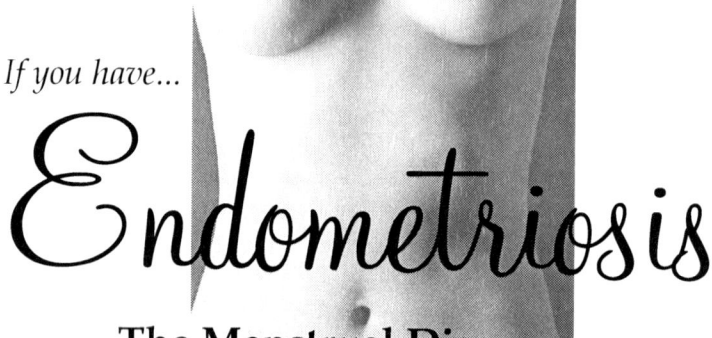

If you have...

Endometriosis

The Menstrual Disease That Can Harm Fertility:
Some Special Advice

For some of you reading this book, getting pregnant will be so fast and easy you'll barely have time to try all of the suggestions before you hear those glorious words " Congratulations you're pregnant!"

For others, it may take a while longer – requiring some "trial and error" experimentation with the various lifestyle changes before you find the solutions that zone in on your specific needs. But once you do I am confident that you too will be pregnant soon.

For some of you, however, having a baby will be just a bit more of a challenge. While it's definitely possible to conceive and have a healthy baby naturally, it may take you a bit more time or some additional work before it happens. This may be the case if you are among a growing number of women diagnosed with endometriosis – a menstrual related disorder that is currently the leading cause of infertility among young women. It's also one of the most under diagnosed conditions in women's health.

In fact, when I first began writing about endometriosis – back in the early 1980's - it wasn't even fully recognized as an illness! I wrote one of the very first books on this disorder (The Endometriosis Answer Book), and when I did the majority of doctors weren't even aware that the problem existed. Women who had the symptoms were frequently told that their problems were "all in their head!"

While today the diagnostic criteria and testing for this condition is light years ahead of the past, I'm sorry to say that many women are still being misdiagnosed, and too often endometriosis continues to go un-recognized and under treated.

For this reason I urge you to keep reading , and listen to your body to discover if any of the symptoms or problems I discuss apply to you. If they do, then sharing this information with your doctor can be instrumental in making sure you get the correct diagnosis, and if necessary, the correct medical treatment.

More often than not, the solutions discussed in this book – and particularly in the remainder of this chapter - will be all you need to overcome most of your fertility challenges. But in the event that you will need more help and a deeper understanding of this condition I recommend that you pick up a copy of up our companion book, *Getting Pregnant: What You Need To Know Now*. Here you will find much more in depth information on endometriosis and the medical and specifically the fertility treatments that can help you conceive.

UNDERSTANDING ENDOMETRIOSIS : WHAT YOU MUST KNOW

When I began to research and write about endometriosis, it was at the height of the feminist movement – a time when women were just beginning to enter the work force at break speed. Because the incidence of this disease was believed to be higher among women who were stressed, it was dubbed "The Career Woman's Disease" – simply because those early days of breaking through the "glass ceiling" were so stressful for women.

But today, every woman is stressed. And from the CEO at the head of a company to the stay-at-home wife and mom who is the head of her household, from young gals in their early 20's to those at the tail end of their reproductive years, we now know that endometriosis affects a wide spectrum of women, from all walks of life.

But what exactly is this curious sounding ailment - and how does it affect you? In simplest terms, endometriosis is believed to be an auto-immune disorder. This is an umbrella term used to describe any number of conditions in which your immune system reacts inappropriately to your body's own tissue.

In the case of endometriosis, problems begin when small bits of uterine tissue lining normally meant to leave your body every month during a menstrual cycle, instead migrate backwards and head into your fallopian tubes. Here the tissue can either lodge, causing blockages, or, as is most often the case, also continue to move through your tubes into your abdominal cavity. Once here, it can land on other organs, including your ovaries, the outside ends of your fallopian tubes (called the fimbria), anywhere outside of your uterus, or even on your bowels. There have also been some reports of this renegade endometrial tissue traveling through the body and land on the lung!

But this tissue migration itself isn't really the problem, because this process actually occurs in up to 90% of all women - and most do not go on to develop endometriosis. That's because in most instances, the body's immune system kicks into high gear and searches out this misplaced tissue and destroys it, thereby stopping any further abnormal activity.

For the approximately 5.5 million women with endometriosis however, the immune system fails to do its job. Instead of recognizing that this uterine tissue is in the wrong place, it views it as normal – so normal in fact it begins to signal the body to produce a series of chemicals to encourage growth! This in turn signals the tissue to implant itself on whatever organ it lands and actually begin growing!

Moreover, like the tissue inside your uterus, this renegade tissue is also hormonally charged. So, month after month, cycle after cycle, it responds to hormone stimulation by becoming thicker and growing larger. In addition, because the original deposits are also joined by new deposits left after every period, eventually these lesions can become so widespread and affect so many organs the entire pelvic cavity is affected. This spread, along with a stretching of the tissue and the development of scar tissue, both of which also occur over time, is what is often responsible for the common "tell tale" sign of endometriosis – which is chronic pelvic pain and discomfort that usually worsens in the days before each new period begins.

ENDOMETRIOSIS: THE SYMPTOMS

- Severe menstrual cramps often starting on the first day of the period.
- Ovulation pain (Mittleschmertz)
- Pelvic pain that worsens just before a period begins.
- Painful intercourse
- Infertility/ Difficulty conceiving
- Recurring bladder infections
- Pelvic cysts and tumors
- Lower back pain, with or without nausea, vomiting and dizziness during each period

It's important to note that the severity of your symptoms doesn't always correlate with the severity of your disease. It is possible to have severe endometriosis with very few symptoms or very little diseased tissue and a lot of symptoms.

Although most women who are eventually diagnosed with endometriosis usually have at least two symptoms, it's important to note that some of those symptoms can also be indicative of other disorders, including ovarian cysts or pelvic infections. This is one important reason why you must have your symptoms diagnosed by a gynecologist. Equally important to note is that for reasons we really don't understand, in some women endometriosis produces no symptoms at all.

Moreover, one of the more frustrating aspects of treating this condition is that there appears to be no correlation between the extent of disease and symptoms that are experienced. Some women who have almost every symptom on the list may have very little disease, while others may have extensive endometrial deposits in every area of their pelvis and feel no outward symptoms. In fact, sometimes the first clue that something is wrong is that they are not able to get pregnant!

HOW ENDOMETRIOSIS AFFECTS FERTILITY

When it comes to getting pregnant, having endometriosis can present some unique challenges. Often, the degree to which this disease has affected you, and the length of time you've been affected are two key points in determining just how – or even if – your fertility will be affected. That said, when problems do occur, they can impact your reproductive system in several key ways.

- **The Ovaries** – Because the ovaries are a frequent "target" for the misplaced endometrial tissue, they are often a frequent site of problems. Among the most common are the formation of what are called "chocolate cysts". Filled with old blood (the reason for the chocolate color) these cysts can dampen ovarian function, often to the point where egg growth, development and release are affected.

- **The Fallopian Tubes** – Another popular place for endometrial tissue to take hold and begin growing is inside the fallopian tubes, as well as outside, on the ends called the fimbria. When this occurs, blockages and scar tissue can develop which can keep sperm from getting to your egg, or stop a fertilized egg from getting to the uterus.

- **Uterus** - In some severe cases of endometriosis, the misplaced tissue can invade the muscular wall of the uterus resulting in a problem known as adenomyosis. Similar to a fibroid tumor these growths can interfere with embryo implantation or make it difficult for your baby to grow properly within your uterus. The result is frequently very early stage miscarriage.

- **Hormones** - In addition to causing structural damage, endometrial lesions can also emit a hormone-like substance known as "prostaglandin". This can cause contractions anywhere within the reproductive system, including not only your uterus, but also your fallopian tubes. In my experience, should these spasms occur early on in your conception they can be strong enough to push your newly fertilized egg down your fallopian tube too quickly, before your uterus is ready for implantation. When this occurs, again, miscarriage is often the result.

While any of these fertility consequences are possible in any woman who has endometriosis, most problems occur in those who remain undiagnosed and untreated. In truth, endometriosis is the leading cause of infertility in young women – but it's important to remember this is only the case when the condition is not properly treated.

Once you do receive proper care – and the earlier the better – your odds of getting pregnant go up dramatically, often to the point where your risk of infertility is only slightly higher than that of women who don't have this disease. Of course for some, the fastest and easiest route to conception is a laboratory assisted pregnancy - and when this is the case please remember there are many options and many new medical treatments available to help - including the new Green IVF natural cycle procedure you'll read about later in this book.

But that said, I would venture to guess that for many of you with endometriosis, getting pregnant on your own is not only possible, but very likely – if you take just a few simple precautions and follow a few simple rules.

To this end, I am happy to tell you that virtually all of the information you have read in this book thus far will be helpful to you. But there are also a few specific suggestions just for you – some extra guidelines and a few additional steps you can take to enhance the effects even more.

As such, what follows is some key advice for the easy and natural steps you can take to increase your odds of getting pregnant, beginning right away!

DIET AND ENDOMETRIOSIS:
THE FOOD SECRETS THAT CAN CHANGE YOUR LIFE

One of the more important studies on endometriosis to recently emerge is an analysis conducted by a group of Italian researchers. What makes this report so extraordinary for me is that it is among the first pieces of research to solidly and scientifically connect all the dots between diet and endometriosis.

Certainly I have always believed that food as well as nutrients play an essential role in controlling this condition – particularly in regard to fertility. And I have always recommended dietary changes as a means to improve symptoms. Still, I am always very excited to discover that another one of my theories is proven through meticulous scientific analysis.

This was the case a few years ago thanks to research conducted by doctors at the University of Milan and published in the journal *Human Reproduction*. Here researchers validated one of the "secrets" behind why so many of my patients with endometriosis were able to not only get pregnant, but give birth to wonderful, happy, healthy babies.

So what is the secret ? A diet high in fresh fruits and vegetables, and a reduction in the consumption of animal fat, red meat, ham and beer . How can this help?

First, in strictly physiological terms, a diet high in animal fat – including red meat - increases production of prostaglandin, a collection of unsaturated fatty acids which control smooth muscle movement and can have a direct influence on how well your ovaries function, particularly in regard to ovulation.

Moreover, endometriosis is also linked to hormonal factors, particularly an abundance of unopposed estrogen – which is estrogen without the benefit of sufficient progesterone for balance. When you eat a diet high in animal fat , it increases the production of more fat cells, which as you read earlier, contributes to the production of estrogen. But it also does something else that's key to endometriosis: It incrases *the circulation* of all that extra estrogen being produced. And so, the more animal fat you consume, the more estrogen your body produces *and the*

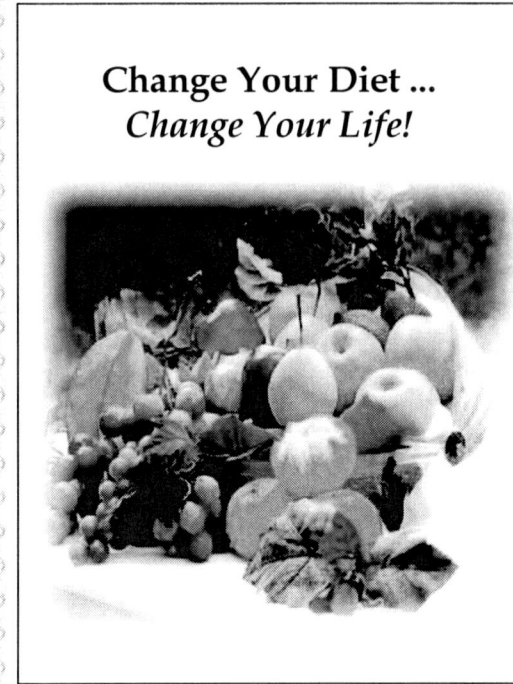

> **Change Your Diet ... *Change Your Life!***
>
> *Changing your diet so that it includes less red meat and more fruits and vegetables is one important step you can take to control your endometriosis. Not only will you feel better and experience fewer symptoms, but it will help you to get pregnant faster.*

more of that that estrogen circulates through your body. Ultimately, that's a set up for the kind of hormonal imbalance that not only contributes to endometriosis, but also dramatically increases the risk of infertility.

What can help? A diet rich in fruits and vegetables, particularly those containing the antioxidant nutrients such as vitamin C, carotenoids, folic acid and lycopene. All can help protect your body by keeping the growth of endometrial implants at bay.

So, the more fruits and vegetables you eat – and the less animal fat you consume - the harder it becomes for the misplaced endometrial tissue to grow. And that means less endometriosis to interfere with your fertility, and better baby-making chances overall!

Fanning the Flames:
How Inflammation Effects Endometriosis

In addition to the reasons I just gave for avoiding foods high in animal fat, there is yet one more concern - and it has to do with "inflammation".

As you read in an earlier chapter, inflammatory foods are those which are linked to the production of chemicals which can cause inflammation body-wide. This inflammation not only increases your risk of heart disease, high blood pressure and even cancer, but it also exacerbates fertility related conditions including endometriosis and PCOS (poly cystic ovarian syndrome, which you'll learn more about in the next chapter).

Moreover, since inflammation, in and of itself ,can also influence the ability to get pregnant, a diet high in inflammatory foods can set your fertility up for a double whammy!

So, what are the inflammatory foods that impact endometriosis the most?

Not surprisingly, at the top of the list is :

- Animal fat,
- Red meat
- Ham

As you may recall, these are the very same foods found in the Italian study to increase the risk of endometriosis! But the "danger" list also includes a few more foods you might not think of as harmful!

Some of these foods include:
- Bagels
- Corn flakes
- Most commercial baked goods including donuts & packaged cookies
- French fries and tortilla chips
- Yams, corn oil, walnut oil, grape seed oil
- Bananas, cherries, cranberries, grapes, and peanuts.

The good news however is that there are also foods that can help you! Indeed, we now know that just as there are foods that increase inflammation, so too are there foods which help decrease the production of these inflammatory chemicals. Known simply as "anti-inflammatory" foods, these are the staples that encourage wellness in women with endometriosis and even counter some of the damage caused by the inflammatory foods you do eat.

So what are these healthy "anti-inflammatory" foods?

At the top of this list are "healthy fats", including Omega-3 fatty acids, nutrients found in foods such as cold water fish like salmon or mackerel, as well as in flax seeds and walnuts. You can also purchase foods enhanced with these important fatty acids – including eggs, beverages and yogurt - and they can help as well

But in addition to "healthy fats" there are also a variety of fruits and vegetables that have anti-inflammatory properties. These include onions, lettuce, garlic, celery, cauliflower, cabbage, broccoli, peaches, papayas, cantaloupe, honeydew, nectarines, apricots and cashew nuts.

But as important as it is to include these anti-inflammatory foods in your diet, I don't want you to simply eat these items and nothing else!

Indeed, many of the foods which are linked to inflammation – such as certain whole grains, some fruits, and even red meat – can offer other important health and fertility benefits, so you should not exclude them entirely.

The best solution is to strike a balance between inflammatory and anti-inflammatory foods. While this is good advice for any woman trying to get pregnant, it is especially important if you are dealing with any inflammatory condition, particularly endometriosis.

If you want to learn more about inflammatory foods I invite you visit FertilityDietGuide.com where you will find important news and information on the foods that impact fertility – including more on the links between inflammation, food and fertility.

THE TEN BEST FOODS TO EAT IF YOU HAVE ENDOMETRIOSIS

- Wild salmon
- Tuna
- Chicken White Meat
- Onions and garlic
- Lettuce (all types) and celery
- Cauliflower, broccoli, cabbage, Swiss chard
- Strawberries and grapefruits
- Papayas
- Honeydew and Cantaloupe Melons
- Cashew nuts, sunflower seeds

FOODS TO AVOID IF YOU HAVE ENDOMETRIOSIS

- Red Meat
- Ham
- Foods high in trans fat such as commercial baked goods
- Potatoes, especially French fries
- All soy foods (they stimulate estrogen production)
- Any foods containing Soy Protein Isolates
- Cherries
- Bananas
- Grapes
- Corn Flakes
- Corn Oil, Canola Oil, Grape seed Oil

ANTIOXIDANT POWER & ENDOMETRIOSIS: YOUR HEALTH WARRIORS

Certainly, all of the supplement advice you have read in this book thus far can help you. But if you are diagnosed with endometriosis there are some special considerations – and some additional nutrients that are key to not only helping you to get pregnant, but controlling your disease overall.

Among the most important are found in the group of vitamins known as antioxidants – including vitamins A, C, D, and E.

Why are they so important? First, these vitamins are your key warriors when it comes to beating down oxidative stress – a type of imbalance that results when your body's ability to repair damaged cells is outpaced by the damage itself. That damage can be the result of anything from environmental stressors such as chemical exposures or even too much sun, to a poor diet (one high in trans fats and animal fat, for example), or any other number of factors that can put your health at risk.

While everyone experiences oxidative stress to some degree, women with endometriosis appear to be at greater risk. In fact, the medical literature now suggests that oxidative stress may actually play a role in the development and progression of endometriosis. This sets up a kind of domino effect wherein the susceptibility to damage becomes a leading cause of damage , and both increase your susceptibility to harm.

But again, you can take steps to stop the cycle of damage – and the first and best place to start is by increasing your intake of these antioxidants. The importance of taking this step was recently underscored in a very important study conducted by a group of Mexican researchers. Reporting in the journal *Reproductive Biology and Endocrinology*, the researchers documented how women with endometriosis have a much lower profile of antioxidants in their blood to begin with.

Moreover the doctors found that by putting these women on a diet that is super packed with antioxidant nutrients, they were able to turn their antioxidant profiles completely around, bringing their levels up to speed *in just two months time!*

The nutrient level intakes used to achieve this included:

- 1050 units daily of Vitamin A (150% increase of the recommended daily intake)

- 500 mg of Vitamin C daily (660% of the recommended daily intake)

- 20 mg of Vitamin E (133% of the recommended daily intake).

Perhaps most significant was that all of these increases came not from supplements, but from natural foods! Vitamins A and C were garnered primarily from 3 portions per day of vegetables including Swiss chard, broccoli, spinach, tomato and carrots as well as 5 portions per day of fruits including strawberries, guavas, kiwi, lemons, cantaloupe, oranges, papaya and grapefruit. Vitamin E was garnered from sunflower seeds and peanuts.

What is equally important is that not only were these foods able to increase the blood levels of these key antioxidant fertility nutrients, but doing so dramatically reduced the markers for oxidative stress and raised the levels of other protective biochemical factors. So, when the threat of damage goes down and the increase in protection goes up, you have the best – and the healthiest – of all worlds!

While the study ended too soon to know for certain if the reduction of oxidative damage resulted in an increase in fertility in these particular women, but that said, other studies have shown that when oxidative stress goes down, ovulation improves, egg production is better and in general, pregnancy occurs more easily.

Moreover my personal experience treating thousands of women with endometriosis indictates that an increase in antioxidant vitamins, plus the addition of copper and zinc supplements (the women in the study were also found to be deficient in these minerals) will not only ameliorate symptoms and in some instances reduce the growth of endometrial lesions, but also dramatically increase the chance for a successful pregnancy.

The bottom line: By adding more fruits and vegetables to your diet you can absolutely help reduce your symptoms of endometriosis while at the same time boosting your fertility!

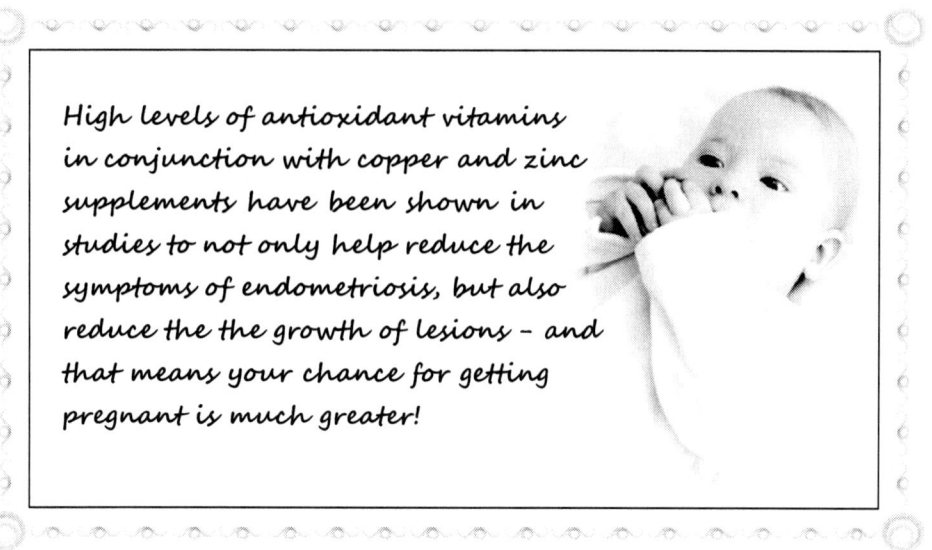

> *High levels of antioxidant vitamins in conjunction with copper and zinc supplements have been shown in studies to not only help reduce the symptoms of endometriosis, but also reduce the the growth of lesions – and that means your chance for getting pregnant is much greater!*

INCREASE YOUR DEFENSES WITH SUPPLEMENTS

Although I firmly believe in the power of a healthy diet as key to increasing fertility, I also know that for many of you, eating all the "right" foods can be sometimes difficult. For this reason I always recommended that all my fertility patients take a high potency multi-vitamin – and for those of you with endometriosis this is "MUST ! In fact, I cannot stress often enough the importance of taking just this one step when it comes to overcoming any of the difficulties you may have in getting pregnant.

That said, I also want you to remember that vitamin supplements are just that – supplements, and not meant to replace a healthy diet . So, it's also key that you continue to eat as many fruits and vegetables as you can.

When deciding on what supplements to take, I'm certain that for most of you, a good multivitamin will give you a solid foundation - or you can look to a prenatal vitamin, which also contains high levels of all of the most important nutrients your body needs at this time.

As to additional levels of support I suggest that you follow the vitamin and mineral recommendations featured throughout this book. Indeed, whatever is good for fertility is even better when you have endometriosis! In addition however, there are also a few specific supplements that science has shown can help not only reduce the symptoms of endometriosis, but also encourage fertility at the same time.

The most important of these supplements for you to take are:

- **OMEGA-3 ESSENTIAL FATTY ACIDS** – In one study researchers from the University of Western Ontario found that fish oil containing two specific Omega-3 compounds - EPA and DHA - can relieve pain associated with endometriosis by decreasing levels of an inflammatory chemical called prostaglandin E2. Other research found fish oil slows the growth of endometrial tissue. In terms of fertility, much like the foods containing high levels of Omega-3 , supplements increase blood flow to the uterus and in doing so ensures a healthy implantation and healthier pregnancy when conception does occur.

- **EVENING OIL OF PRIMROSE** – This supplement has been around for a long time, with mostly anecdotal reports of its effectiveness. However, there are a few medical studies to show it may help reduce the pain of endometriosis, and in doing so help decrease some of the inflammation thought to interfere with conception.

- **BEE PROPOLIS** - Though it's often confused with bee pollen, propolis is actually a resin that is extracted from trees by bees – much the way pollen is extracted from flowers. But how can this help women with endometriosis? Early research has shown that propolis appears to have strong anti-inflammatory effects. Since one theory tells us that pain associated with endometriosis is part of the body's inflammatory response to the misplaced tissue, anything that decreases that inflammatory response, decreases pain – which in turn cuts the cycle of increasing inflammatory responses. But it's not just the pain of endometriosis that propolis can help. Indeed a study published recently in the journal *Fertility and Sterility* found it may also improve fertility. In this research women with endometriosis who were not able to get pregnant for at least two years were given 500 mg of bee propolis twice daily for nine months. The rate of pregnancy was then compared to another group of women, with endometriosis, taking a placebo. The result: A whopping 60% of the women taking the bee propolis got pregnant , compared to just 20% who were taking the placebo. While it's not clear how the propolis influenced fertility, it is my guess that the same inflammatory activity that helps endometrial pain, also helps reduce inflammation linked to infertility.

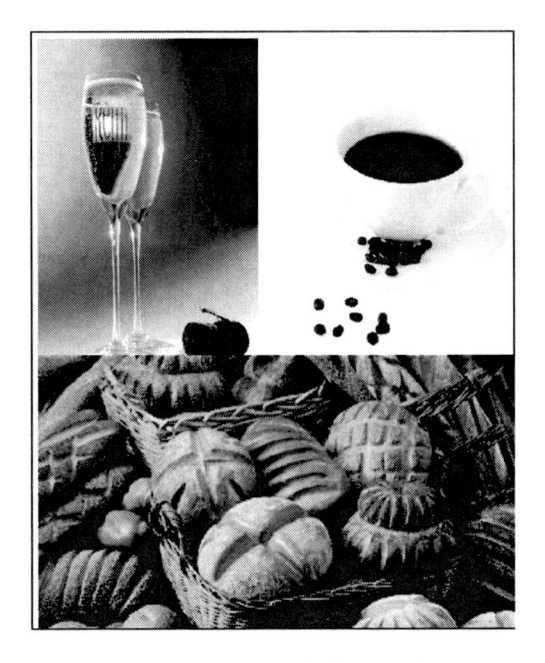

Alcohol, Caffeine, and Bread:

Links to Endometriosis You Should Not IGNOre

Among the more controversial links between endometriosis and food, are those surrounding consumption of alcohol, caffeine and wheat products, including most breads. What's the connection?

In terms of alcohol, there is no solid evidence that drinking will increase endometriosis. But there is good evidence that alcohol promotes inflammation – so in this respect I believe that cutting down consumption is a good idea. Moreover, since we know that alcohol can also impact your fertility, avoiding it may offer you double protection.

In terms of caffeine, the link is a little clearer Studies show that high levels of caffeine may influence the production of estrogen. Since endometriosis is associated with estrogen dominance, you want to avoid any food or drink that increases estrogen production. I recommend no more than the caffeine found in three cups of coffee daily – and less if you can swing it!

Perhaps the newest food link to endometriosis comes in the form of a gluten sensitivity – or otherwise known as a "celiac disease".

According to nutritionist Dian Mills, who specializes in treating women with endometriosis, if you are sensitive to gluten then removing wheat from your diet will not only reduce some of the pain associated with this condition, but may also encourage fertility. So, how do you know if you have a gluten sensitivity?

Symptoms usually include constipation, diarrhea, cramps and bloating, particularly following meals that contain wheat. And remember, this is not only bread, but any product that contains wheat including pastries, cake, pasta, muffins, cookies, even crackers (See Chapter 7 for more information on celiac disease and infertility).

What's important to note, however, is that the incidence of gluten sensitivity is on the rise. Many believe it may be due to the genetic manipulation of the proteins found naturally in wheat, some of which are being altered to increase the heartiness of the stock or shorten the growing season. The result has caused many women who never had problem with these foods to suddenly develop one.

To see if this might be the case for you, you should eliminate all sources of wheat from your diet for two months. If your symptoms clear, and particularly if your endometriosis symptoms lessen, then cutting wheat out of your diet may be an important step towards getting pregnant.

Remember, however, you still do need whole grains, so be sure to substitute brown rice, corn, oats, quinoa, or other whole grains in place of wheat, to keep your diet healthy and well balanced.

STRESS, ENDOMETRIOSIS & GETTING PREGNANT:
WHAT YOU MUST KNOW

As I mentioned earlier, one of the reasons that endometriosis was first known as the "Career Woman's Disease" was because the links to stress are so profound.

Indeed, at a time when women were fighting the hardest to not only break through the glass ceiling but to simply get their foot into the door of big business, the stress was indeed enormous. In many ways and in many career venues this pressure continues – so it's no wonder than stress related diseases are now attacking women in record numbers.

And this includes endometriosis. So what's the specific connection to stress? As you read earlier, when your body is under stress it produces a number of chemicals and hormones that can impact a wide variety of systems body-wide – including the hormones involved in getting pregnant. Moreover, the production of stress hormones also increases inflammation body-wide. Yes, there's that word again, inflammation!

So, in addition to inflammatory foods, situational conditions such as chronic long term stress, even at a low level, can contribute to the production and eventual build up of these same harmful inflammatory chemicals, and in doing so not only increase your risk of fertility problems, but also symptoms related to your

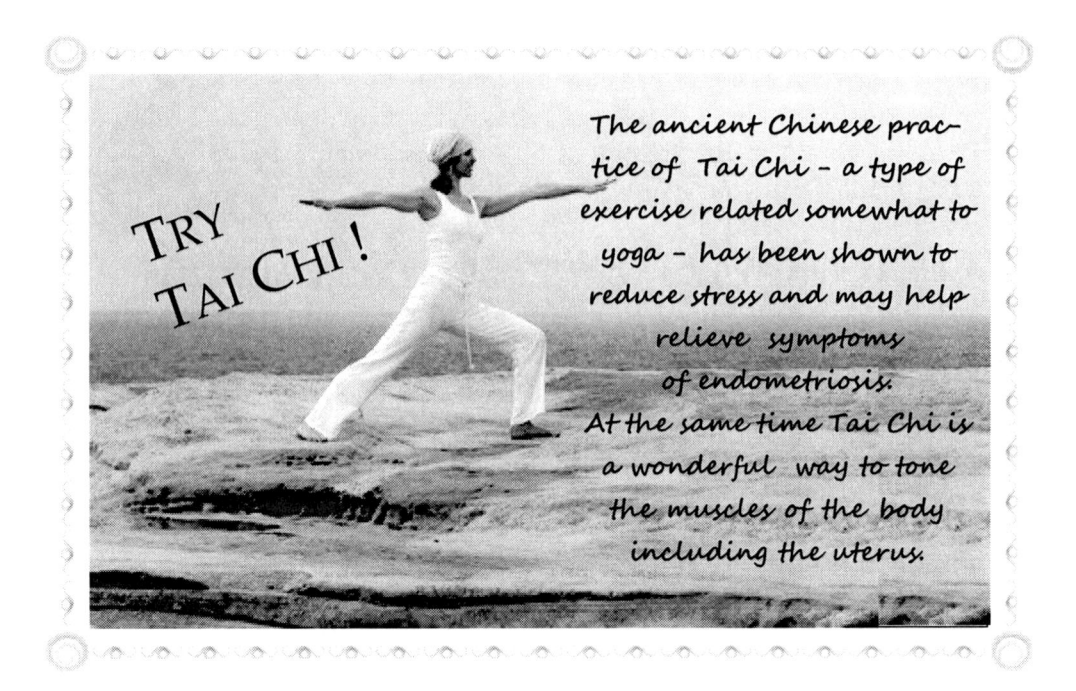

> **TRY TAI CHI!**
>
> The ancient Chinese practice of Tai Chi – a type of exercise related somewhat to yoga – has been shown to reduce stress and may help relieve symptoms of endometriosis. At the same time Tai Chi is a wonderful way to tone the muscles of the body including the uterus.

endometriosis. In some instances, if the stress is significant enough, it may even contribute to the development of the disease itself.

For all these reasons it's imperative for any woman diagnosed with endometriosis – or even those at risk – to make it a point of including some time for relaxation in your life.

In fact, I can't emphasize enough the importance of making time for yourself to chill out and relax *at least once a day.* For some it's best in the early morning, on rising, a time when many of my patients tell me it's easiest to grab 15 or 20 minutes for a "centering" session that helps induce a sense of calm that can last for hours.

For others it can be at bedtime – a way of unwinding and calming down, letting go of the day's tensions and entering into a restorative's nights rest.

For still others it's that mid-day or early evening break when a yoga class, meditation, chanting or even a mild exercise routine will do the trick. While there is no one "anti-stress" activity that is right for all women, what's important is that you find the stress-reducing activities that work best for you – and do them regularly. While it's not always possible to eliminate the causes of our stress, the one thing we can do is counter the effects by taking time to distress and relax. Not only will doing so aid in the treatment of your endometriosis, but it can also benefit your fertility and your overall health as well.

A Final Word: It's Your Life and Your Fertility

Certainly all of the lifestyle advice featured in this book – particularly the information found in the chapters on lifestyle and the environment – are important for all women who want to get pregnant. But I urge those of you diagnosed with endometriosis to pay special attention to this information – and to take as many steps as you can to reduce your exposure to any of the lifestyle and environmental factors mentioned as harmful in earlier chapters.

This is especially important when it comes to chemicals categorized as "hormone disrupters" - in particular those classified as "xeno estrogens. As I explained earlier, these are chemicals that, once inside the body begin to act much like hormones, throwing your reproductive biochemistry into a tailspin. This isn't healthy for men or women, but for those of you already battling a hormone-related condition such as endometriosis these exposures can be even more worrisome.

In fact, it's possible that one of the factors influencing the findings of the Italian researchers I referred to earlier was that one of the sites from which they recruited study subjects is very close to Seveso, Italy, where, in late 1970's there was a massive chemical accident . That accident caused a release into the environment of multiple chemicals linked to endometriosis – including dioxin. As such these spills may have not only influenced the number of women afflicted with endometriosis, but may have also further sensitized their bodies so that they became more susceptible to the dietary risk factors.

Ultimately, it may not be possible to eliminate or even avoid many of the environmental factors capable of affecting your health and your fertility. But certainly paying strict attention to the ways and means in which you can reduce their impact on your health – including following the dietary and nutritional advice featured in this book – can go a long way in not only reducing the severity of whatever exposures you do encounter, but also provide a layer of protection as well. In fact, by following the advice in this book, and working with your doctor to help control or even eliminate your endometriosis, you will not only feel better, but you will dramatically increase your chances for conception.

One final point I'd like to re-emphasize again is the importance of having your symptoms properly diagnosed, and making sure you receive proper treatment. As I said earlier, while today endometriosis is a recognized disorder, and diagnosis is easier, but sadly, women are still getting misdiagnosed and mistreated every day.

Indeed, according to the Endometriosis Association there is often a delay of up to ten years between the onset of symptoms and getting the correct diagnosis and treatment. Even today many women are still being routinely told by their doctors that their symptoms, particularly severe menstrual pain, are the result of "psychological problems" and all " in their head."

If this is what has happened to you, and if, despite your prevalence of symptoms your doctor fails to recognize that something is wrong, do not give up. Instead, seek the care of another doctor – if possible one who specializes in the treatment of endometriosis . Oftentimes a university hospital or medical center can give you a referral to such an expert.

You can also visit **EndometriosisAssociation.org** where you will find a lot of terrific reference materials and advice on finding treatment and care in your area.

I also want to remind you that if you want more information on getting pregnant when you have endometriosis, please visit me on the web at **GettingPregnantNow.org** or pick up a copy of my fertility treatment book, *"Getting Pregnant: What You Need to Know Now",* which is available in bookstores nationwide and in most libraries.

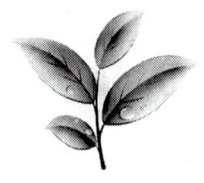

CHAPTER SEVENTEEN

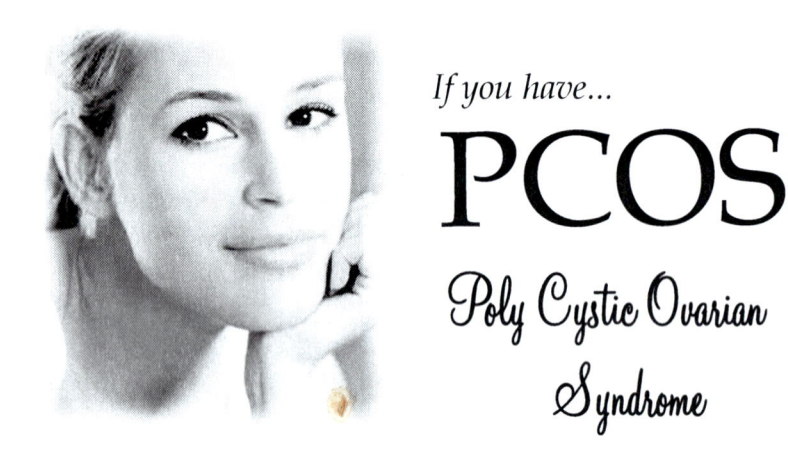

If you have...
PCOS
Poly Cystic Ovarian Syndrome

How It Affects Fertility & What You Can Do!

Although I had been a fertility doctor for more than two decades, with every new patient and every new infertility story they told, my heart never stopped aching for those who wanted desperately to have a baby and could not do so.

But of all the stories I heard, perhaps none were more touching than those told to me by patients suffering with not just infertility, but a cacophony of troubling symptoms that were turning their lives upside down. Irregular menstrual cycles, heavy bleeding, acne breakouts, unwanted facial or body hair and frequently, a battle with obesity that, despite their best efforts, they just could not win.

These were also the same constellation of problems that seemed to be affecting more and more women. As I looked into their faces I could often see the tears welling in their eyes as they asked "Doctor, what is wrong with me?"

Of course I always took all the necessary tests in order to make a diagnosis. But more often than not I knew instinctively from that very first meeting these women had PCOS – poly cystic ovarian syndrome, a potentially devastating condition that impacts not just the ovaries but the entire reproductive and endocrine systems. Not coincidentally, it has also become a leading cause of infertility among young women.

But what exactly is PCOS – and how and why does it harm your fertility? It all begins with understanding a little something about how your ovaries function – and what can get in the way.

Indeed, under normal circumstances each month your ovaries produce a number of egg follicles – tiny little fluid filled "cysts" packed with hormones, particularly estrogen. While the number of follicles produced each month can vary, key to getting pregnant is that one or two of them grow stronger than the rest and eventually develop into an "egg".

As your egg "ripens" and eventually reaches its "peak", it pops from its shell, leaves your ovary and flows down into your fallopian tube. It is this activity that helps trigger a variety of hormonal secretions – including estrogen and progesterone – which work together to prepare your body for pregnancy.

If your egg meets up with your partner's sperm (usually in your fallopian tube) conception occurs and a pregnancy happens. If sperm and egg don't "hook up" then your egg travels solo to your uterus – which in turn signals hormone levels to drop, and a menstrual cycle to begin.

But when PCOS occurs all this activity changes.

Alterations in hormone production cause the ovaries to over produce follicles – so many, in fact, that they line up and drape the inside of the ovary in a kind of "pearl necklace" formation. The problem, however, isn't just that there are too many follicles, but due to a variety of hormonal upsets, almost none of them are able to develop into an egg. This in turn means there is very little chance for ovulation or any of the normal hormonal activity that follows. And that means getting pregnant is very difficult.

Moreover, as time goes on, these follicles continue to collect in the ovary. Not only does this cause the formation of painful cysts, but also the development of "hard shell" around the outside of your ovary. So, even if an egg does happen to develop, it usually can't make its way out of the ovary. And that means getting pregnant naturally becomes pretty much impossible - one reason why PCOS is a leading cause of infertility.

SYMPTOMS OF PCOS

The following are the most common symptoms of PCOS. Because, however, they can also be symptoms of other problems, it's important that you see your doctor if you regularly experience any of the following:

- Highly irregular periods or no periods.
- Infertility.
- Abnormal hair growth on the face and body.
- Weight gain even with dieting and increased exercise.
- Going for months without a period, then heavy bleeding for days.
- High blood pressure
- Elevated testosterone, prolactin, and DHEA
- Abnormal ratio of LH to FSH
- Depression

You may also experience fatigue, tiredness after eating sweets, unusual thirst or hunger - all signs related to the underlying blood sugar conditions associated with PCOS.

PCOS: Why It Occurs

The medical condition known as PCOS was first identified in the 1930's. At the time it was called Stein-Leventhal syndrome after the two doctors who pioneered the research and first categorized the symptoms into a single condition - which is now believed to be the most severe form of this disease.

Back in the 1930's - and for many years going forward, doctors believed PCOS was strictly an ovarian problem, affecting only a small number of women.

Today however research has shown PCOS in a whole new and different light. Not only do we now know that many more women are affected than originally believed, but today virtually all endocrinologists and gynecologists concur that the ovaries are simply one area of the body affected by PCOS - *but not the cause.*

So what is behind this ailment?

Many believe it is linked to insulin resistance – a condition closely linked to type 2 diabetes.

As you read in an earlier chapter, insulin is a hormone secreted by the pancreas in response to eating food. Its purpose is to transport the resulting sugar from the food you eat out of your bloodstream and into your cells. In essence, the insulin acts like a kind of "door knocker" that asks the cells to open up and let sugars in.

The condition known as "insulin resistance" occurs when your cells become "resistant" to that "knock on the door". In an effort to convince your cells to respond, your body begins producing greater amounts of insulin. And for a while, this works.

Eventually, however, your cells *stop responding* – no matter how much insulin is produced. When this occurs sugar remains in your bloodstream and a condition known as type 2 diabetes occurs.

In women who are susceptible, however, insulin resistance causes still another problem, this one related to ovarian function.

Indeed, when there is a continuing excess of insulin being released, the ovaries respond by amping up production of testosterone - the "male" hormone which is normally produced in a woman's body in very tiny amounts. As testosterone levels rise, it becomes difficult for follicles to develop into an egg- which in turn means there is no ovulation. When follicles continue to be stimulated but no eggs develop it causes a series of hormonal and other biochemical events that come together to produce many of the symptoms associated with PCOS.

While today a good portion of the female population is *insulin resistant* – it is one of the fastest growing ailments among both young men and young women - *not every woman with insulin resistance develops PCOS*. Why? No one knows for certain but it appears as if heredity plays a key role.

In short, if your mother, grandmother or sister has PCOS, there's a strong chance you will as well.

Interestingly, new research has revealed that when a woman has PCOS her brothers are at higher risk for developing insulin resistance and type 2 diabetes.

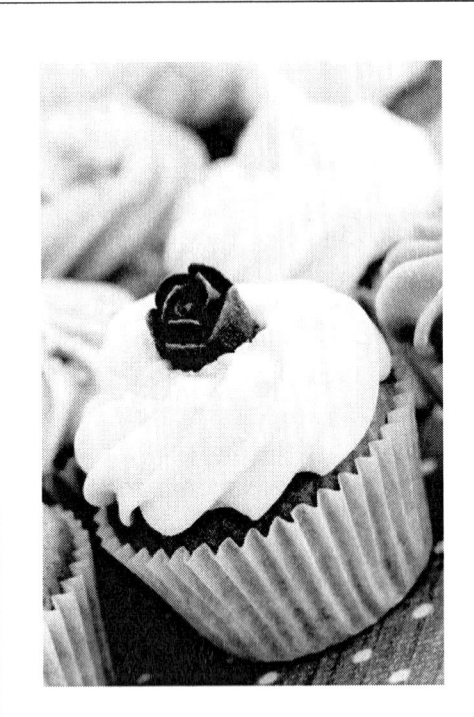

Q: I have a strong craving for sweets & I'm always thirsty. My mom says that's one of the reasons I can't get pregnant. Is she right?

A: This time, mother may know best! The symptoms you describe can be early warning signs of insulin resistance - which can interfere with your ability to get pregnant. If you also have any of the other symptoms of PCOS, then you should talk to your doctor about a 6 hour glucose tolerance test to see how your body handles sugar. You should also talk to your gynecologist about an ultra sound of your ovaries. Together this should give you some good information about your fertility.

PCOS: Hope and Help for Getting Pregnant

As devastating as PCOS can be, there have been great strides made in not only treatment, but also in resolving the fertility-related consequences. Among the most important is the use of the medication Metformin – a prescription drug that helps increase the body's responsiveness to insulin and in doing so can help turn PCOS around.

When the egg-stimulating drug Clomid is also added into the mix, I'm happy to report that most women with PCOS can successfully get pregnant!

But in addition to these medical treatments, there is also much that every woman can do on her own to help reduce the fertility related consequences of PCOS and in the process also help overcome many of the symptoms of this condition.

Among the most successful ways to accomplish both is via change in diet. In fact, if there is any group of women for whom a change in diet is critical, it is women with insulin resistance and PCOS.

How Diet Affects PCOS - And Fertility

While all foods contain some sugars, it is simple carbohydrates, foods like white bread, pasta, cake, and candy, plus starches like white potatoes and white rice which contain the most. So, they require the greatest surges of insulin in order to move the resulting sugar out of your blood and into your cells.

As such, when your diet consists of mostly of these simple carbs and starches, your pancreas is really working overtime. And this not only increases your risk of insulin resistance, but also many related ovulatory problems.

In fact, this is a good time to remind you of the study of some 18,000 women mentioned earlier in the book. Here, a group of Harvard researchers found that women whose diets consisted largely of simple carbohydrates were 92% more likely to experience ovulatory problems – not unlike the kind experienced by women with PCOS.

So, it's easy to see how a diet high in these same foods will not only impact your fertility, but the symptoms of PCOS as well.

But if you're thinking the path to better health means cutting out all your carbs, think again. Because in order to maintain your overall health and your fertility, you do need some carbohydrates in your daily diet. So what's the answer?

Fill your plate with what is known as *"complex carbohydrates"* – which includes most fruits and vegetables and lots of high fiber grains. In short, these are the type of carbohydrates that burn slowly rather than quickly – and therein lies one key to controlling those insulin spikes linked to PCOS. How does this work?

First, the high fiber content of these foods slows down the release of sugars into the blood stream – so you don't need a lot of insulin to be released all at once. But complex carbohydrates, especially fruits and vegetables also contain a number of nutrients that work with your body to *stabilize* blood sugar levels and keep insulin within a more normal range.

But while cutting down on simple carbohydrates and adding more complex carbohydrates and fiber to your diet can help, it doesn't stop here.

More than any other group of women, those with PCOS need "healthy fats" – particularly the Omega-3 fatty acids known as eicosapentaenic acid (EPA) and docosahexanoic acid (DHA). Found in foods such as cold water fish, as well as flax seed and walnuts, they can be a major help for women with PCOS. Why?

When insulin is overproduced it kicks off a host of other biochemical snafus, including the production of inflammatory chemicals, some of which ignite some symptoms of PCOS – including difficulty losing weight. As you read earlier, Omega-3 fatty acids are essential to combating inflammation – so in this respect they can be immediately helpful in combating some of the symptoms of PCOS, as well as encouraging ovulation.

In fact, in one study published in the *Journal of Clinical Endocrinology and Metabolism* researchers found that simply adding supplements of Omega-3 fatty acids to the diet of women with PCOS was enough of a boost to kick start ovulation!

In this instance, no drugs were necessary to get the reproductive system back on track. (See the nutrient list later in this chapter for more information on Omega 3 supplements).

But as helpful as these good fats can be, a diet high in "bad fats" can have the opposite effect. Indeed, foods high in saturated fa(such as most commercial baked goods and snacks) not only increase inflammation but in the process trigger a cascade of biochemical activity that directly impacts ovulation.

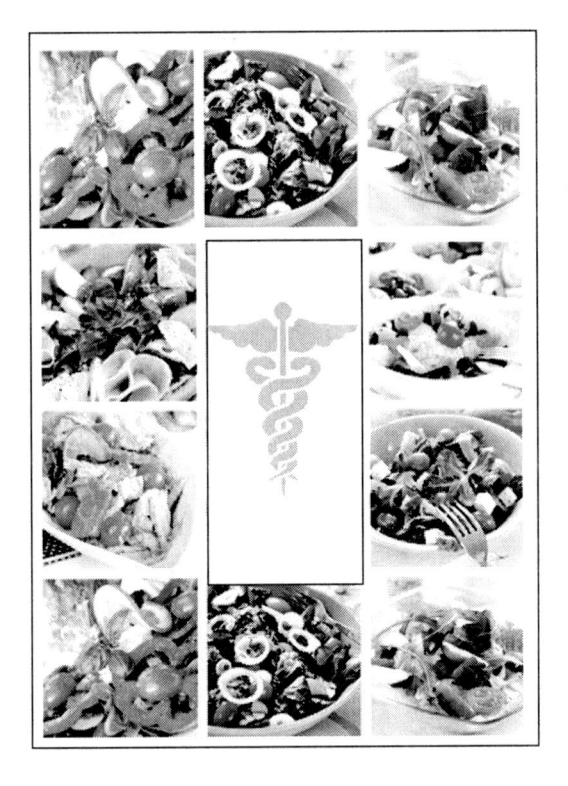

What to Eat If You Have PCOS

Today, most experts agree that the best diet for women with PCOS is one that consists mainly of foods that are "low "on the "glycemic index". As you read earlier, this is a system of rating foods based on how quickly they are metabolized into sugar – and the impact they have on both insulin secretion and sugar levels.

Foods that have a "high" glycemic index - such as white bread, pasta, white rice and most commercial baked goods - cause your blood to be flooded with sugar, which in turn causes a quick and voluminous release of insulin.

Meanwhile, foods with a "low" glycemic index - such as whole grain breads and cereals, pretty much all vegetables and many fruits, as well as meat, poultry and fish - are metabolized at a much slower pace. This means that blood sugar won't take a huge jumps up following these meals - and that in turn means your body won't need to pump out as much insulin.

But it also means that when blood sugars are stable -and not subjected to these rapid ups and downs - your entire endocrine system works more efficiently - including the hormones involved in getting pregnant.

In my book Eat, Love, Get Pregnant, I give you the glycemic index rating of over 200 foods known to improve fertility – and I help you plan a diet that can target your specific fertility problems and help you get pregnant faster.

But for right now what follows is my quick "hit list" of some of the best foods for PCOS – *as well as those foods you should avoid.* I urge you to use these lists as a guide to planning your meals and finding the meals that work best for you.

Top 10 Must Have Foods for PCOS

1. Salmon or tuna
2. White meat chicken or turkey
3. Beans
4. Whole grain/whole wheat bread or pasta
5. Brown rice
6. Nut butters
7. Yogurt (unsweetened)
8. Broccoli, Kale, Cabbage, cauliflower, lettuce, red peppers
9. Apricots, nectarines, peaches, strawberries, blueberries, watermelon, cantaloupe, honeydew
10. Green tea, decaffeinated tea or coffee

Top 10 Foods to Avoid If You Have PCOS

1. Anything made from white flour including bread, pasta, cakes, cookies, pies.
2. Commercial baked goods particularly those high in trans fats
3. French fries, white potatoes
4. Candy
5. Cookies – except those made from whole grain flour
6. All soft drinks
7. All fruit juices
8. Coffee (with caffeine)
9. Processed meats (ham, bologna, salami, etc).
10. Artificial sweeteners

The Nutrients for PCOS:
What to Take To Support Your Fertility

As you already know from reading this book, I firmly believe that the best way to get all your nutrients is via a healthy diet. When you "eat" your way to a healthier body you not only get all the vitamins and minerals you need, you also get fiber as well as many other factors found in whole foods that are beneficial to your health. Plus, the more healthy foods you consume, the less room you will have for the "junk" foods that can harm your health – so eating well is a big win all the way around!

At the same time I also know that many of you probably don't eat as healthy as you wish you could. Sometimes cost is a factor – and unfortunately some of the healthiest foods, like fish or even some fruits and vegetables, can be expensive, particularly if you live in an area where these items have to be imported.

Of course, one easy solution is to **"eat local"** - which really is another way of saying eat *"in season"*. When you concentrate on the fruits and vegetables that are in season in your area, you will save a ton of money plus get a healthy variety of foods throughout the year.

But when that's not possible, I do recommend that you take vitamin and nutrient supplements – with the firm understanding that these are "supplements" meant to augment a healthy diet, not replace it!

To this end, all of the suggestions for vitamins and minerals made in this book thus far will not only help those of you with PCOS, in many instances they can be a true life –line, or should I say "fertility-line", working to get your body ready for conception, even under adverse conditions.

In addition, however, there are a few nutrients that are particularly important if you have PCOS – and I'd like to take a few moments to tell you what they are and how they can help.

Of course the best place to start is with a good multi vitamin, and build from there – so I am going to encourage each of you to make certain you use this as your nutrient foundation.

I believe that adding to this with the following additional nutrients can go a long way in helping to "feed" your body and replenish your fertility, while reducing some of the consequences of PCOS.

The 7 Key Nutrients for PCOS

Nutrient # 1: Chromium

This is an essential trace mineral that plays a key role in insulin activity, and is necessary for the metabolism of carbohydrates, proteins and fats. Studies show that achieving optimal chromium levels can reduce insulin resistance and improve blood sugar control, as well as reduce the risk of both type 2 diabetes and heart disease. In one small study of women with PCOS, a 1000 mcg chromium supplement used daily for just two months improved insulin sensitivity by as much as 35%, while reducing actual insulin levels by 22%. Other research has found chromium supplements can reduce triglycerides and total cholesterol, which, if you are overweight, may be above normal for you. Perhaps most important, developing a chromium deficiency may be easier than you realize. Why? Studies have shown that in those who have diabetes and/or insulin resistance, the level of chromium is naturally lower – suggesting a possible defect in the ability to either pull chromium from food or to maintain levels once it's ingested.

Recommended Dosage: The typical dosage for chromium supplements is 200 mcg daily. That said, if you are looking for a therapeutic effect you will likely have to go as high as 500 mcg twice daily before blood sugars are affected.

Important: Because chromium levels can impact blood sugar, you must let your doctor know if you are taking these supplements, and the amount. You should also monitor your sugar levels more often if you are taking Metformin or any other insulin sensitivity medications, since chromium could cause your sugar levels to fall too low.

Also be aware that you should not use high levels of chromium longer than 3 to 4 months without your doctor's approval. There are no long term studies to assess safety data when high levels are used for a long period of time. And finally be aware that most multivitamins already contain about 200 mcg of chromium so be sure to figure in the amount you are getting in your multi, before deciding on the strength of your supplement. To help increase absorption, always try to take chromium in conjunction with a vitamin D - and if you can find the two in one supplement, that's the way to go!

NUTRIENT # 2 : D-CHIRO-INOSITOL

Related to the family of B vitamins, inositol is a nutrient found in the membrane or outer covering of every cell in your body and it is important for the transmission of information from one cell to another. There are several different chemically related types of inositol used by the body including d-chiro inositol, pinitol (which is converted by the body into d-chiro inositol) and myo-inositol, which is often referred to as simply "inositol". Each type plays a slightly different role in the body.

In terms of supplements the form known as D-Chiro-Inositol appears to be the most important for women with PCOS. Why? This nutrient can play a key role in ovarian function including regulating testosterone production in a woman's body. And evidence shows women with PCOS may either be naturally deficient in D-Chiro-inositol or they have a defect in their ability to metabolize all inositol.

The good news is that supplements of D-Chiro-Inositol appear to help. In one study involving 44 obese women with PCOS, 1,200 mg of D-chiro-inositol daily for 8 weeks decreased testosterone levels by some 55% while also improving ovarian function - most likely by impacting insulin activity. Moreover, 86% of the women taking the supplement were able to ovulate compared to just 26% of women taking a placebo.

While the most impressive study results have been linked to D-Chiro-Inositol, even supplements known simply as "inositol" may help. In one double blind study conducted at the University of Perugia in Italy, 23% of women diagnosed with PCOS who took 100 mg of inositol twice a day for 14 weeks were able to ovulate - compared to just 13% of the group taking placebo. Moreover, the women taking the inositol supplement ovulated once every 24 days, while the women taking the placebo did so only every 42 days. Additionally the researchers noted that the number of women who failed to ovulate at all was much higher in the placebo group.

Interestingly, the women taking the inositol also experienced significant weight loss and a reduction in the appetite hormone "leptin", while the group taking the placebo actually gained weight. Since excess weight increases the risk of insulin resistance, this is another way this supplement can help.

Although there are several different types of inositol on the market, if possible, do try to seek out the D-Chiro-Inositol for best results.

RECOMMENDED DOSAGE : 200 mg to 1,000 mg of D-Chiro Inositol daily appears safe. However, if you are taking medication for depression, or insulin resistance, check with your doctor on the right dosage of inositol for you. There is some very limited evidence to suggest that in high amounts inositol may increase the risk of uterine contractions, so if you are bleeding heavily stop inositol supplements. You should also stop them as soon as you know you are a pregnant.

NUTRIENT # 3: NAC (N-ACETYL-CYSTEINE)

This nutrient is a derivative of the amino acid known as "cysteine". It has powerful antioxidant properties and it is required by the body to manufacture "glutathione", another antioxidant necessary for protecting cells from damage. Because it's not available in any foods, NAC is necessary as a supplement – particularly if you have PCOS. Why?

Research indicates it may play a key role in increasing a cells responsiveness to insulin. In one recent study women diagnosed with PCOS used daily supplements of NAC for 6 weeks. This resulted in a reduction in insulin resistance and a significant drop in testosterone levels. What was key here, however, is that the dosage appeared to be linked to weight. Thin women only needed about 1.8 grams of NAC daily to achieve the desired result, while obese women needed up to 3 grams daily to see results.

NAC is also important because it may reduce some of the side effects associated with certain medicines used to treat PCOS – including Metformin. Indeed, one side effect of Metformin is elevated levels of the amino acid homocystine, an increase of which has been linked to an increase of coronary artery disease, heart attack, chronic fatigue, fibromyalgia, cognitive impairment, and cervical cancer. Studies show that adding NAC to your Metformin regimen can reduce risks by reducing levels of homocysteine.

To help women with PCOS turn follicles into eggs, we frequently prescribe the fertility drug Clomid. Unfortunately, however, some women simply do not respond to this medication. When this is the case, NAC may help by increasing the body's sensitivity to Clomid, thereby enhancing its effects. In one study of a 150 PCOS patients, those who were considered "Clomid-resistant" added NAC to their drug regimen. The result: Some 49% ovulated and 1.3% became pregnant. In the Clomid-only group just 21% ovulated and there were no pregnancies.

The study was repeated in a second, much larger group of nearly 600 women. In this study 52% of the women taking Clomid plus NAC ovulated compared to just 18% in the Clomid-only group. The study authors conclude that " N-Acetyl cysteine is proved effective in inducing or augmenting ovulation in polycystic ovary patients."

RECOMMENDED DOSAGE: Start with up to 600 mg of NAC once daily and talk to your doctor before increasing dosages to those used in the studies. Also talk to your doctor before taking NAC if you are currently being prescribed either Metformin or Clomid. If you get pregnant, you can safely continue to take NAC. In fact, studies show it may be helpful in protecting your unborn baby from environmental toxins including exposure to second hand smoke.

NUTRIENT # 4: SAW PALMETTO

It's likely you may have heard of saw palmetto as a treatment for enlarged prostate in men. But the very reason that it works for this problem, also makes it a viable treatment for women with PCOS. Why? In men, the prostate becomes enlarged due to high levels of testosterone, which the body converts to a more potent hormone known as dihydrotestosterone or DHT. In women with PCOS, both testosterone and DHT levels are elevated above normal. In fact, it is high levels of DHT believed to be responsible for some of the symptoms of PCOS including unwanted body hair growth as well as a thinning or loss of scalp hair.

In both men and women saw palmetto works by inhibiting the production of 5-alpha-reductase, an enzyme which allows the body to convert testosterone to DHT. When levels of 5-alpha-reductase are low, the conversion does not occur as readily - and that can help keep DHT levels low.

This is important since not only do women with PCOS have higher-than-normal levels of both testosterone and DHT, but a recent study conducted at the University of Birmingham in England found they may also have increased activity of 5-alpha-reductase. This means it is easier for your body to convert testosterone to DHT, thus increasing your likelihood of symptoms.

RECOMMEND DOSAGE: Since there is no recommended dosage for women, it's best to use the male dosing regimen as a guideline. Commonly men are advised to take 320 mg per day of saw palmetto standardized to contain a minimum of 0.2 – 0.4% sterols. Results are expected in about 6 weeks and if improvement occurs men are advised to continue the medication indefinitely.

I suggest women start with about half that dosage – about 150 mg per day if you are slim and about 200 mg per day if you are overweight or obese. However, please note that saw palmetto can interfere with birth control pills, some hormone treatments, and a number of medications so do not take this herb until you clear it with your doctor.

> **Q:** Are there any herbs to increase male fertility?
>
> **A:** There are! Among the most popular are believed to be Ginseng, Saw Palmetto, Astragalus and Macca Root.
>
> Nutrients for male fertility include zinc, folic acid, selenium, and the amino acids L-arginine and L-Carnetine,
>
> Read more about all of this in Chapter 15 on Male Fertility!

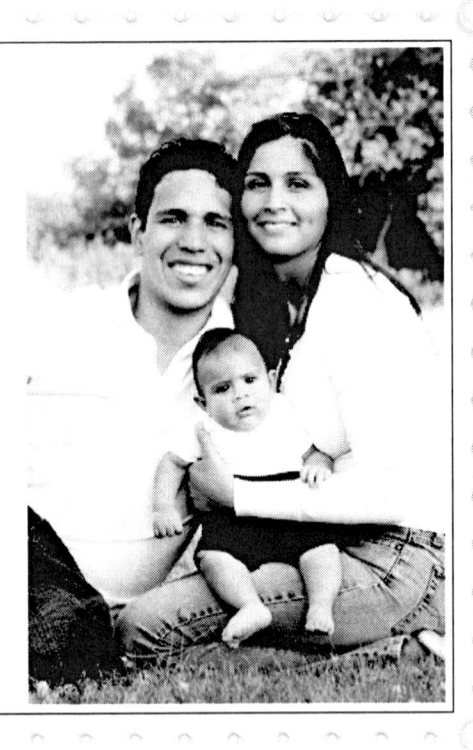

NUTRIENT # 5: VITEX (CHASTE BERRY)

As you read earlier, Vitex has been used by women for centuries to help balance hormones, and encourage a healthy menstrual cycle. It works by acting directly on the brain to increase production of LH (luteinizing hormone) and inhibit FS (follicle stimulating hormone) while also shifting the balance of estrogen to progesterone. Ultimately all this helps regulate the menstrual cycle.

Because in women with PCOS luteinizing hormone (LH) is often abnormally high, while FSH is abnormally low, at first glance it would seem as if this herb would not be of much help. However, another property of vitex is that it reduces levels of a hormone known as prolactin, which, in women with PCOS is abnormally high. Indeed, when proloactin reaches a certain level, fertility can be completely blocked.

In one small but significant study, Vitex not only reduced prolactin levels in women with PCOS, but it also initiated a menstrual cycle in every study participant - even those who had great difficulty menstruating in the past.

So, in this respect it appears as if the impact of Vitex on the menstrual cycle is the over riding factor that helps women with PCOS. Moreover Vitex has also been found to reduce the incidence of ovarian cysts in women with PCOS, another reason it can be helpful.

Recommended Dosage: Every woman is different – and every case of PCOS is different, so if possible, it's best to take this medication under the recommendations of a licensed naturopathic physician.

That said, the general guideline for daily dosing is 60 drops of Vitex (if you are using a tincture), standardized to contain 0.6% of agusides or 175 mg or more daily of Vitex extract standardized to contain 0.6% agusides. You can safely take this drug daily for up to 18 months, providing you are not pregnant. Follow up treatment lasting as long as nine years has been reported as safe.

Important warning: If you are taking prescription medications of any kind, talk to your doctor before adding Vitex to your regimen. This is particularly important if you have been prescribed any hormone medications, including Clomid.

NUTRIENT # 6: VITAMIN D

It's known as the "sunshine vitamin" – because your body makes vitamin D from a chemical reaction that occurs when skin is exposed to sunlight. But since most of us don't get enough sunlight, Vitamin D supplements are essential.

In terms of getting pregnant, Vitamin D acts as a fertility booster for *all women*, but those of you with PCOS may need the help so much more. Why? Studies show that PCOS patients are more likely to be deficient in Vitamin D - with some evidence that the deficiency itself may be one underlying factor in this condition.

The good news: Increasing your intake of vitamin D can have a major impact, on all your symptoms – including infertility. What's more it doesn't long to see the results!

In one small but significant study of women with PCOS, treatment with 50,000 IUs of vitamin D plus 1,500 mg of calcium (necessary to absorb the vitamin D) up to twice weekly helped normalize menstrual cycles within two months for more than 80% of the participants. Nearly 25% of the women in the study were able to get pregnant! Dysfunctional uterine bleeding – including long and heavy menstrual cycles – also resolved and normalized within the 2 month time period.

In other studies, low vitamin D levels have also been linked to insulin resistance problems, so clearly it can help PCOS from this respect as well. In fact, in one study researchers found that the lower the level of vitamin D, the more insulin resistance there was – even in healthy, young adults.

Recommended Dosage: According to the Food and Nutrition Board of the National Research Council, up to 2,000 units daily of vitamin D 3 is safe. I routinely recommend this amount for all women trying to get pregnant and I believe you can safely take up to 4,000 units a day, particularly if you have PCOS.

You can also augment the amount of Vitamin D you get from supplements by spending up to 20 minutes per day in the sun - without wearing sunscreen. Studies show that this amount of time is not only safe but can have some enormous health benefits. If you are going to be in the sun longer than 20 minutes, do make sure to apply sunscreen liberally.

> **Q:** *I have heard that spending time in the sun is also good for sperm – is this true?*
>
> **A:** It is true! Just like women, men also need vitamin D to produce healthy sperm. In one study spending just a few hours a week in the sun - just long enough to get a light tan - men were able to dramatically increase a very low sperm count! The effects of vitamin D on both male and female reproduction is one reason why so many couples get pregnant after spending a relaxing vacation in the sun!

Nutrient # 7: Omega-3 Fatty Acids

As you read earlier in this chapter – and earlier in the book – among the most important nutrients for fertility are essential fatty acids – particularly those that fall under the heading of Omega-3 fatty acids. Although they are necessary for health - and mandatory for fertility - they are the only nutrient your body cannot make on its own. You must get Omega-3 fatty acids from foods or supplements. While food sources are best, supplements are also helpful. What can they do?

Studies show that among women with PCOS, Omega-3 fatty acids can reduce harmful levels of inflammation, reduce the severity of insulin resistance, play a role in encouraging ovulation and increase your chances for a healthier pregnancy. In fact, many Chinese medicine doctors believe that when the body is low on Omega-3 fatty acids, eggs will not be healthy enough to fertilize.

While fish oil capsules are the best form of Omega-3 supplementation, there are products made from other sources including flax seed oil that can help. Be certain, however, to read the section on choosing an Omega-3 supplement found in Chapter 11.

Recommended Dosage: My personal recommendation for women with PCOS is 1,500 to 2,000 mg or up to 2 grams of EPA and DHA once daily. According to the FDA you can safely take up to 3,000 mg (or 3 grams) daily with no adverse effects, but I definitely would not go above that amount without talking to your doctor first. In fact, because this supplement can have blood thinning effects, you should definitely check with your doctor before taking it in any amount.

Q: *I've heard that fish oil is dangerous – because of all the pollutants in the water. How can taking fish oil supplements be safe or helpful?*

A: Certainly, some fish is tainted - and depending on what waters they come from, levels of contaminants can be quite high. So, one way to ensure the safety of your fish oil supplements is to look for those that come from fish caught in pristine waters - such as those off the coast of most Scandinavian countries. The other solution is to seek out products that have been put through a filtration process called molecular distillation that removes all the harmful contaminants. Look for this designation on product labels.

PCOS MEDICATIONS: SOME IMPORTANT WARNINGS

In addition to Metformin used to control insulin levels, there are two additional medications that are sometimes prescribed to combat some of the symptoms of PCOS including unwanted hair growth, oily skin and acne.

These two medications are spironolactone (Aldactone), and finasteride (Propecia, Proscar). You may recognize finasteride as the men's hair growth drug "Rogaine".

How do these drugs work? Both spironolactone and finasteride inhibit production of 5-alpha-reductase, which as you just read helps convert testosterone to DHT. So when levels of 5-alpha-reductase are low, you will have less DHT in your body – and that means fewer symptoms, particularly less growth of unwanted hair, and less scalp hair loss.

That said, while the drugs work they are not without their side effects. Spironolactone, for example, has been associated with an increase in irregular bleeding, as well as nausea, indigestion and fatigue.

The problems with finasteride are much more serious, and studies show this drug should never be used by any woman who is not on birth control. If you are trying to get pregnant not only should you never take this drug, your partner should not use it for hair growth while you are trying to conceive. Why? Studies show that even traces of finasteride in a woman's body during pregnancy can lead to severe birth defects – and those traces can get there via the semen of men using this medication.

If you are currently being prescribed finasteride for your PCOS, be certain to tell your doctor you want to get pregnant so you can discuss alternative treatment options. If your partner is using finasteride – which I will remind you again is the hair growth drug "Rogaine"- make certain he stops using it at least one month prior to when you want to get pregnant. And by the way, this last piece of advice applies to the partners of all women trying to conceive, not just those with PCOS.

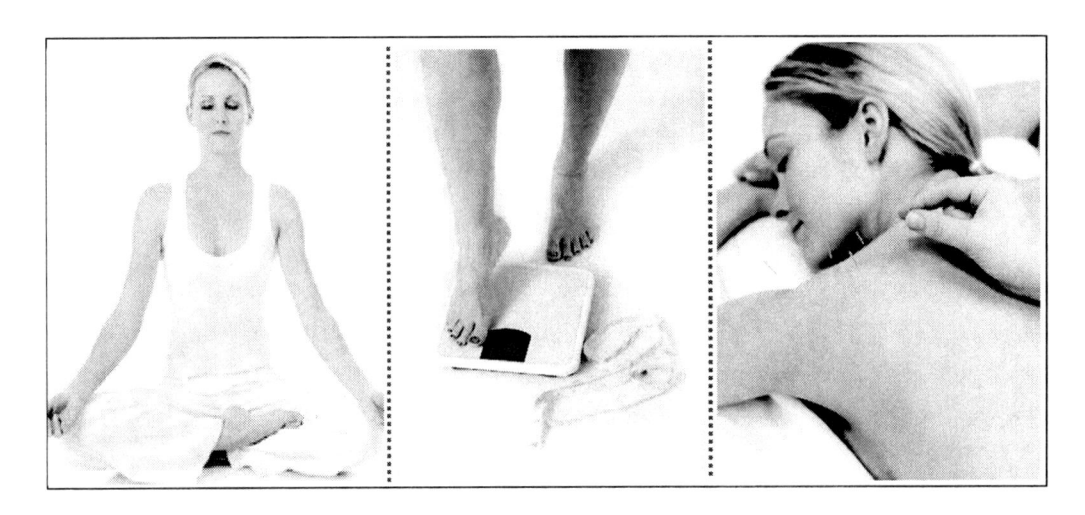

Exercise, Weight Control & Acupuncture:
The Magic Triad for PCOS

One of the more frustrating aspects of living with PCOS is that the combination of hormonal imbalances and insulin resistance can often add up to weight gain – with weight loss a very difficult task, even for those who diet virtually all the time.

If you're also trying to get pregnant, this puts a kind of "double whammy" on your fertility. Not only can the PCOS make it harder to conceive, but, as you read in an earlier chapter, excess weight carries its own set of fertility challenges. For many women it is this conundrum that delivers the final one-two punch to their parenting hopes and dreams. But this doesn't have to be the case!

First, if you follow the advice found in this chapter, and continue to work with your doctor on medical solutions for your PCOS, your insulin resistance will eventually come under control - and this will make it a whole lot easier to control your weight. In fact, many patients who struggled for years with weight problems could not believe just how easy it was to diet and lose those extra pounds once we got their sugar levels under control.

But equally important, research shows that the ancient Chinese treatment known as "acupuncture", can, alone or in combination with exercise, control symptoms of both PCOS and insulin resistance, while it boosts fertility! How does this work?

Acupuncture is the science of using either needles or mild electrical currents to stimulate various nerve points along the body. Among the many things it can accomplish is a reduction in activity of the sympathetic nervous system – which is the system our body uses during the "fight or flight" response. So what does this have to do with fertility – and specifically PCOS?

Research has shown that in women with PCOS, activity of the sympathetic nervous system is often elevated – and that this elevation may, in fact, be partly responsible for the over production of insulin, and an increased incidence of insulin resistance – as well as related conditions including diabetes, obesity, heart disease and stroke.

By reducing the activity of the sympathetic nervous system not only can acupuncture reduce risks of all these conditions, but in the process also decrease menstrual irregularities, which in turn increases fertility.

And that is exactly what one study of 20 women diagnosed with PCOS reported in a recent issue of the *Journal of The American Physiological Society.* Here, researchers from the University of Goteborg in Sweden found that by using a combination of both acupuncture and exercise – which is also known to decrease sympathetic nervous system activity – they were able to jump start the menstrual cycles of women with PCOS – and in some instances even encourage a pregnancy!

To put the study in motion doctors divided the women into the following three groups:

- Nine women received 14 acupuncture treatments over 16 weeks, with stimulation points located in the abdominal muscles, and the backs of the knees, which, according to Chinese medicine are the points that correlate with ovarian activity.

- Five women were instructed to engage in vigorous exercise (brisk walking, cycling or aerobic movement) for 30 to 45 minutes at least three days per week. The goal was to maintain a pulse above 120 beats a minute for this duration of each exercise session. They received no acupuncture.

- Six women received information on the importance of exercise and healthy diet but were not assigned to do anything specific. This was the "control" group and they also received no acupuncture.

Researchers measured the activity of the sympathetic nervous system in all the women both at the start of the study and again at the conclusion of the 16 week trial.

Here is what the study found:

- Both the women in the acupuncture group and those in the exercise group experienced a similarly significant decrease in muscular sympathetic nerve activity compared to the control group.

- The acupuncture group also experienced a drop in waist size, reported fewer menstrual irregularities and experienced a significant decrease in testosterone levels – all key to overcoming PCOS. However, the women in this group did not lose weight or alter their BMI – the measurement of body fat which also plays a role in PCOS.

- The exercise group showed no change in waist size and reported no improvement of menstrual irregularities or reduction in testosterone – but they did experience a drop in weight and a decrease in their BMI.

As such, researchers conclude that the combination of acupuncture and exercise hits all the bases in terms of the factors most important in controlling the symptoms and the consequences of PCOS.

PREVIOUS STUDIES FOUND SIMILAR RESULTS!

This finding dovetails perfectly with the results of a previous study published in the *Scandinavian Journal of Obstetrics and Gynecology* several years earlier. Here, doctors documented that after 10 to 14 treatments of electro-acupuncture administered over the course of two to three months, 38% of women with mild to moderate PCOS began to experience regular ovulation.

THE BOTTOM LINE: If you aren't already engaged in an exercise program I urge you to begin right now. And the best way to start is with a regular walking program. You should begin with a half mile at a time, twice a day if you can swing it, and work your way up to one mile and eventually three miles. Once you are "in stride", you can add hand weights (to increase the rate at which your whole body works) and you can engage in power walking, which not only means moving along at a faster clip, but also swinging your arms and moving your upper body as you walk.

If you can add acupuncture to your regimen, so much the better – but if you do, be certain to seek out a licensed acupuncture doctor and one who has experience treating either infertility patients or gynecologic conditions. Also be sure to inform your gynecologist that you will be undergoing acupuncture treatments. If you experience any negative results - either during or following any treatment, including heavy bleeding, abdominal pain, or general pelvic pain - stop, and see your gynecologist right away.

You can read more about how acupuncture can help all women increase their fertility in Chapter 19.

Getting Pregnant With PCOS:
When More Help Is Needed

For many women with PCOS, getting pregnant will require nothing more than a change in diet, a higher intake of nutrients, and a regular exercise program. In fact, I can tell you without hesitation that many of my PCOS patients were able to begin ovulating, and go on to get pregnant, by using just these few simple measures.

For some women, however, this won't be quite enough. This is particularly true if you are overweight and living with PCOS for some time, and especially if your condition remained undiagnosed for many years. When this is the case, some medical help may be necessary to turn your reproductive odds around.

As I mentioned to you earlier, two of the most commonly used drugs are Metformin (to increase cell sensitivity to insulin), and Clomid, (to stimulate the production of eggs within the ovary). Used either alone, or more often together, this powerful combination gives your ovaries the "one-two" punch that can restore hormonal balance and get you ovulating. And that means your chances for a natural conception dramatically improve!

Ovarian Drilling: Another Treatment Option

If, however, still more help is needed – or if your body does not respond to Clomid – a medical procedure known as "ovarian drilling" can help.

Although this sounds a little frightening, let me assure you it is a relatively simple procedure that involves just one or two tiny incisions into your abdomen for a surgery known as a "laparoscopy". Into these tiny incisions your surgeon will insert thin rods which will hold instruments, or sometimes laser equipment. This is used to make tiny holes in the surface of your ovaries, or sometimes, to actually burn away part of the ovarian tissue.

How can this help? Researchers believe that making small holes in the ovaries helps to "damage" some of the tissue which produces testosterone, thus lowering levels of this and other related hormones blocking egg development and ovulation.

In well over a dozen studies ovary drilling was found to be up to 92% successful in promoting ovulation – although the women who responded best were those at or near their ideal body weight. Women who were obese had a much lower success rate with this surgery – most likely because other factors related to their weight – such as a hormonal imbalance – were continuing to impact ovulation.

For those women who did not spontaneously begin to ovulate after the surgery, a good portion of them did so after stimulation with the egg producing drug Clomid – even if they had not responded to this , or insulin lowering medications tried prior to the egg drilling.

The one major risk involved in this surgery is that if the drilling is not done in a precise manner, or it occurs in an area of the ovary too close to the fallopian tube, scar tissue can result, which can block the tubes and result in another type of infertility.

That said, a skilled surgeon who is experienced in ovarian drilling is likely to have great results. Most often this procedure is done on an outpatient basis, with no hospital stay required and only minimal pain on recovery.

If you have failed to respond to the natural regimens as well as the insulin regulating and egg producing medications, then ovarian drilling is an option you should discuss with your doctor.

CATCHING YOUR FERTILITY THIEF : A FINAL WORD

There is no question that PCOS can present a challenge to any woman trying to get pregnant. Not only can your symptoms affect the way you feel, both physically and emotionally, certainly they can make getting pregnant harder than it has to be.

But what is key, however, is that *once diagnosed this is a relatively simple condition to get under control.* And the best part is you can play a major role in keeping your symptoms and your fertility problems at bay.

Certainly, having your condition accurately diagnosed is the most important first step. And if your doctor determines that you need medication to control blood sugar, it will definitely help overturn some of the fertility problems linked to PCOS. But what's really important is that you also pay careful attention to your diet and lifestyle. In doing so you will not only make a significant difference in your symptom profile, but also impact how quickly and easily you get pregnant. In fact, more so than any other group of women, I can promise that those of you with PCOS who follow the dietary and nutrient suggestions detailed in this book, will definitely see a boost in your overall reproductive health and in your chances of conceiving.

At the same time you must also realize that reproductive change doesn't happen overnight, so be patient with yourself, and give your body time to heal and restore itself. I believe you will begin to feel better within a month of starting the diet and lifestyle changes I recommend – and even sooner if you work with your doctor on finding the right medications.

But if it takes a little bit longer, don't despair and do not give up! PCOS is a treatable condition – and with the right care you will catch your fertility thief sooner than you think!

And remember if you need more information on the fertility treatments that can help you get pregnant, be sure to visit **GettingPregnantNow.org** and pick up a copy of our complete fertility treatment guide *"Getting Pregnant: What You Need To Know Now. "*

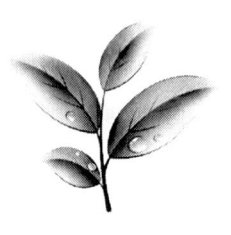

CHAPTER EIGHTEEN

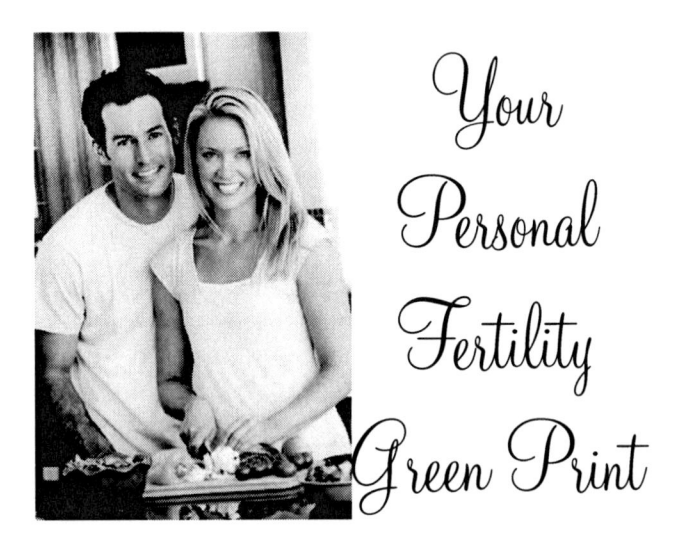

Your Personal Fertility Green Print

A Six Month Countdown Guide To Help You Get Pregnant!

By now I hope you have come to see just how many ways you can naturally influence your fertility – and in doing so dramatically increase your chances for getting pregnant.

In fact it is my hope that you have at least started to implement some of the lifestyle changes I have already recommended – and if so, you should begin to see some results in the very near future. Remember, you have to give it a little bit of time and have some patience ...but I'm very certain you will see results! But that said I also want to once again remind you that if, you are under age 35 and you have not conceived after a year of following the suggestions in this book, or if you are over 35 and pregnancy does not occur within 6 to 8 months, then you and your partner should have some baseline fertility testing. If it turns out that you do need some additional medical help getting pregnant, remember, the earlier you seek that help, the quicker and easier it will be to get pregnant!

More importantly, I'm happy to tell you that getting medical help also doesn't mean you have to abandon your *green fertility* goals! As you will read in the final chapter of this book, there are many new and wonderful fertility treatments that are quite "green" in their approach. There is even a brand new natural form of "GREEN IVF"!

Moreover, I'm even happier to tell you that all of the green fertility advice you've read thus far works equally well, whether you get pregnant on your own, or if you need some additional medical help conceiving. In fact, if you follow the suggestions in this book I can promise that any medical treatment you might need will work better and faster, and ultimately cost less because your health and your fertility will be optimized.

But regardless of whether your pregnancy is all natural, or *Mother Nature* needs a little coaxing from *Father Medicine*, to help ensure that your efforts are successful, I've condensed the most important information in this book into the following 6 month plan. I like to refer to this as my *"Green Print For Pregnancy Success"* - an all-natural system that lays out step-by-step the actions you and your partner need to take – and when to take them – beginning six months prior to when you want to conceive.

To illustrate how it works I've chosen February for the target conception date. The months in which you take these steps will depend on your target date . To chart the correct time frame for your pregnancy simply count backwards six months from the month you want to conceive – and that will be the month you start your *Green Print for Pregnancy Success.*

Also, don't be concerned if you can't complete the steps in the time allotted. Remember this is only a suggested outline so you and your partner should work at your own pace to accomplish as many of the steps as you can prior to conception.

Your Green Print for Pregnancy Success Personal Planner

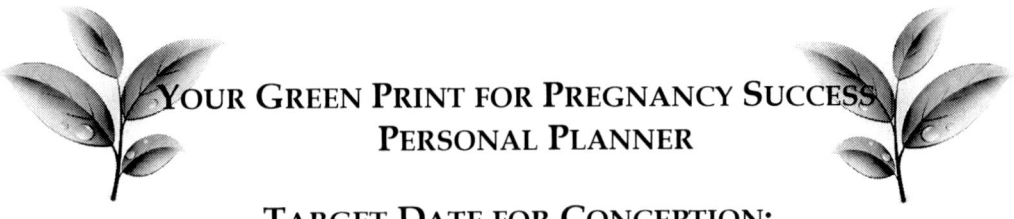

Target Date for Conception: April

Pre Conception Month Six: October

Green Fertility Goal: To begin cleansing your body of as many toxic substances as possible. The goal here is to prepare your body for a healthy conception and give your baby the best possible start in life.

Natural Strategy: Begin reducing exposures to all toxic chemicals over which you have some control. Try not to go outdoors when lawns are being doused with growth chemicals and weed killers, and try avoid the use of chemical pesticides both in and out of doors. When possible look to natural pesticides such as citronella to fight off mosquitoes or boric acid or black pepper to do away with ants and spiders.

If you or your partner smoke, this is the time to begin a program to help you quit. If either of you use alcohol (more than 4 drinks a week) now is the time to begin cutting down. If you use social drugs, you should stop beginning this month. This is also the time to begin cutting out all artificial sweeteners and limit your sugar intake as well.

Mother Nature Suggests: Begin adding as many fruits and vegetables to your diet as you can. If you can't get fresh produce, then your next best choice is frozen. If you choose canned veggies, look for those without added salt. Canned fruit should be packed in water – with no additional sugars. If you can't find these, then choose the "lightest" syrup you can find and then rinse the fruit in water before eating. Do not choose canned fruit that is artificially sweetened.

PRE CONCEPTION MONTH FIVE: NOVEMBER

GREEN FERTILITY GOAL: To achieve the best weight possible before conception. This will have a huge impact on how quickly and easily you conceive. This is also the month to begin a regular exercise program – or to start cutting back if you are working out more than 5 days per week.

NATURAL STRATEGY: Your weight can be a major factor in determining how quickly or how easily you get pregnant. In fact, being overweight or underweight can cause a shift in hormones that interferes with your ability to conceive. At the same time, a shift in weight that is too sudden – either a quick loss or gain – can throw your hormones into even more of a tailspin. For this reason you should begin working towards your fertility weight goals at least 5 months prior to when you want to conceive – and *do so slowly*. A gradual change in weight is always the healthiest, particularly for your fertility.

If you don't already have a regular exercise program, this is the month to start! At the same time, if you are working out more than 5 days a week, or more than 1 hour 3 to 4 days a week, this is the time to cut back just a bit. As you read in an earlier chapter, when it comes to fertility, too much exercise is as bad as no exercise! The ideal workout schedule for fertility is 30 to 45 minutes 3 to 4 days per week. If you are working out more, and particularly if your periods are light, scanty, or irregular, you definitely need to start cutting back on your workouts.

MOTHER NATURE SUGGESTS: If you need to lose weight, you must avoid crash diets (they wreak havoc with hormones) diet pills, fasting, starvation or total liquid diets. Instead look to increase your intake of fresh fruits and vegetables and eat more high - fiber complex carbohydrates to keep you feeling fuller longer. If you need to gain weight, add up to 500 calories a day over what you are eating now. You can easily do this by adding a between-meal supplement drink or by increasing your intake of healthy fats.

In terms of exercise, walking is one of the greatest things you can do for your fertility! You should begin with ½ mile a day and work up to two to three miles two to three times per week. If you are working out too hard and too long – and your menstrual cycle is irregular – try cutting back on some of your more strenuous routines and replace them with a vigorous walk!

Pre Conception Month Four: December

Green Fertility Goal: To overcome nutritional deficiencies linked to infertility.

Natural Strategy: If you have not already started to change your diet, this is the month when change must begin! The best place to start is with the food suggestions explored in Chapter 7 – which will give you a good basis for an overall healthy meal plan. You should also begin eating as many of the "fertility foods" listed in this same chapter as possible – and don't forget to have your partner join you in these healthy meals! Indeed, many of the same foods that impact your fertility will impact his as well. Plus when you help and support each other in meeting your nutritional fertility goals you also work together towards getting pregnant and having a healthier baby!

But this is also the month when you should begin taking a daily pre natal vitamin or add extra folic acid to your multi vitamin. This will not only help boost your fertility but also help ensure a healthy conception, reducing the risk of fetal abnormalities and miscarriage.

Mother Nature Suggests: To help encourage your fertility even more, begin taking the herbal supplements explored in Chapter 11. Since most of these products take at least 8 to 12 weeks before you see a significant difference, the earlier you begin using them prior to conception, the more likely you are to see results.

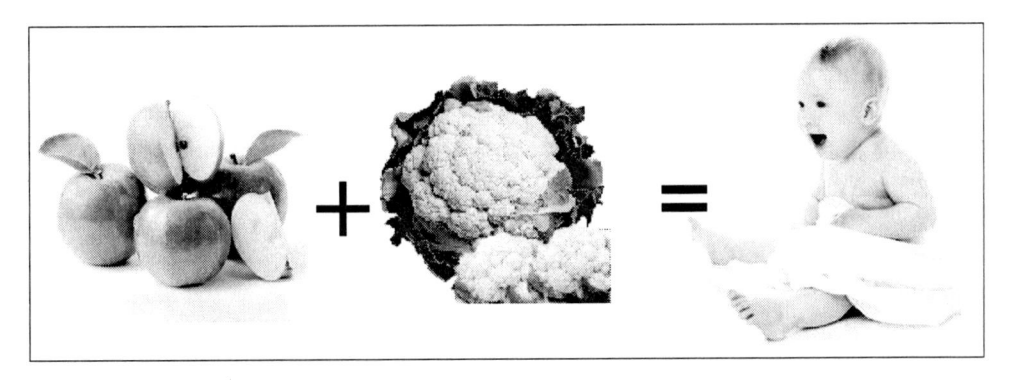

Pre Conception Month Three: January

Green Fertility Goal: To avoid fertility or pregnancy – related complications that may arise from medication or birth control pills; to reduce exposure to fertility robbing environmental factors.

Natural Strategy: If you have been using birth control pills you should stop them this month and switch to a barrier method of contraception until you are ready to get pregnant. Since it can take up to three cycles for some women to begin ovulating normally after stopping the Pill, it's important that you take steps now to help normalize your cycle beginning at least 3 months prior to when you want to conceive.

This is the month you should also begin limiting the use of any unnecessary medications, including both prescription and over-the-counter drugs. This includes cold remedies, pain relievers, sinus medications, cough medicines, diuretics, tranquillizers and antibiotics.

Remember however the key here is "unnecessary" medications. If you are using any of these drugs for a chronic condition, this is the month to talk to your doctor about whether or not the medications you are using can interfere with fertility or pregnancy – and if so, discuss what other treatments can be substituted. If you make the switch now, your fertility will not be compromised. This advice also applies to your partner since there are a number of medications that can impact sperm production as well.

Mother Nature Suggests: If you can't stop or reduce the use of certain medications, you should be extra vigilant about taking your prenatal vitamins and adding some extra Vitamin C, D and B complex. These are the nutrients that help bolster your immune system and reduce toxic overloads linked to infertility. This is the month your partner should take steps to ensure the production of healthy sperm. In addition to reducing the use of unnecessary medications, he should begin this month to avoid hot tubs, hot baths, and tight underwear and to limit the use of his laptop computer *on this lap.* (Working on a table or desk is fine!). He should also stop all use of recreational drugs.

PRE CONCEPTION MONTH TWO: FEBRUARY

GREEN FERTILITY GOAL: To ensure your reproductive health, make certain all chronic medical problems are under control, including thyroid disorders and blood sugar; to ensure that you and your partner are free of any fertility-robbing infections; to begin charting your natural fertility signs.

NATURAL STRATEGY: Begin this month with a pre conception exam. If you are using an IUD, this is the time it should be removed, and you should be tested once again for the presence of any "silent" fertility robbing infections such as chlamydia. You should also have a pelvic exam to ensure that no fertility-robbing problems have arisen since your last check up. Certainly any obvious conditions such as a yeast infection or even a vaginal irritation must be treated now. If you have either a thyroid problem or blood sugar issues this is also the time to get symptoms under control – so make sure your doctor runs any necessary routine tests.

This is also the month to begin charting your ovulation. Using a combination of methods described in Chapter Three , keep written records of temperature and other signs of ovulation so you will begin to know exactly when in your upcoming cycles you will be the most fertile.

MOTHER NATURE SUGGESTS: If you haven't already begun stress reduction activities, this is the month to start. Be it meditation, yoga, deep breathing or simply relaxing with a good book, you must make time to unwind each and every day. As you learned in Chapter Six, stress is a major fertility thief. And, while you may not be able to remove the stressors from your life, you can certainly help your body to deal with the consequences by making time every day, to unwind and relax.

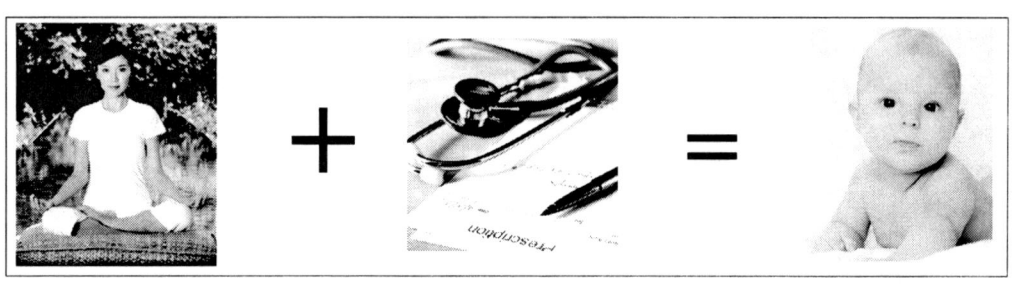

PRE CONCEPTION MONTH ONE: MARCH

GREEN FERTILITY GOAL: To achieve maximum fertility potential

NATURAL STRATEGY: This is the month when you need to get really "serious" about the lifestyle changes that have a direct impact on conception. During this month you and your partner should dramatically restrict alcohol consumption, and avoid the use of all recreational drugs. If you have been dieting to lose weight, you can taper off on this month – eating a super healthy diet and getting proper nourishment is much more important at this point then losing one or two more pounds.

While I don't mean that you should toss caution to the wind and eat anything you like, but this is the month when you can lighten up a bit and concentrate more on eating healthy than counting calories.

If you are on a regular exercise program you should also cut back a bit this month – making certain to work out no more than 20 to 30 minutes 3 days a week. The one thing you don't want to do this month is work your body too hard - particularly if you have been using several of the ovulation prediction methods described earlier to track your most fertile time. Working out too much could throw those predictions off – so don't make any dramatic changes in your routines this month.

Finally, try to relax as much as possible this month – and maybe even increase your "me" time a bit each week. If you have been setting aside two hours a week for stress reduction, increase it to four hours per week during this preconception month. I can promise it will pay off in terms of helping you conceive faster and easier. During this extra time be sure to do something that is not only healthy and relaxing, but something you enjoy

MOTHER NATURE SUGGESTS: If you can afford to take some time off from work, this is the month to cash in on those saved up vacation or sick days. If you are saving up your vacation for your actual conception month – also a good idea – then try to cut back on some of your work – load this month, so that you don't find yourself working at home evenings and weekends. Again, it's extremely important that in the month prior to conception you spend as much time relaxing as you can.

YOUR TARGET CONCEPTION MONTH: APRIL

GREEN FERTILITY GOAL: To have a quick, easy natural conception – and get pregnant fast!

NATURAL STRATEGIES: If you are using an ovulation prediction kit, a fertility monitor or any of the natural ovulation prediction strategies mentioned earlier in this book, this is the month to pay close attention.

As the time draws near, plan to start making love as often as possible starting five days before you expect ovulation to occur. To help make the most of these efforts, many couples find that taking a few vacation days is great way to ensure you have both the time, and a stress-free environment in which to relax and make love whenever the mood strikes you!

If you can also sneak away to romantic get-a-away - even better! If not, doing what you can to make your home fires burn as romantically as possible is also a plus.

You should also pay extra close attention to vaginal health and hygiene during this month, and if you see any signs of infection – including abnormal discharge, see your doctor before you attempt conception. Also try not to use any vaginal lubricants, deodorants, or other types of intimate creams or lotions in the days prior to attempting conception.

MOTHER NATURE SUGGESTS: Approach this time frame radiating love and affection for each other – and don't just concentrate on making a baby! Truly enjoy each other – and when you can expand your love making sessions to include lots of romantic foreplay.

When you concentrate on the happiness you feel being together, and the love you have for one another, you set the stage for the kind of happy hormonal harmony that definitely increases your chance of conception. At the same time, feel confident in your ability to get pregnant and believe with your whole heart that your parenting dreams will come true!

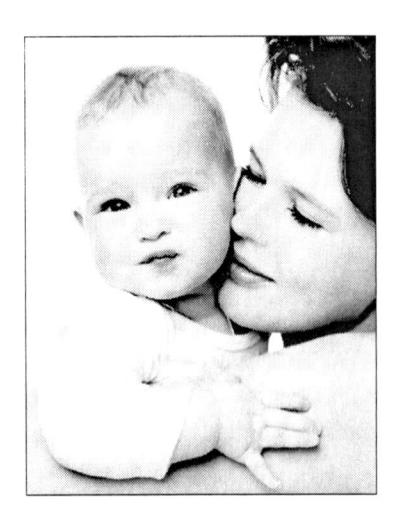

Ten Natural Ways to Increase Your Pregnancy Odds – Right Now

Several days prior to when you want to conceive start doing the following:

1. **PRIME YOUR MUCOUS** – Take one to two teaspoons daily of Robitussin Chest Congestion with guaifenesin beginning three to four days before you want to conceive. This will help thin vaginal mucous and make sperm transport quicker and easier. Be certain however to use only the Chest Congestion formula. You want to avoid the ingredient dexthromathoraphene, which can be harmful to fertility.

2. **MAKE LOVE OFTEN!** While doctors once believed that making love too often would decrease a man's potency, we now know this isn't true! As long as your partner is healthy, making love as often as you like during your fertile window is the best way to increase your chances of conception.

3. *KEEP YOUR COOL!* You and your partner should avoid hot tubs, very hot showers, saunas or steam rooms, particularly during the days you are trying to conceive.

4. **SLEEP PER CHANCE TO DREAM!** - Make certain you get at least 7 to 8 hours of sleep for two nights in a row before attempting conception. This can have an amazing restorative power on your entire body as well as boost your fertility!

5. **LOAD UP ON VITAMINS!** In addition to your prenatal or multi vitamin with extra folic acid, as your most fertile time approaches increase your vitamin C intake by 500 mg and your B Complex by 50 mg. Your partner should do the same.

6. **TRY A FERTILITY MASSAGE!** This is something you can do on your own – or together with your partner. To begin, place your hands palm down on your tummy and begin lightly rubbing your hands in a clockwise circular motion around your belly button.

   Gradually widen the circle so that you are gently stimulating blood flow towards your bikini line and beyond. Do this for up to 10 minutes at a time, up to 3 times a day. Additionally, you may also want to gently massage the center of your big toe on each foot. In Chinese medicine this point correlates with the pituitary gland and may help stimulate the production of hormones related to conception.

ONCE YOU BEGIN TRYING TO GET PREGNANT:

7. **LIMIT MOVEMENT AFTER INTERCOURSE -** By remaining in a prone position for up to 30 minutes after intercourse you will help encourage sperm to travel towards your uterus. You should also put a pillow under your pelvis, slanting your V zone backwards, to further help facilitate the movement of sperm in the right direction!

8. **HOLD SPERM IN YOUR VAGINA** – Lightly press together the outside lips of your vagina as soon as your partner withdraws - and hold it closed for several minutes. This will also help ensure that every possible sperm makes its way inside.

9. **USE FAST WITHDRAWAL -** Studies show that if your partner withdraws his penis immediately following the first ejaculation, sperm concentration is increased and chances for conception improve.

10. **THINK ABOUT MAKING LOVE** – not about making babies! Stay positive and focused, don't stress and don't worry! And most of all don't turn conception into a "chore"! Enjoy the process, enjoy each other, and never forget the secret ingredient is "LOVE" !

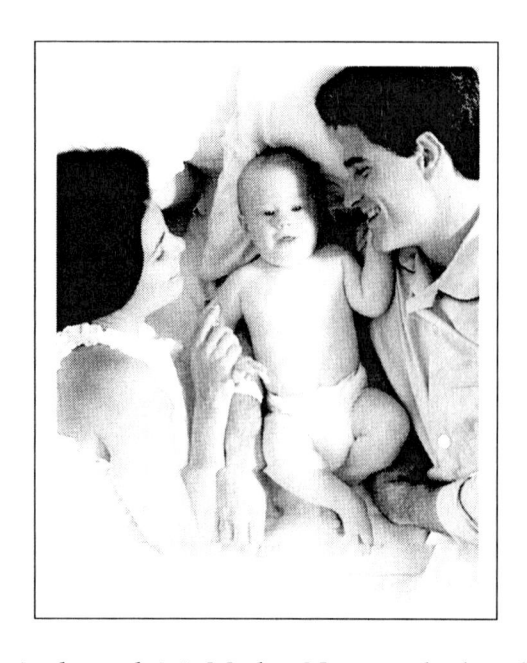

IF CONCEPTION DOES NOT HAPPEN RIGHT AWAY ....

While for some of you following my Green Fertility Plan conception will occur during your target month – on the first try! That said, depending on your age, and the age of your partner, as well as many individual variables, most couples will require at least 3 to 6 months of trying before conception happens.

It's also important to remember that it can take up to one year to get pregnant, even if you and your partner are young and in perfect health! Indeed, as a fertility doctor I am often reminded that in the end, it is Mother Nature who has the final say – and sometimes a pregnancy simply takes a bit longer to achieve, even when all conditions are perfect. In fact, statistically speaking the rate of pregnancy in normal, healthy couples is only 14 percent – with just three pregnancies possible for every 25 acts of intercourse performed during the most fertile time.

So, if in fact you don't get pregnant right away, don't worry and don't get stressed! Just keep following the Green Fertility Plan, and continue to repeat the suggestions for your target month and I am quite certain that before long you will get pregnant!

That said I would be remiss in my care of you if I did not mention yet one last time, that if you are under age 35 and have not conceived after 12 months of regular, unprotected intercourse during your most fertile times, or if you are over 35 and conception does not occur within 6 months, you should have a baseline check up with either a fertility specialist, or any obstetrician or gynecologist who has a background in fertility testing. And your partner should have some basic sperm testing as well.

This is important even if you have both already had the preconception check up exams that I recommended at the start of this book, since sometimes factors which influence fertility can change over time. So, even if you were in great shape in

January, for example, by the following September problems could have arisen which might be keeping you from conceiving.

If, in fact, your tests show that everything is okay, then you can feel free to continue following the advice in this book and to keep on trying, confidant that nothing is wrong!

However, if a another year passes and you are still not pregnant, then it is time to seek a more in-depth analysis of your fertility profile.

It doesn't automatically mean something is wrong – but it could mean a problem may have been overlooked, or that you may need a little medical help to make your parenting dreams come true.

If this turns out to be the case, then don't become worried or fearful and never give up hope! There are are many new and wonderful medical treatments available, at least some of which utilize a truly green and natural approach to helping you get pregnant.

If you read on to the final chapter in this book, you will see just how far fertility medicine has come since little Baby Louise – the first IVF baby – was born in 1978 – and just how easy it can be to *get pregnant naturally*, with just a little help from your doctor!

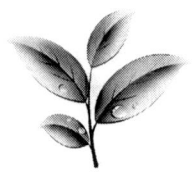

Chapter Nineteen

Getting Pregnant:

When Science & Nature Combine...
Miracles Can Happen!

There is no doubt in my mind that for most of you reading this book, the natural solutions and diet and lifestyle changes featured throughout will be all the help you need in achieving your parenting dreams.

While some of you may need to make more changes than others, and some may take longer to get pregnant, once you find your "fertility zone" you'll know exactly what needs to be done right now, and each and every time you want to conceive in the future.

But as a fertility specialist for more than two decades I also know that for some of you there may be fertility problems that go beyond what can be "fixed" by a simple change in diet or lifestyle.

If there is damage to your to fallopian tubes, for example, as the result of scar tissue or infection, if your ability to ovulate good eggs has been compromised, or if your partner has serious sperm making problems, lifestyle and dietary changes simply can't take you the whole way there.

And that is where some of the newer medical technologies may be able to give you that extra helping hand so that you can get pregnant faster and easier.

Moreover, some of the newest technologies combine medicine and nature in a way that not only allows for a more natural conception, but in the process also reduces some of the costs, so that getting fertility help is now much more affordable than ever before.

In my best selling book *"Getting Pregnant: What You Need To Know"* we explore many of these newer technologies in great detail. And if you are having problems getting pregnant we hope you'll consider reading this book as well – it has already helped tens of thousands of couples get pregnant and I am quite certain it can help you as well!

In the meantime, however, I've prepared the following short guide to some of the very newest and most natural ways your doctor can help you get pregnant faster and easier, including the new **"GREEN IVF"** - a natural cycle fertility treatment that is as close to nature as science can get! I hope you will use this information to open a discussion with your doctor, and that together you can find the treatments that work best for you and your partner.

Additionally, I also want to urge you to keep following all the advice in this book thus far - not only in regard to changes in diet and lifestyle but also the recommendations in terms of vitamins, herbs, supplements, exercise and stress reduction techniques.

The truth is, anything that encourages natural fertility, also encourages the success of *all fertility treatments*.

So in the event that you will need some type medical treatment to help you conceive, I can promise that everything you have learned in this book will help ensure that your treatments will be more successful, and you will get pregnant faster and easier!

Getting Pregnant: The Newest Natural Technologies

Among the most popular of all fertility treatments worldwide involves a process known as IVF or in vitro fertilization. While there are many different varieties of IVF and varying techniques that are used, the basic premise remains the same: To allow fertilization to take place outside the body in an environment that is medically created to optimize the chance for conception.

The newest and most exciting form of these technologies is something I like to call GREEN IVF - because it is one of the most natural of all the new ways your doctor can help you get pregnant. In a few moments I'll tell you why – and how it differs from traditional IVF. But in order to fully understand and appreciate those differences, I want to take just a few minutes to help you understand how traditional IVF works.

Understanding IVF

The traditional IVF process involves using a series of medications to prime your body to manufacture multiple eggs, and then extracting those eggs from your ovary in a procedure called "egg retrieval". Your eggs are then placed into a laboratory dish filled with a special fluid designed to encourage healthy development. When this occurs – in anywhere from 12 to 48 hours – a specific amount of your partner's sperm is added to the dish, turning it into a kind of "glass fallopian tube". Much the way it would happen in your own fallopian tube, here sperm and egg "find" each other. When this occurs, your partner's sperm penetrates one or more of your eggs and once joined, an embryo is created - just as it would be naturally inside your body. When your embryos reaches a certain size up to three are transferred into your uterus where they will hopefully implant and begin to grow. And voila ... pregnancy begins! The remainder of your gestation will be the same as if conception had occurred inside your body.

This traditional form of IVF is best when you have a problem ovulating, if you have damage within your fallopian tubes (from a previous infection for example, or extensive endometriosis), or if your partner has low sperm quantity or quality.

In an increasingly popular form of IVF known as ICSI (intracytoplasmic sperm injection) your partner's sperm is injected directly inside your egg. This not only

Traditional IVF

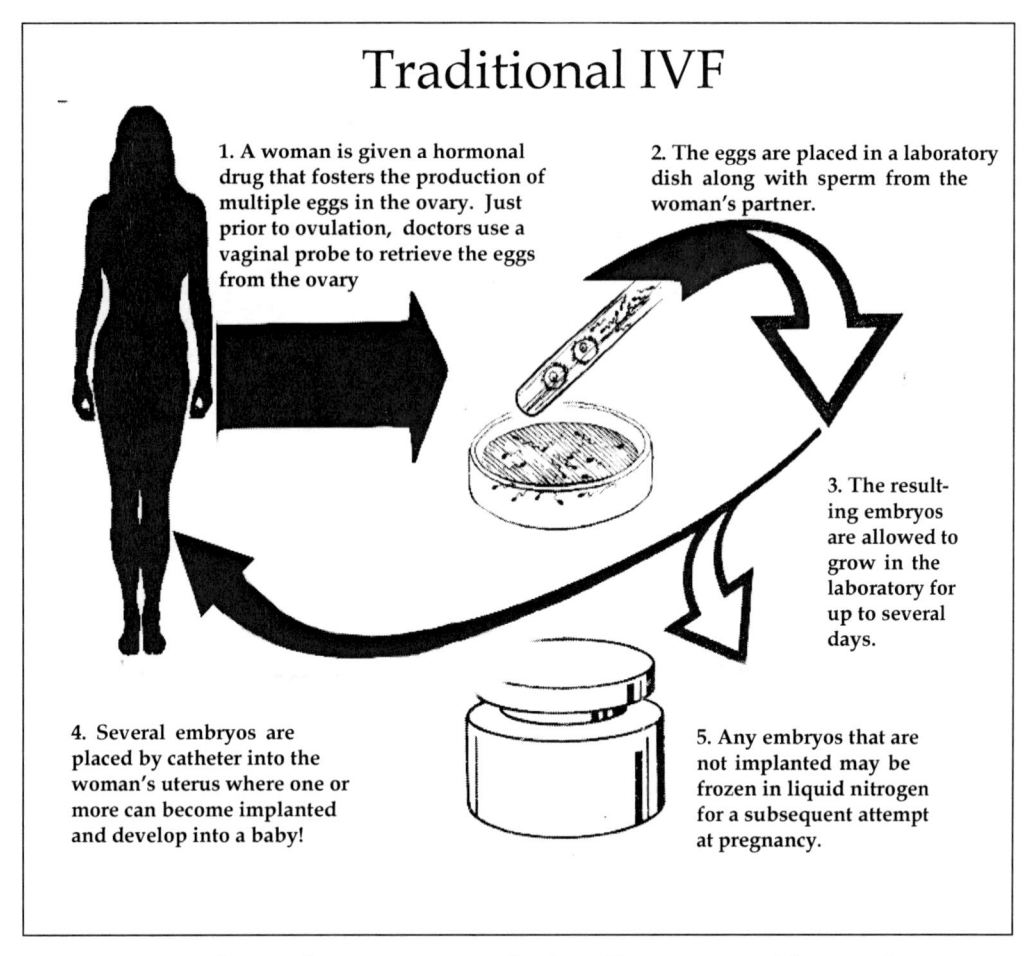

1. A woman is given a hormonal drug that fosters the production of multiple eggs in the ovary. Just prior to ovulation, doctors use a vaginal probe to retrieve the eggs from the ovary

2. The eggs are placed in a laboratory dish along with sperm from the woman's partner.

3. The resulting embryos are allowed to grow in the laboratory for up to several days.

4. Several embryos are placed by catheter into the woman's uterus where one or more can become implanted and develop into a baby!

5. Any embryos that are not implanted may be frozen in liquid nitrogen for a subsequent attempt at pregnancy.

increases your chance for pregnancy, it also allows men with very few sperm to father a child much more easily. This procedure is best when male fertility factors are prominent, or when issues within your body prevent sperm from reaching your egg.

In still another variation of IVF known as GIFT (gamme intro fallopian tube transfer) your eggs and your partner's sperm are loaded into a catheter and injected into your fallopian tube, where a natural conception is allowed to take place inside your body.

The GIFT procedure is often used when a woman's tubes are in good health, but ovulation does not occur regularly or something blocks the eggs from leaving the ovary. It can also be helpful if sperm are not as plentiful as they should be.

The New Green IVF

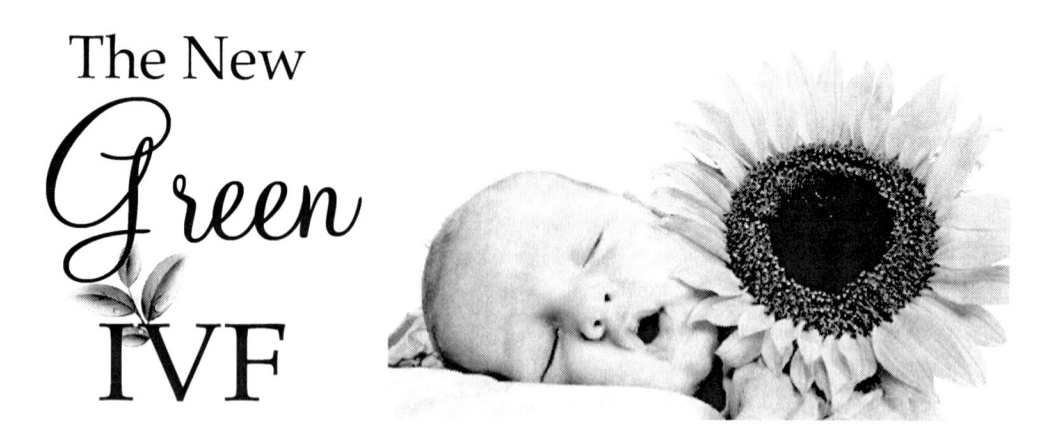

From almost the time IVF began - the first birth took place in 1978 - one of the key factors allowing this procedure to work as well as it has, is the use of fertility drugs. These are medications designed to encourage the growth and development of multiple eggs while also allowing doctors to manipulate your hormones and in a sense "take control" of your fertility cycle.

The result: Instead of making and ovulating just one egg, a woman can make many eggs; instead of pregnancy occurring from one embryo, multiple eggs are combined with lots of sperm resulting in multiple embryos. Instead of just one fertilized embryo making it's way to a woman's uterus, multiple embryos are transferred into her body. All of this increases the chance for pregnancy.

The most common egg-making medications are clomiphene citrate (Clomid, Serophene), follicle stimulating hormone (Follistim, Gonal-f), human chorionic gonadotropin or HCG (Ovidrel, Pregnyl, Novarel), GnRH Agonists like Antagon and Cetrocide, and sometimes leuprolide (Lupron, synthetic gonadotropin inhibitor). And for many couples these, and medications like them, become the deciding factor that allows conception to occur. This is particularly true for women whose fertility problems are related to egg production and ovulation, as well as for those over age 40 – a time when not only natural egg production declines, but so does the quality of each egg that is produced.

That said, the use of these medications are not without problems. Some involve the need for painful injections, while others are riddled with side effects that can impact a woman both emotionally and physically. As such, as time went on research also began to suggest that at least some of these medications may actually be increasing a woman's health risks later in life, including the risk of some hormone - sensitive cancers.

And of course, most fertility drugs are also costly, sometimes accounting for up to one half of the cost of the cycle. Moreover, whether used in conjunction with IVF - or even on their own- fertility drugs almost always result in a multiple birth, most often twins.

As all of these issues came together, a group of brilliant new fertility pioneers began to look for what might be a better way to combine science and nature - one that does not involve the use of these medications. Their thought: That the less medicine interferes with nature, the better the outcome might be!

The result of this thinking eventually led to the development of what I like to call 'GREEN IVF' - a natural cycle fertility treatment that relies primarily on the workings of a woman's own body to lay the groundwork for the IVF procedure.

So, instead of bombarding your body with medications designed to force your system to produce an abnormally large number of eggs in a given cycle, Green IVF allows your body to do what it does naturally - i.e., grow, mature, and develop just one egg, the " right " egg, the "best" egg for fertilization. That one egg is then harvested, combined with sperm, and the *single resulting embryo* is placed back into your uterus - in almost the exact same way it would be if your conception had occurred naturally inside your body.

According to Drs. DiMattina and Gordon, who have pioneered this procedure in the Washington, DC area, when it comes to selecting the best egg for fertilization, a woman may know best - or at least her body does!

Indeed, by allowing the body to naturally select the egg that will be fertilized, doctors who perform GREEN IVF believe they are joining together the best of mother nature with the best of science for a combination that simply can't be beat!

"With Natural Cycle IVF we are essentially going back to the future: one egg, one embryo and one baby," writes Dr. DiMattina on his website at DominionFertility.com

ARE YOU A CANDIDATE FOR GREEN IVF?

Certainly, the traditional form of IVF is still among the most popular and the most widely used laboratory assisted pregnancy techniques throughout the world. But for a special group of women, the new GREEN IVF may be just what the doctor ordered! So who is the best candidate for GREEN IVF?

According to John Zhang M.D., Ph.D., director of the New Hope Fertility Clinic in New York City, and one of the true pioneers of natural cycle IVF, this procedure is " Ideal for women who choose to live a drug-free and chemical-free lifestyle or for women who, because of age or poor fertility health, are less likely to produce multiple eggs even if heavy IVF drugs are administered."

Indeed, in one study published recently in the journal *Fertility and Sterility*, a group of reproductive experts from Rome, Italy found that in women who did not previously respond well to fertility drugs, natural cycle "GREEN IVF" was able to help them achieve a successful implantation at a rate nearly three times higher than those who underwent traditional IVF with drug stimulation. Moreover, the younger the women were, the higher the rate of pregnancy.

And so it's clear that this procedure not only works, but for some women may actually be a much better alternative than even traditional IVF.

As to some of the specific criteria for success, many who perform GREEN IVF believe the following is important:

- You have fairly normal and regular menstrual cycles.

- You are ovulating on a fairly regular basis

- Day 3 or Day 10 your FSH should be under 20

- Day 3 levels of E2 (estrogen) are less than 70.

I believe you should also consider GREEN IVF if you have been told that one or both fallopian tubes are blocked, you have experienced chronic early stage miscarriage, or your partner has less than optimal sperm.

GREEN IVF FOR WOMEN OVER 40

If you are over age 40, the success of GREEN IVF varies from center to center. In some, like Dominion Fertility, natural cycle IVF is not encouraged for women over 35. But in Dr. Zhang's center, for example, women over 40 are regularly treated with natural cycle IVF. So, if you are turned down by one center, keep looking before you give up on the idea of GREEN IVF. You should get at least 3 opinions before deciding if this is the procedure for you. If you visit GreenFertility.com you'll find a listing of the most popular centers around the US offering the new GREEN IVF. Or send us an email and we'll help you locate a center in your area.

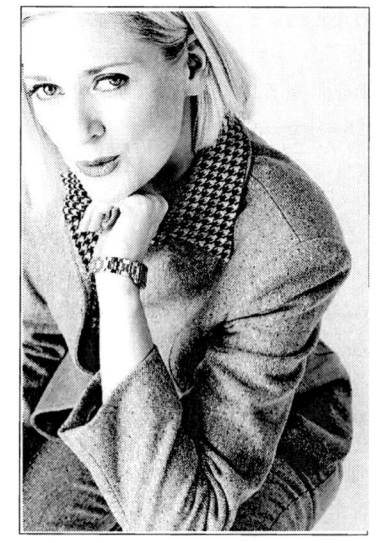

GREEN IVF: THE SUCCESS RATE

If you are like most of my patients, among your primary concerns – with any fertility treatment – is the success rate. Or, more simply put how many pregnancies result from this procedure when compared to the number of times it has been tried. In the case of traditional IVF we have reams of data from years of experience that tells the story.

But GREEN IVF is new, and the number of clinics around the world performing this treatment is still small by comparison. So that means we don't have anywhere near the kind of "numbers" we do with traditional IVF. But the good news is that though somewhat limited, the data we do have reveals astounding results!

In fact, based on information reported in the medical literature, along with the success rates of centers like New Hope Fertility, Dominion Fertility, and others, patients who undergo between two and three GREEN IVF procedures have a cumulative success rate that is equal to, or exceeds, that of traditional IVF – which is about 35%. Pregnancy rates for natural conception for couples who are young and healthy is roughly 25% per each menstrual cycle.

Of course there is criticism of GREEN IVF – most often based on the idea that it may take many cycles before a pregnancy is achieved. I, however, don't believe this is necessarily true. For example, in a research paper recently submitted and accepted by the American Society of Reproductive Medicine, one clinic reports that 64% of patients undergoing GREEN IVF got pregnant on the first try, while 21% got pregnant on their second try. This is equal to or better than the success rate of traditional IVF!

Indeed, at the University of Southern California, where doctors were among the first to pioneer all forms of IVF, natural cycle IVF has been an area of interest for more than two decades. Here, studies conducted as early as 1992 found that although the pregnancy rate was half compared to cycles where drugs were used, *the per embryo implantation rate was much higher* in the women undergoing natural cycle IVF, making it overall, the more successful treatment!

According to the experts at USC, now that the success rate of the typical IVF pregnancy is so much higher than in 1992, they anticipate the success rates with natural cycle IVF will be much higher now as well - one reason they are among the first university fertility programs to undertake a major study of natural IVF.

What's also important to remember however, is that if indeed, you require more than one cycle of GREEN IVF to get pregnant, because no drugs are being used, these repeat cycles are generally far less demanding, physically, emotionally and financially, then repeated cycles of traditional IVF.

> Remember ....
> how you get
> pregnant doesn't
> matter ... your
> baby will love
> you just the same!

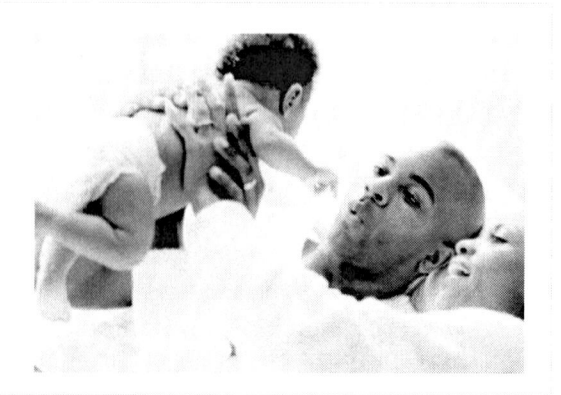

A New Twist on GREEN IVF

If you are one of millions of women battling PCOS – poly cystic ovarian syndrome – or if you have any problems ovulating - a new twist on the "GREEN IVF" might give your fertility an extra boost! The procedure is called "immature oocyte retrieval". Here, doctors use a trans-vaginal ultra sound to help guide them to the inside of your ovary where they harvest un-stimulated, still immature egg "follicles".

Once the follicles are removed, they are placed into a special solution allowing them to develop into fully matured eggs – much the way they would in your ovary. As they mature and ready for conception, they are mixed with sperm using traditional IVF techniques, and eventually the resulting embryo is placed into the uterus.

This procedure is wonderful if you do have PCOS, since often times this condition precludes you being able to actually manufacture your own eggs. But thanks to this procedure, as long as your body is making the *egg follicles,* you can still get pregnant!

But it's not just women with PCOS who can benefit from this procedure. Because there is no need for eggs to actually grow and develop, there is no need to use egg –producing drugs, or to use medications to stop ovulation so the eggs can be harvested.

So this procedure is another way of performing a drug-free GREEN IVF.

Of course as with most fertility treatments, timing is everything! Indeed, in order for the natural hormonal stimulation which follows ovulation to naturally prepare your uterus for a healthy conception, follicle retrieval must take place at the right time in your cycle – early enough to "catch" the follicles before they start to develop, but late enough in the cycle so that the natural hormonal stimulations still occur and your uterus can be ready and waiting to receive your embryo.

What can help is "priming" the body with small doses of natural estrogen, equal to what you would be making on your own, if your eggs were developing in, and ovulating from, your ovary. The supplemental estrogen helps the lining of your uterus to more fully develop in anticipation of receiving a fertilized embryo.

ACUPUNCTURE:
A DRUG FREE ANCIENT CHINESE FERTILITY SECRET THAT REALLY WORKS!

If headlines are any indication of what's hot and what's not, it's easy to believe that infertility treatment is strictly a modern day science, made possible solely through the courtesy of high-tech medicine.

But as good as modern science is, many couples trying to get pregnant find themselves turning to an age-old treatment for help -- one so steeped in tradition it's about as far from life in the 21st century as one can get.

That treatment is acupuncture, and today, even high-tech reproductive specialists are looking to the somewhat mysterious world of Chinese medicine to help those fertility patients for whom western science alone is not quite enough.

"Most of our patients are referred to us by reproductive medicine specialists -- they are usually women who have failed one or usually more than one attempt at IVF (in vitro fertilization), and their doctor is looking for something to help implement the success of their treatment, over and above what the protocols alone can accomplish," says Raymond Chang, MD, the medical director of Meridian Medical and a classically trained acupuncturist as well as western-trained medical doctor.

Acupuncture is an ancient Chinese medicine treatment that relies on the painless but strategic placement of tiny needles into a "grid-like" pattern that spans the body, from head to toe. The needles are used to stimulate certain key "energy points" believed to regulate spiritual, mental, emotional, and physical balance. And, for many women, it's often just what the doctor ordered.

Moreover, many believe it can allow you to cross the line from **infertile** to **fertile** by helping your body function more efficiently. For many women, this extra "boost" is all they need to get pregnant naturally, on their own.

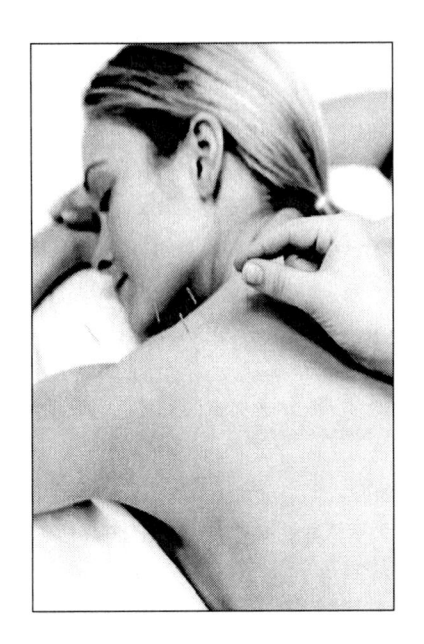

> **Q:** I'd like to try acupuncture but I hate needles — & I'm wondering if it hurts?
>
> **A:** No, it doesn't hurt! Acupuncture is an ancient Chinese medicine treatment that painlessly places a series of tiny needles just under the skin in a specific grid-like pattern. While some women report feeling a slight "Twinge" when the needles are inserted, most say they feel no pain at all! In fact, many women report the treatment is relaxing and calming helping them to feel fully rejuvenated!
>
> But if even the thought of needles sends shivers up your spine, you may be a candidate for the new "electronic acupuncture - an innovative technique that uses minute electronic pulses on the surface of the skin to simulate the same points as the needles. This generates a slight feeling of vibration but is thought to be virtually pain-free. Many Chinese Medicine doctors now off this alternative method of acupuncture as well as the traditional form.

When this isn't the case, acupuncture has also been shown to increase the success of many modern reproductive treatments, including IVF.

Indeed, in a study of 160 women, published April 2002 in the reproductive journal *Fertility and Sterility,* a group of German researchers found that adding acupuncture to the traditional IVF treatment protocols substantially increased pregnancy

In this study one group of 80 patients received two, 25-minute acupuncture treatments -- one prior to having fertilized embryos transferred into their uterus, and one directly afterwards. The second group of 80, who also underwent embryo transfer, received no acupuncture treatments.

The result: While women in both groups got pregnant, the rate was significantly higher in the acupuncture group - 34 pregnancies, compared with 21 in the women who received IVF alone.

More recently, two Colorado physicians teamed up on several studies that offered similar results.

Dr. Paul C. Magarelli, an infertility doctor at the Reproductive Medicine & Fertility Center in Colorado Springs, Colorado, and Dr. Diane K. Cridennda, a licensed acupuncturist with a master's degree in Oriental medicine studied 147 women all believed to be "poor responders" to traditional IVF.

By adding acupuncture treatments to their fertility regimen, the doctors found they were able to increase pregnancy rates by a whopping 40%, with 11% more babies born to the women treated with acupuncture!

In still another study released by Magarelli and Cridennda, acupuncture appeared to increase the overall pregnancy rate by a significant 24%, over women who did not receive the acupuncture treatments.

ACUPUNCTURE: WORKS FOR NATURAL PREGNANCIES AS WELL!

While increasing the odds of IVF is an important milestone for acupuncture treatments, it's not the only way this ancient Chinese mystery can help. Chang says acupuncture also works to stimulate egg production in women who can't -- or don't want to -- use fertility medications to help them get pregnant.

"When you compare the pregnancy rates for an egg producing drug such as Clomid to acupuncture alone, the rates are equal to those undergoing IVF - a 50% chance of pregnancy in three months for general patients," says Chang.

I believe that if you also follow the diet, exercise and supplement guidelines in this book, acupuncture may help you even more! Indeed, whether you are getting pregnant naturally, or using one of the new GREEN IVF procedures, it's clear that acupuncture can increase your chances for conception - and for some couples, quite dramatically!

How Acupuncture Helps You Get Pregnant

According to the traditional Chinese medicine explanation, acupuncture stimulates and moves Qi (pronounced "Chee") a form of life energy that ancient wisdom says must flow through the body unhampered from head to toe, 24/7. When it doesn't, illness or malfunction - including infertility - arise.

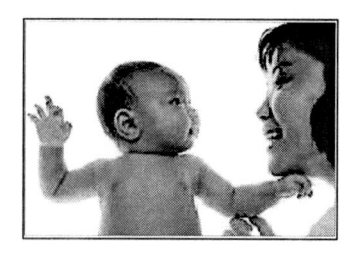

"Acupuncture works to restore the flow of Qi - your essence, your body energy - so with regards to infertility, treatment has a calming, restorative effect that increases a sense of well-being and ultimately helps the body to accept the creation of new life," says acupuncturist Ifeoma Okoronkwo, MD, a professor of medicine at New York University School of Medicine.

By placing the needles at key energy meridians linked to the reproductive organs, Okoronkwo says acupuncture increases, and more importantly, moves the flow of Qi from areas where it may be too abundant, to areas that are deficient, all in a direction that encourages fertility.

To get your fertility Qi up to snuff, most experts say you will need about two, 30 minute treatments a week, sometimes for several months, before the effects can be seen.

However, a slightly more Western way of looking at the effects points less to the mystical Qi and more towards the solid science of brain chemistry.

In studies published in the journal *Fertility and Sterility* in 2002, researchers found a clear link between treatment and the brain hormones involved in conception. More specifically their research noted that acupuncture increases production of endorphins, the body's natural "feel good" brain chemical that also plays a role in regulating the menstrual cycle.

Chang says acupuncture also appears to have a neuro-endocrine effect, impacting a three-way axis between two areas of the brain involved with hormone production (the hypothalamus and the pituitary glands) and the ovaries. And, say experts, it's a constellation of activity that ultimately impacts egg production and possibly ovulation.

In still another research paper published in the journal *Medical Acupuncture* in 2000, Sandra Emmons, MD, assistant professor of obstetrics and gynecology at Oregon Health Sciences University, reports that acupuncture may directly impact the number of egg follicles available for fertilization in women undergoing IVF.

"My guess is that acupuncture is changing the blood supply to the ovaries, possibly dilating the arteries and increasing blood flow, so that ultimately, the ovaries are receiving greater amounts of hormonal stimulation," says Emmons, who also uses acupuncture in her traditional medical practice.

Chang says acupuncture may also help when the lining of the uterus is too weak to sustain a pregnancy - a problem that is also known to increase the risk of chronic miscarriage.

By increasing blood flow to this area, the lining may be better able to absorb the nutrients and hormones necessary to help it grow strong enough to hold onto an implanted embryo, says Chang.

Is Acupuncture Right For you? How To Tell !

As good as it sounds, acupuncture is clearly not the panacea for all fertility problems. If, for example, a structural defect exists -- such as a blocked fallopian tube or a fibroid tumor - on it's own, acupuncture won't help you get pregnant.

Likewise, once past a certain age, no amount of tickling your Qi is going to increase necessary hormones that have long gone out of production.

For this reason, I strongly recommend that you have at least a basic fertility workup before attempting acupuncture treatment, particularly if you are approaching, or you are over, the age of 40.

If it turns out you have structural problems that require a traditional medical approach, then the sooner you find that out and get the proper treatment, the more likely it will be that you can get pregnant.

At the same time Dr. Chang believes - and I agree - that if you are young, in your early to mid -thirties, you might want to consider acupuncture first, before investing in more costly treatment regimens.

"Sometimes a few months of acupuncture will be enough to help you get pregnant on your own," says Dr. Chang. And in fact, this has been my experience as well.

If, in fact, you do seek acupuncture treatment be aware that not all protocols are equal.

"There is tremendous variability within the field -- with many different techniques and a great deal of the success dependant upon how much the acupuncturist knows about the treatment of infertility," says Okoronkwo.

Costs can also vary dramatically, ranging from several hundred dollars to $1,000 or more, depending on how long you are treated, and who is doing the treatment. And while many insurance companies now cover the cost of acupuncture treatments, some don't when treatment involves infertility, so check your policy carefully.

ACUPUNCTURE : NEW HOPE FOR MALE FERTILITY TOO!

Although we most often hear about the benefits of acupuncture on female fertility, new research has shown that men may benefit as well with some surprising and important effects on sperm production and motility!

In one small but significant study recently published in the journal *Fertility and Sterility* doctors used acupuncture to treat 28 men all diagnosed with "unexplained infertility".

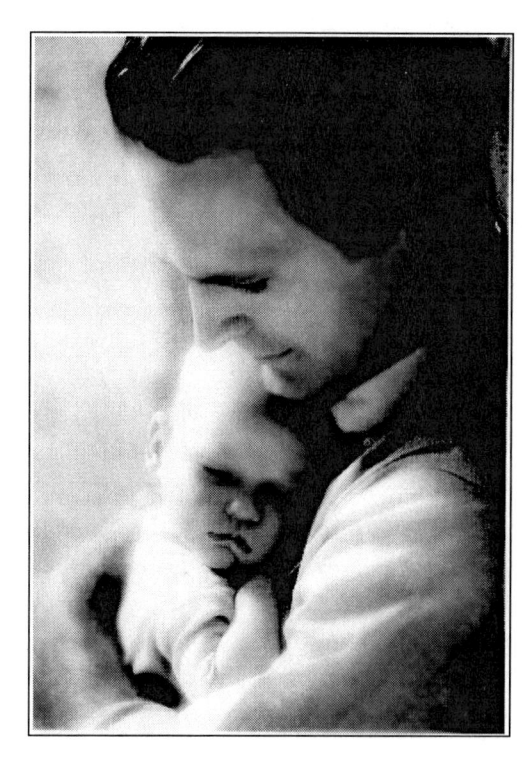

At the start of the study each of the men were asked to abstain from sex for three days and then provide a sperm sample which was analyzed for both the percentage of healthy sperm and sperm motility. Following this each of the men received acupuncture treatments lasting 35 minutes twice a week for a period of 5 weeks and a total of 10 treatments. After the final treatment the men were asked to once again provide another sperm sample.

The Result: After comparing these 2 sets of semen samples with 2 sets taken from 12 men who did not receive any treatments, doctors saw a dramatic difference.

Indeed, while the control group saw just a modest 5% increase in the rate of sperm motility (how fast sperm can swim) between the two samples, the group who underwent the acupuncture treatment saw a dramatic rise of between 44.5% and 50% in their "before" and "after" samples.

Moreover, the amount and the percentage of healthy sperm also increased dramatically in the group receiving the acupuncture! *Indeed, the number of healthy sperm in the acupuncture group increased by 4-fold after treatment, up from 40,000 healthy sperm to a whopping 200,000 per ejaculate!*

But there was still more good news for the men in the acupuncture group.

Prior to receiving treatment, only 22.5% of the sperm contained normal "acrosomes" - the head of the sperm which helps penetrate the eggs outer shell so fertilization can take place. After treatment, the percentage of sperm with normal acrosomes jumped to 38.5% thereby increasing the chance for conception by a significant margin.

Although the acupuncture treatments were astounding in terms of the overall increase in quality and general health of sperm, they did not work quite as well in helping immature sperm become mature - which is a common cause of male infertility.

Still, based on the findings the authors concluded that acupuncture is a viable treatment for male infertility, certainly able to reduce a number of sperm abnormalities and increase overall fertility in not only men whose partners are undergoing IVF, but also in couples who are trying to get pregnant naturally!

It is my personal belief that if you and your partner have been diagnosed with unexplained infertility, or if you have been unsuccessfully trying for more than a year to get pregnant, then both of you may benefit from acupuncture treatments. Indeed, as part of my overall program for achieving optimum pre-conception health, I believe that acupuncture can not only work on specific fertility-related issues, but also increase your overall health in ways that will benefit your fertility. That said, it's also important to remember that if you are going to participate in acupuncture treatments, you must take some steps to insure that you are in the right hands. And by that I mean not only a doctor who is skilled in acupuncture, but one that is also familiar with fertility treatments.

As such, I've put together the following list of pointers to help guide you to getting the very best treatment available.

SIX TIPS FOR FINDING
SAFE & HEALTHY ACUPUNCTURE TREATMENTS!

1. Seek out a doctor who is adequately trained and licensed in acupuncture, as well one who has a background in treating infertility. An MD who simply practices acupuncture once in a while often has just several hundred hours experience, compared to several thousand hours of training and practice required for a traditional Chinese Medicine doctors who practice acupuncture.

2. Look for an acupuncturist associated with a major academic medical center.

3. If you are undergoing fertility treatments with a reproductive endocrinologist, make certain that your doctor has a working relationship with your acupuncturist, and that they work in harmony to establish a treatment regimen.

4. If you are not seeing a fertility specialist, do have the Pre Conception Counseling Exam detailed in Chapter 3, making certain that your doctor is aware of your acupuncture treatment plan.

5. Although acupuncture often works in harmony with Chinese herbal medicine, if you are undergoing IVF or any traditional fertility treatment, don't take any herbs without the OK of your reproductive medicine specialist and your acupuncturist.

6. If you are undergoing an IVF protocol and acupuncture simultaneously, once you reach the implantation stage it's imperative to get a pregnancy test before proceeding with more acupuncture treatments. If you are trying to get pregnant on your own it is equally important to have your pregnancy verified by an obstetrician as soon as possible. Some of the same points used to stimulate the uterus and increase fertility may also cause a miscarriage - so your acupuncturist needs to know if you are, or could be pregnant.

More Natural Technologies To Help You Get Pregnant

In addition to GREEN IVF , I am happy to tell you there is another fertility technology that can also be done "drug free". It's called Artificial Insemination – but trust me when I tell you there is nothing artificial or unnatural about the pregnancy that results! During this procedure your doctor will retrieve a sample of your partner's sperm and put it through several laboratory procedures known collectively as "sperm washing" .

The purpose here to sort out the "good" sperm from the not so good, and concentrate the very best and healthiest to use for insemination.

The insemination itself is a procedure that injects your partner's sperm into one of several areas of your reproductive tract . Done around the time you are ovulating, sperm find their way to your egg by swimming naturally. When contact is made conception can take place completely naturally, inside your body.

Originally insemination was developed to help couples where the male partner could not ejaculate or have an erection. Today, however insemination is used for a wide variety of problems including:

- Marginal to low sperm counts

- Poor sperm motility

- To overcome chronic miscarriage in couples with sperm antibody issues

- Hostile cervical mucous – where your mucous is either too thick or of a consistency that makes it difficult for sperm to reach your egg.

- Vaginal, cervical or uterine abnormalities that would make it more difficult for sperm to reach you egg.

Moreover, in the past I have successfully used various types of insemination to treat a great number of couples grappling with "unexplained infertility" – where no reason could be found for their conception problems. In this respect I have always believed that insemination is a great tool for overcoming many minor defects in both partner's reproductive systems and help them get pregnant fast in one of the most natural treatments in the "fertility medicine chest"

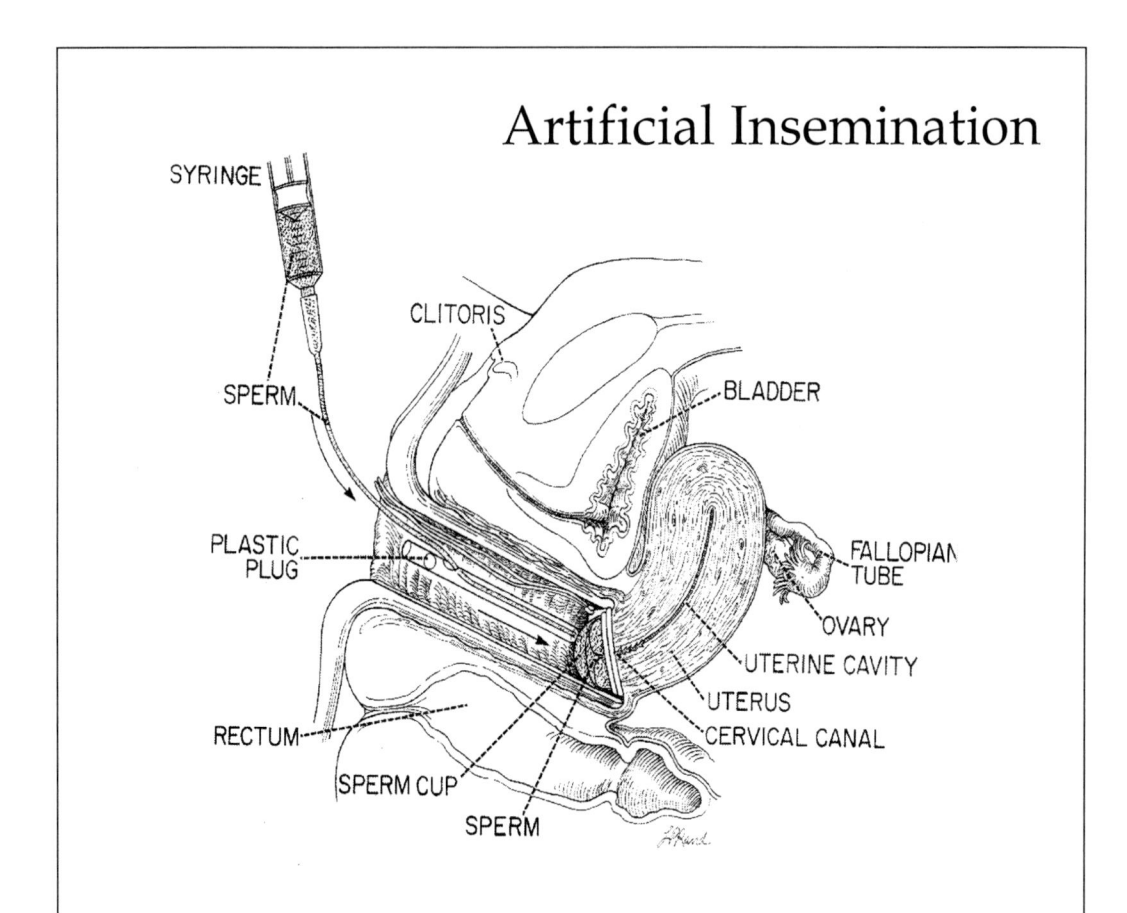

Artificial Insemination

During artificial insemination your partner's sperm will be placed inside a hypodermic needle vial attached to a catheter with a long narrow tube. The tube is inserted into your vagina and using a plunging action the sperm are injected. Sometimes your doctor can insert either a small plastic plug or a "sperm cup" which helps hold the sperm inside, thus increasing the chance for conception.

Not All Inseminations Are Alike

Depending on the reason behind your need for this treatment, your doctor may select one of three different types of insemination procedures – each with a unique slant that can help overcome specific problems.

The three main types of insemination are:

- **Vaginal insemination:** This is the first type of insemination developed and it involves simply placing your partner's sperm inside your vagina around the time you are ovulating. Totally on their own, the sperm swim through your uterus to your fallopian tube where they meet up with your egg so fertilization can occur. This method is best if your partner has ejaculation or erection problems, or if you have 'unexplained' infertility.

- **Intracervical insemination:** This method places sperm a little higher up in your reproductive system, at the very top of your cervix. This is a good method to use if there are problems with your cervical mucous, if you have any vaginal abnormalities, or if your partner has a low sperm count or poor sperm motility. The logic here is that the less distance sperm have to travel the easier it can be to get to your egg.

- **Intrauterine Insemination** – or IUI: This type of insemination bypasses both your vagina and your cervix and places sperm directly into your uterus, very close to the opening of your fallopian tube. This method works very well if you have any problems within your reproductive tract, including not only issues with cervical mucous, but also any scar tissue or other problems related to endometriosis. It's also excellent when your partner has a very low sperm count or very poor sperm motility.

Please not that any of the above mentioned techniques can also be safely and effectively used in conjunction with fertility drugs used to help you manufacture more eggs.

If, however, your goal is to avoid the use of fertility medications, and you want your conception to be as "GREEN" as possible, then it is certainly acceptable to try any of the above types of insemination without the use of any fertility medications.

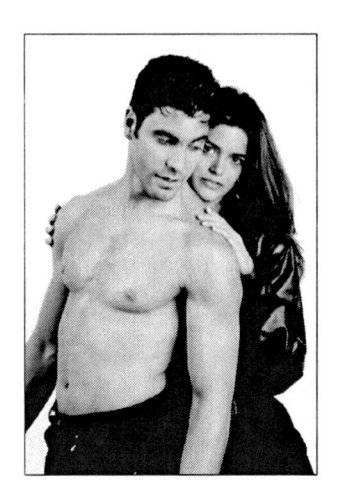

DIY Insemination?

Q: I've recently read about a new DIY – do it yourself – at home insemination kit. I'm wondering if it works...and if it is the same type of insemination I would get at my doctor's office? It seems much less expensive!

A: If you're referring to the new CONCEPTION KIT by Conceivex, the answer is yes, they do work for many couples.

While it's not exactly *the same kind of insemination* you'll get in a doctor's office, I've found it can be very helpful for some patients.

To use the kit your partner slips on a condom-like sperm collector. After making love normally, the contents of the sperm collector is emptied into a small plastic cervical cap which you insert into your vagina, high up close to your cervix. This works to concentrate his sperm and place it at the right entry point. Plus, the cap works to "seal off" the exit, so sperm must go forward swimming towards your uterus. You keep the cap in place for up to 6 hours.

The kit also contains ovulation predictor materials and other aids to help you know the right time to be intimate. It sells for around $349 but most insurance companies offer a co-pay. Learn more about it at:
www.GreenFertility.com

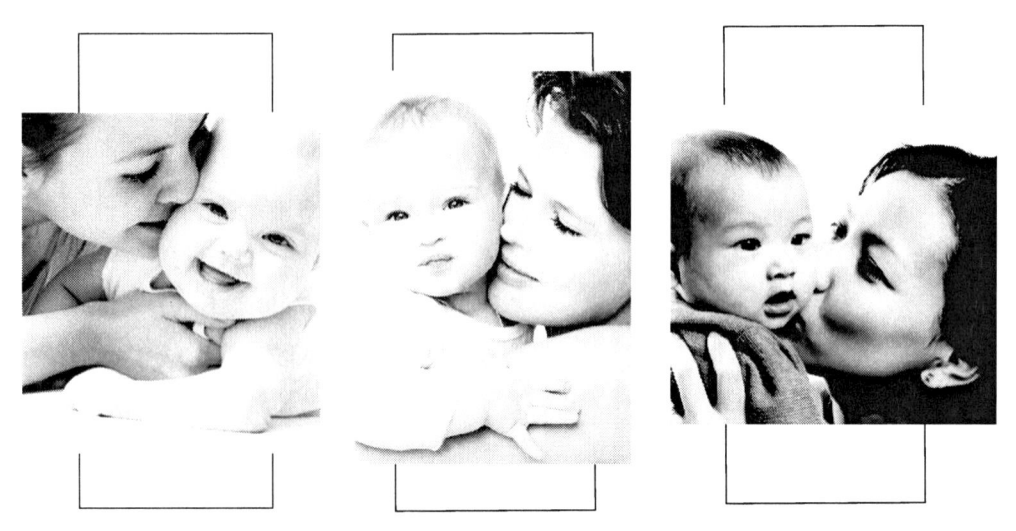

ALL NATURAL WAYS TO INCREASE THE SUCCESS OF ANY FERTILITY TREATMENT

As I mentioned to you earlier, everything you have read in this book thus far- all of the information on diet and lifestyle changes, and certainly all of the advice on herbs, supplements, exercise and even stress reduction - can go a long way in helping any "green" fertility treatment work better and faster, while also giving your baby the best possible start in life.

Indeed, by following the plan in this book you will not only be able to increase and encourage your fertility, but in doing so also improve your overall health. And that, in turn, sets the stage for a healthy conception, no matter how that conception occurs!

At the same time, there are some specific things that you can do to help make any fertility treatment more successful! These are tips and advice that over the years my patients always found helpful - and I believe they can help you as well. In fact, by following this extra advice I can promise you that regardless of the fertility treatment you choose - be it a GREEN IVF, traditional IVF or anything in between - you will have a better chance at success and a better opportunity to conceive and give birth to a healthier baby!

5 WAYS TO GET PREGNANT FASTER!

1. **NEVER OVERLOOK THE POWER OF A PRENATAL VITAMIN!** Just because you are not getting pregnant in a totally natural way does not mean you can forgo this important prenatal step. Indeed, there is some research to suggest the body may have an even greater need for these nutrients if you are undergoing IVF so be sure to take at least *one (and you can take two)* prenatal vitamins daily. I also urge you to follow the fertility diet plan in this book – and for even greater detail on the foods that can help encourage a successful IVF visit FertilityDietGuide.com or pick up a copy of my new book Eat, Love, Get Pregnant.

2. **CONSIDER NATURAL PROGESTERONE SUPPLEMENTS** - Even if you are committed to a drug-free all- green IVF, you can feel good about taking natural progesterone supplements - a bio identical form of the hormone your body makes naturally after ovulation. How can this help? Studies show that progesterone supplements can increase the health of your uterine lining which in turn reduces your risk of miscarriage, insures a healthier pregnancy and offers your baby some clear developmental advantages. You should also ask your doctor about taking 333 mg of the antibiotic erythromycin twice daily for several days following your egg retrieval. I have found this is an excellent way to reduce the risk of infection that can sometimes occur after egg retrieval and eventually impact implantation.

3. **GET LAZY – AND STAY IN BED LONGER!** Following an insemination or the transfer of your embryo to your uterus (the final stage of your GREEN IVF), you should remain in the recovery room, lying down, for at least two hours. When you go home, get into bed, and remain there for up to 72 hours, getting up only to use the bathroom or get a bite to eat. While some IVF programs suggest returning to normal activities within two to three hours, I have always found the extra rest can be extremely beneficial in increasing the success of a pregnancy. This step is especially vital if you have a history of miscarriage.

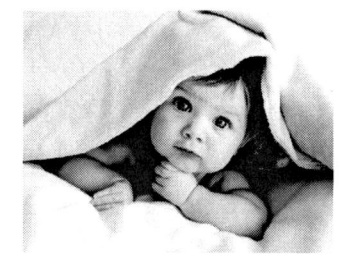

4. **LIMIT EXERCISE -** First, you should not do any type of exercise – even light workouts – for the first 3 weeks following your embryo transfer or insemination, and extend that to 8 weeks if you have a history of miscarriage. Once your pregnancy is confirmed, limit all heavy exercise and heavy physical activity during the first trimester, or first 3 to 4 months of your pregnancy. While you don't have to lie in bed and certainly you can resume work outside the home and/or do light housekeeping, still it's important to the success of our pregnancy that you body is not overly stressed or over heated during this important first trimester.

5. **DO NOT SMOKE – AND AVOID SECOND HAND SMOKE -** Earlier in this book I told you all the ways in which smoking can interfere with fertility and make getting pregnant harder. What I want to emphasize for you now is that smoking, as well as exposure to second hand smoke, can also impact your conception after you are pregnant, and reduce the success of your IVF or insemination procedure. Indeed, according to studies at the Sheba Medical Center in Tel Hoshomer, Israel, smoking decreases estrogen levels, which not only impacts egg development but can also impact how healthy your pregnancy will be. Smoking can also harm your baby and increase your risk of miscarriage. If you smoke, please try to stop smoking prior to seeking fertility treatments – and once you are pregnant, do not smoke and try to avoid as much exposure to second hand smoke as you can.

Taking just a few extra steps following your fertility procedure will help insure it's success!

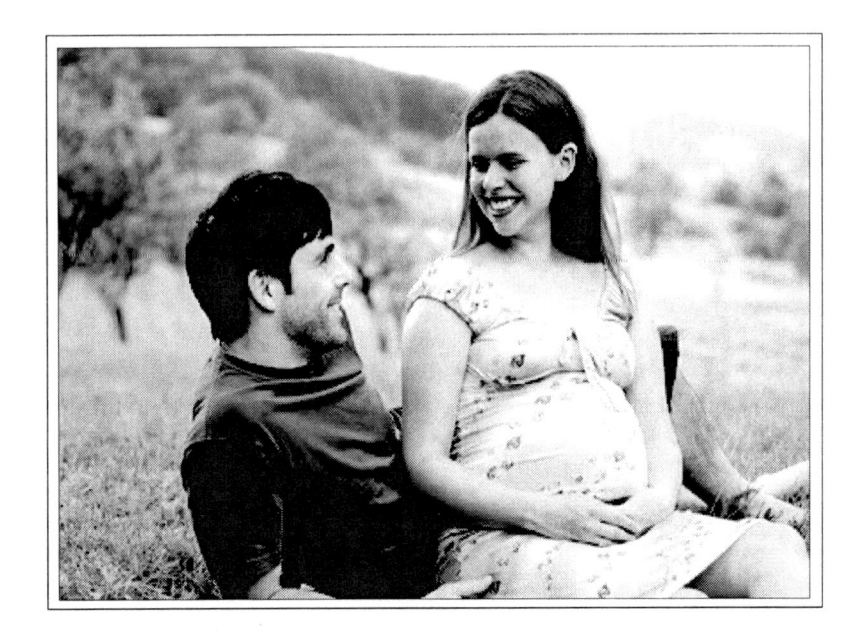

Going Green & Getting Pregnant:
Some Final Advice from Me To You

Certainly it is my hope – and my expectation – that most of you reading this book will be able to get pregnant naturally, on your own, without the need for any medical treatments or interventions.

At the same time, I also want you to remember that if you are under age 35 and have not conceived after a year of trying the suggestions in this book, or over 35 and more than 6 months have passed, you must see a fertility doctor for a baseline check up.

If, at that point, a problem is discovered, oftentimes a number of simple and easy procedures can be performed to correct the problem. In my book Getting Pregnant: What You Need To Know Now I detail many of the simple steps your doctor can take to help you and your partner correct whatever problem is standing in the way of achieving a natural conception.

But if, in fact, you still need more help, I hope you will not only consider these new GREEN fertility medical alternatives, but also keep an open mind about the entire gamut of fertility treatments that are available to help you. If you keep your heart open to all parenting possibilities then I can promise you nearly 100% that your sweet baby dreams will come true!

At the same time, I want to pre-warn you about some opposition to this new GREEN fertility movement – not only the natural solutions mentioned in this book, but specifically the new GREEN IVF procedures I detailed for you in this chapter. Indeed, there are some doctors who simply don't believe in the power of "GREEN" and may in fact try to convince you that only the strictest medical treatments will help - *when in fact this may not be true at all.*

Indeed, I'm a bit sad to report that some within the fertility community are not only small minded, but that some of the opposition to GREEN fertility, and in particular GREEN IVF is part of a negative campaign fueled, at least in part, by some pharmaceutical companies who, quite honestly, stand to lose a great deal of money if *green fertility* treatments *take flight*. In fact, many natural treatments, including not only vitamins and natural hormones but even dietary changes once met with similar opposition, ostensibly because these treatments could not be patented - meaning there was little money to be made.

Today, however, we have much scientific evidence to show the power of many natural approaches, including not only a healthy diet, but also the use of vitamins, minerals, and other supplements to not only help you pregnant faster and easier, but also improve the quality of your health and your life.

GREEN IVF , however, is still relatively new – so it becomes an easy target for those who will not profit from it's development and use. As such, if you go online to research GREEN IVF I am quite certain you will see at least some fertility centers and experts condemning the use of natural cycle IVF – or any form of GREEN fertility treatment or care. At the same time, it's also likely that you will see proponents of GREEN and natural fertility treatments who condemn traditional medical approaches - even to the point of scaring people into believing they are unsafe or even harmful.

So, who is right and who is wrong? Well I have always believed that both science and nature can live peaceably side-by-side, with both Mother Nature and the medical profession, including pharmaceutical companies, each contributing to our well being in their own important ways.

As such I find it difficult to accept or understand any fertility clinic or doctor who condemns the use of Natural or GREEN IVF – just as I have difficulties understanding programs who use only Mother Nature's cures and refuse to even acknowledge when a couple needs extra medical help.

Indeed, I believe the truth is that today, every couple who wants to have a baby, can have a baby – but not every treatment is right for every couple! And while it would be terrific if natural treatments were the best solution for every couple trying to conceive, the truth is, without the help of medical treatments, including fertility drugs, some couples might never know the joy of parenthood.

And so my message to you is this: Whenever possible use Mother Nature to her best advantage – and do all you can to naturally encourage conception. But in the event that this isn't possible, do not close your mind to the options that traditional medicine can offer – including all forms of fertility treatments. When it comes to getting pregnant, it's a wonderful brave new world - and the best part is you have the power to choose what is right for you!

Also remember, you can always get the very latest updates to this book - and the newest most important information about natural fertility at our web site, GreenFertility.com - including a registry of all centers offering GREEN IVF!

You can also visit us at GettingPregnantNow.com where you'll always find the very latest and most important information about all the new medical fertility technologies available to help you conceive!

Lastly, I hope that you will write me with any questions you have - and of course to tell me about your Green Fertility success stories, of which I know there will be many! I wish you the very best of luck and success as you begin or continue your journey to parenthood. I know your children will be blessed to have such wonderful, dedicated and concerned parents.

My Warmest Regards;

Dr. Niels Lauersen

About Dr. Lauersen

In private practice for more than 30 years, Dr. Niels Lauersen founded the New York Medical Center for Reproductive Technology in 1984 to meet the growing needs of the thousands of patients from the United States and abroad who sought his expertise every year.

As a board certified obstetrician/gynecologist, as well as a surgeon, Dr. Lauersen became world-renowned for his expertise in the management of high risk pregnancy, the treatment of endometriosis, PMS, & hormone imbalances as well as the development of fertility - sparing surgeries to avoid hysterectomy.

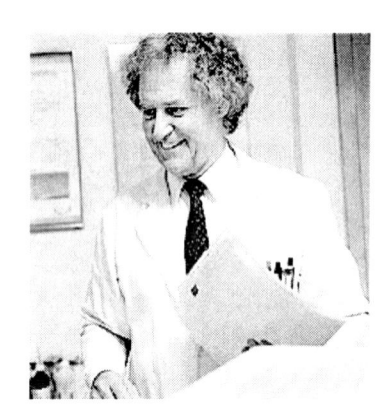

As a fertility expert, he was a founding member of the New York Society for Reproductive Medicine and among the first private physicians in the New York area to offer a full range of infertility treatments, including IVF, GIFT, and the newest ICSI, at his prestigious Park Avenue fertility center.

Educated in his native Denmark, Dr. Lauersen received his American medical training at New York Hospital-Cornell Medical Center, where he continued to do research and clinical patient management and held a professorship in Obstetrics and Gynecology. His academic career expanded, to include professorships at both the Mt. Sinai School of Medicine and New York Medical College. In addition to his private practice, he was also on the clinical staff of Mt Sinai Medical Center, Lenox Hill Hospital, and St. Vincent's Medical Center, all in New York City.

During his active practice career, Dr. Lauersen was a Fellow of the American College of Obstetrics and Gynecology, and a member of the American Medical Association, the Society For Gynecological Investigation, The American Fertility Society, and the NY Obstetrical & Gynecological Society.

As the author of 10 books on women's health care, including the international best selling fertility book *Getting Pregnant,* Dr. Lauersen has published more than 100 hundred scientific medical papers, and wrote and edited several medical textbooks. He has lectured extensively throughout the world and appeared on numerous national television and radio shows including those hosted by Oprah Winfrey, Joan Hamburg, Regis Philbin, Phil Donahue, Sally Jessy Raphael, Maury Povitch and Geraldo Rivera. He has been featured in articles in newspapers and magazines worldwide including Time Magazine, The New York Times, New York Magazine, The NY Daily News, People Magazine, The Los Angeles Times and others.

Currently, he is the medical director of GettingPregnantNow.org, one of the leading fertility and pregnancy web sites as well as a principal in a medical publishing firm. He also a consultant on the use of natural treatments in both men and women's health.

Dr. Lauersen also holds a European medical license for practice throughout the European Union.

About Colette Bouchez

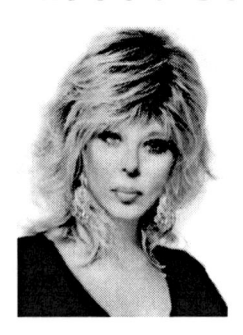

As the author of 9 books on women's health, including an international best seller, a Women's Wellness Health Pro on Wellsphere.com and the creator of the phenomenally popular RedDressDiary.com weekly health column, Colette Bouchez has become one of the most widely read journalists on the Internet. There are currently more than 100,000 pages of references to her work in major search engines, resulting in tens of thousands of individual articles and book excerpts.

As the Editorial Director of ElleMediaNetwork, she is responsible for the editorial content and production of 14 web sites on health, beauty and style, each month programming more than 3 million page views.

As the former content producer for WebMD's women's health, Ms. Bouchez was responsible for conceptualizing and creating content for some 35 million new and unique website readers every month. In March 2007 her WebMD report on anti aging received more than 725,000 hits - and became one of the all-time most read articles on WebMD.

As a journalist Ms. Bouchez's work has been honored by many major medical organizations including:
The American Cancer Society, The American Academy of Dermatology, The American College of Colon Surgeons, The Coalition of Breast Cancer Organizations, The Multiple Sclerosis Society, and Columbia School of Journalism for her health coverage following the aftermath of 9-11. In 1996 she was the writer on the award winning WNBC TV team that produced a seven day report on breast cancer, taking the Emmy for best news documentary. In 1997 she was one of only a small number of journalists ever to be offered a fellowship at the University of Virginia College of Medicine.

In both 2004 and 2005 her articles received the WebMD Reader's Choice for the top ten most read articles of the year. In 2004 the Physician Editors of WebMD chose Ms. Bouchez's reports on fertility as one of 10 most important articles of the year.

In addition to her professional journalism memberships, in 2001 Ms. Bouchez became one of only a select few journalists to be admitted to the prestigious AMWA -American Medical Women's Association -the division of the AMA (American Medical Association) that honors female physicians and researchers.

Her experience in reporting medical news spans more than two decades and includes 14 years as senior medical reporter for the NY Daily News , founding member of the Health Day News Service , an active member of WebMD through 2008. She continues to be a contributing editor to major media including The NY Daily News, The LA Times, The Washington Post, MSN-NBC, WABC News.com,FOX NEWS Network, USA Today.com, and many other news sources.

Ms. Bouchez is also a medical/legal consultant for the prestigious law firm of Gerald Shargel and Associates where her medical research and data has often been used during high profile murder trials.

CONTACT INFORMATION:

NIELS LAUERSEN, M.D., PH.D.
Web Address
www.NielsLauersenMD.org

Direct Email:
DrLauersen@NielsLauersenMD.org

COLETTE BOUCHEZ
Web Address:
www.ColetteBouchez.com

Direct Email:
ColetteBouchez@aol.com

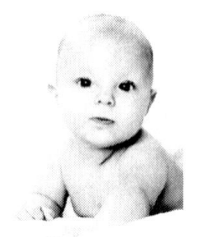

Visit Our Websites:

Our Blog: Fertility-Pregnancy.org

www.GettingPregnantNow.org

www.GreenFertility.com

www.PamperingMom.com

www.EatLoveGetPregnant.com

www.FertilityDietGuide.com

Join us on Facebook at: GreenFertility
Or join our Facebook Natural Fertility Community!

INDEX

A

acid balance 70
ACOG (American Congress of Obstetricians and Gynecologists) 173, 216-17, 222, 225, 229, 237, 255, 258
ACTH 116
acupuncture 11, 433-6, 462-9
acupuncture treatments 434, 464, 466-9
acupuncturist 467, 469
adipocytes 79
alcohol 206, 218, 229, 307, 319, 356-7, 385, 409
Allergies, Sex and infertility 318
almonds 134, 168, 200, 205, 242, 254
alpha-amylase 120
alpha linolenic acid 290
American Association of Oriental Medicine 277
American Congress of Obstetricians and Gynecologists (See ACOG)
American Fertility Society 480
amino acids 282, 285, 287, 295, 382, 388, 426
ancient Chinese medicine treatment 463
anemic 39, 257-8
Annals of The NY Academy of Science 384
anovulation 88-9
anthocyanin 190
anti-fertility workouts 8, 110
anti inflammatory fertility foods 168
Anti stress foods 133
antioxidant protection 184, 259, 376
antioxidant vitamins 17, 187, 241, 347, 379, 406-7
antiphospholipid antibody syndrome 154
appetite 94-5, 225, 238, 377
Archives of Andrology 384
aromatherapy 135, 306
artificial insemination (see also IUI) 470-1

aspirin 212-13, 229, 260, 267, 315-16
astragalus, and male fertility 388, 428

B

Baby Aspirin 316-17
baby-making chances, better 401
bacteria 68, 71, 334, 372
Bacterial vaginosis (and Vitamin D) 235
balance 39, 92, 97, 106, 145, 162-3, 167, 178, 184, 219, 222, 249, 251, 253-4, 265, 269-71
basal body temperature (see also BBT) 48, 58, 281, 296
BBT 48, 50, 58
beans 76, 251, 257-8, 309, 375, 422
beer 10, 157, 202, 307, 357, 366-7, 400
bees 282-7, 408
belly fat & infertility 8
Bernat, scented yarns 306
beta carotene 187, 192-3, 215-18
birth, premature 36, 115, 161
birth weight babies, low 151, 235
Bisphenol A 323-4, 337, 367, 369 (see also BPA)
black cohosh 272-4, 279-80
blood pressure 37, 134, 160-1, 171, 190, 249-50, 286, 372
blood sugar 94, 133, 147, 173, 180, 220, 276, 372, 416, 421, 424, 437, 445
blueberries 148, 168, 185-6, 190-1, 194-5, 282, 379, 422
BMI 8, 80, 84-6, 89, 111, 380-1, 435
body fat 81, 84, 86, 88-91, 110-11, 159, 435
body mass index 84-5, 97, 380
Body Mass Index 84-5, 97, 380
body temperature
 basal 48, 58, 296
 normal 359
body temperature changes 51
Bouchez, Colette 3-4, 7, 481

boxers 10, 359, 361
BPA (Bisphenol A) 323-9, 337, 367-9
Breakthrough Fertility Hormone 8
breast 38, 126, 198, 222

breast cancer 38, 197, 481
breathing 108, 123-4, 128, 139, 445
breathing techniques 107, 109
burn fat 97-8

C

cabbage 136, 148, 196-7, 403-4, 422
caffeine 10, 209, 308-10, 381, 409, 422
cake 94, 144-8, 157, 170, 409, 419, 422
calcium 76, 134, 152, 232-4, 246-51, 378-9, 430
Calcium ascorbate (see also Vitamin C) 230-1
Calcium Fertility Snapshot 248
calcium supplements 231, 247, 250-1, 378
cantaloupe 148, 193, 213, 215, 217-18, 379, 403, 406, 422
carbohydrates 143-4, 147-8, 150, 159, 178, 180, 419-20, 424
 complex 144, 147, 180, 388, 420, 442
 simple 145-7, 264, 419-20
carotinoids 189, 192-3, 215, 379
catecholamines 120
cauliflower 148, 196-7, 403-4, 422
Celiac disease 149-52, 154, 157, 213, 224
Celiac Disease and Infertility 150
cell phones 10, 112, 115, 343, 360-1
cervix 22, 24, 52-4, 66, 76, 284, 472-3
Chang, Lyndon, MD 464-7
chanting 129-30, 411
chasteberry 269-72, 295, 297 (see also Vitex)
cheese 76, 170-1, 218, 237, 378
cherries 190-1, 402, 404
Chinese Fertility 277
Chinese Fertility Cocktail 10
Chinese medicine doctors 277, 431
chlamydia 41-2, 445

chocolate 76, 133, 143, 205, 254, 309, 312
cholesterol 218, 237, 241-2, 286, 376
Choosing Fertility Supplements 10
chromium 261-2, 264, 424
cigarettes 301-3, 305, 338, 354-5
citrus 136, 189, 310, 312, 329
Cleanwell 334-5, 370
Clear-Blue Easy Fertility Monitor 61
Clomid, fertility drug 426
cocaine 319, 362-3
Cocktails and infertility 307
coffee 136, 209, 308-10, 375, 381, 385, 409, 422
computers 115, 187, 236, 342-3, 360-1
conception 12-14, 23-7, 29, 39-40, 45, 62-5, 67-70, 75-6, 138-40, 143-5, 252, 358-9, 362, 440-3, 446-50, 470-2
 healthy 18, 34, 41, 55, 81, 115, 192, 252, 441, 443, 461, 474
conception problems 13, 27, 120, 140, 175, 380, 391, 471
cookies 144-7, 157, 202-3, 209, 409, 422
copper 231, 252-4, 406-7
CoQ10 294
corpus luteum 22, 192, 216
Corresponding Cervical Changes 53-4
cosmetics 321-2, 333, 338
coumadin 275-6
Counseling Exam, new pre-conception 33-4
Crohns Disease 224
CRP 83, 103

D

D-Chiro-Inositol 175, 425
daidzein 175 (see also SOY)
dairy products, high fat 170-2
dancing, to increase fertility 102, 105, 110, 122, 138-9
decreased semen quality 337-8
defective sperm 153, 349, 358, 375, 377
defects, luteal phase 228, 269, 278, 296

depression 155, 213, 219, 222, 225, 342-3, 363, 416, 425
DHA 160-1, 163-4, 287, 289-90, 408, 420, 431
DHEA 10, 292-3, 416
DHT 427, 432
diabetes 15, 36, 39, 78, 82, 95, 103, 113, 142, 162, 164, 212-13, 225, 261, 417-18, 424
diet 15-18, 92, 101-2, 141-2, 145-7, 150-1, 156-7, 161-3, 165-7, 183-5, 191-4, 196-8, 202-3, 400-3, 409-10, 419-21
diet and endometriosis 400
dieting 91, 416, 446
dioxins 322, 333, 340-1, 366
diseases
  fertility-robbing 103, 371
  transmitted 36, 38, 42, 371
DNA 20, 72, 181, 186-7, 198, 350, 354, 374
docosahexaenoic acid (DHA) 161, 420
Domar, Alice 114, 123
Dominion Fertility 459-60
Dong quai 275-7, 280, 389
dopamine 135, 205, 219
douching 70-1, 341
douching & fertility 8
drilling, ovarian 436-7

E

East - west fertility solution 389
egg production 64, 79, 88, 90, 100, 106, 113, 145, 152, 165, 169, 175, 190, 219-20, 293-4, 464-5
eggs
  developing 24, 227
  donor 228, 292
  healthy 27, 146, 180, 194, 227, 267
  immature 461
  making 40, 72, 80, 116
  matured 21, 461
  multiple 454-6, 458
  ovulated 22, 25, 192, 228
eicosapentaenoic acid (EPA) 161, 420
ejaculates 68, 70, 351, 375, 385, 390, 468, 470

embryo 20, 23-4, 74, 88, 118, 161, 182, 184, 192, 194, 211, 215, 223, 228, 454-7, 461
  - fertilized 270, 276, 456, 461, 464
endocrine disrupters 365-6, 376
endometriosis 11, 28, 39, 47, 81, 103-4, 153, 160-1, 165, 182, 190, 198, 201, 210, 256, 394-413
  - pain of 408
  - symptoms of 406-8, 410
environment 10, 15, 185, 187, 321, 323, 330, 333, 336, 342, 345, 412, 454
Environmental Working Group 322, 325, 328, 331-2
enzymes 120, 205, 219, 282, 350, 362, 427
EPA 161, 287, 289-90, 331, 408, 420, 431
erection 63, 318, 356, 371-2, 390, 470
essential fatty acids 160-2, 164, 287, 291-2, 386, 408, 431 (see also EFAs, Omega 3, Omega 6)
Ester C 230-1 (see also Vitamin C)
estrogen 21-3, 40, 53, 57, 59, 79-80, 171-2, 176, 202-3, 246, 269-70, 279-80, 286, 308, 324, 400-1
  - xeno 323, 332, 365, 375, 412
estrogen levels 22, 54, 57, 61, 80, 191, 202, 274, 280, 286, 476
estrogen production 246, 308, 401, 404, 409
Evening Oil of Primrose 10, 291-2, 408
EWG 326, 328
exercise 8, 11, 35, 87, 91, 97-8, 101-11, 124, 126, 171, 210, 263, 391, 433-6, 442, 476
  breathing 123-4
exercise program, regular 100, 442, 446

F

factors, environmental 390, 412, 444
fallopian tubes 13, 21, 23-8, 39, 44, 49, 53, 57, 66, 71, 76, 396, 398-9, 415, 453-5, 472
False unicorn root 279
fat cells 79-83, 90, 97-8, 103, 167, 190, 362, 366, 400

fats   9, 82, 84, 86-7, 110, 143, 150, 157, 159, 164, 169-71, 178, 200, 241, 285, 359
  good   159-60, 164, 167, 170, 200, 420
  healthy   160, 176, 201, 403, 420, 442
fatty acids   160-3, 200, 203, 282, 286-90, 376, 386, 403, 420, 431
  essential   160-2, 164, 287, 291-2, 386, 408, 431
female fertility   153, 224, 226, 240, 252, 254, 262, 319, 336-8, 343, 365, 373, 375-6, 384, 391-2
feminine deodorants, and fertility   73
FertilAid for Women   297
FertilAid for Men   389
fertile time, most   46, 49, 52, 62, 446, 450
fertility
  impaired   320, 378
  improved male   378
  man's   240, 349
  natural   17, 453, 479
  partner's   79, 208, 349
  reduced   337-8, 351
  reduced male   349
  scent of   73
  woman's   29, 342
fertility and fitness   111
fertility benefits   108, 391, 403
Fertility Blend   272, 295-8, 389
Fertility Blend for men   389
fertility blood tests   7, 39
fertility booster   119, 429
fertility-boosting brownie   177
fertility boosting herbs   269, 272
fertility centers   108, 478
fertility chanting exercise   130
fertility clinics   13, 74, 127, 392, 479
fertility cocktail   277
fertility cycle, natural   456
fertility doctor   85, 137, 414, 450, 477
fertility drugs   175, 456, 458, 472
fertility foods
  most common   167
  super   185, 200
fertility formulations, natural   296
fertility herb   275, 279, 291

fertility hormones, re-balancing   281
fertility and hugging   126
Fertility Intuition   7
fertility massage   449
fertility metabolism   8, 101
fertility minerals   249, 252, 255, 259, 261 (see also individual minerals)
fertility monitors   61-2, 447
fertility nutrients   160, 187, 203, 294, 357 (See also individual nutrients)
  key antioxidant   406
fertility pelvic exam   7, 38
fertility problems   15-16, 27, 29, 33, 40, 43, 63, 85-6, 88-9, 97, 316-17, 349, 354-5, 384-5, 391, 437-8
  male   182, 356, 360
fertility proteins   173
fertility Qi   465
fertility robbing   235, 390, 444
fertility robbing chemicals   336-7
fertility-robbing conditions   262, 324
  insulin-related   146
fertility-robbing infections   201, 445
fertility scents   136
Fertility Society of Australia   384
fertility specialist   13, 29, 33, 37, 224, 268, 450, 452, 469
fertility supplements   272, 277, 294, 298
  mixed herbal   272
  natural   266
  over-the-counter   35
  pre-packaged   298
fertility thief   321, 437-8
fertility treatments   30, 108, 119, 169-70, 214, 224, 226, 228, 243, 267-8, 355, 375, 391, 453-4, 474, 478-9
  GREEN   7, 18, 478
  high tech   244, 268
  natural   478
  natural cycle   453, 457
  new male   353
  traditional   469
fertility weight   8, 97
fertility work up, basic   466
fertility yoga   109
FertilityDietGuide.com   177, 185, 475

fertilization 21-5, 45-6, 54, 187, 192, 200, 256, 275, 291, 303, 354, 362, 376, 454, 457, 466
  In vitro 19, 108, 355, 454, 462
fertilization process 27, 216
fertilized egg 22, 28, 71, 81, 88, 120, 182, 201, 216, 223, 228, 252, 274, 278, 292, 398-9
fiber 35, 134, 147, 177, 196, 202, 206, 265, 299, 375, 378-9, 420, 423, 442
fields, electro magnetic 342-3
finasteride 432
fish 76, 163, 173-4, 256, 258, 260, 288-90, 421, 423, 431
fish oil 167, 287-90, 408, 431
fitness 8, 30, 35, 96-9, 101, 103-7, 109-11, 358
Five Deep Breathing Fertility Exercises 124
flame retardants 330
flavonoids 189-91, 199, 270, 273
flax 160, 163, 167, 290-1, 420
flowers 282-3, 408
folic acid 206, 211-14, 221, 223, 225, 295, 375-7, 383, 385, 401, 428, 443, 448
folic acid fertility snapshot 213
follicles 20-2, 41, 57, 80, 219, 270, 415-17, 426, 428, 456, 461
follicular fluid 182, 192, 199, 215, 227
foods 75-6, 92-3, 133-4, 141-5, 147-8, 156-7, 159-68, 170-2, 184-5, 187-9, 203-4, 256-8, 264-5, 329, 402-4, 419-24
  aphrodisiac 205
  fast 164, 166
  inflammatory 9, 167, 402-3, 410
  soy 175-6, 191, 404
foot massage and fertility 137
free radical damage 9, 180-3, 226-7, 241, 379, 383
free radicals 180-4, 227, 294, 361
French fries 148, 157, 159, 166, 172, 402, 404, 422
Fruit 135, 144, 148, 178-80, 184-90, 193-95, 204-5, 218, 231, 254, 264-5, 272, 279-80, 290, 373-4, 379, 401, 403, 406-7, 420-3, 441
  (see also individual fruits by name)

fruit extract 272
FSH (Follicle Stimulating Hormone) 21, 40, 57, 80, 90, 100, 102, 116, 118, 152, 175, 219, 233, 270, 428, 458

G

garlic 198, 260, 264, 374, 376, 403-4
gender, baby's 74-5
genistein 175, 280 (see also Soy)
Getting Pregnant 10-11, 16, 20, 76, 220, 262, 395, 413, 438, 452-3
Gleicher, Norbert MD 201
glucocorticoids 119
gluten 149-50, 152-3, 155-8, 409
gluten allergy 150-8
gluten intolerance 152-4, 158
gluten sensitivity 153, 156, 213, 409-10
glycemic index 421
glycemic load 143-4
GnIH 118-19
GNIH 118-19
GnRH 116, 118-19
grains 94, 134, 144, 147-8, 157-8, 180, 189, 258, 260, 264, 377-8, 403, 410
grapes 160, 189-91, 254, 374, 402, 404
GREEN 11, 31, 345, 440, 459, 472, 477-8
Green Fertility 1, 3-4, 7, 12, 336, 370, 472, 474, 476, 478
green fertility advice 440
GREEN fertility medical alternatives, new 478
Green Fertility Shopping List 370
GREEN Fertility Treatments 19
GREEN IVF 31, 440, 453-4, 457-62, 470, 474-5, 478-9
  new 19, 399, 458-9
green leafy vegetables 217, 258
Green Print for Pregnancy Success 440
green tea 134, 185-6, 190-1, 199-201, 295, 389, 422
GreenFertility.com 157, 333, 335, 373, 459, 479
gum, nicotine 158, 304

H

hand sanitizers   331, 333-4
Harvard   114, 123, 146, 170-1, 174-6, 419
Hasselbeck, Elizabeth   151
health
  baby's   91, 173, 211
  good   38, 104, 160, 232, 243, 262, 265, 268, 275, 328, 343, 350, 382, 455
Health scientist Maureen McKenzie   195
healthy diet   162, 228, 243, 245, 260, 265, 268, 283, 299, 407, 423, 434, 478
healthy sperm (See also Sperm, healthy)
healthy sperm, production of   351, 354, 356, 373-4, 378-9, 388, 444
heart disease   15, 36, 78, 82, 96, 104, 113, 142, 159, 162, 164, 167, 189-90, 203, 233, 241
herbal supplements   35, 158, 267-8, 443
herbs   199, 258, 265, 268-80, 287-8, 292, 295-9, 382, 387-8, 427-8, 453, 469, 474
HGH (human growth hormone)   363
home (healthy)   33, 48, 112, 165, 209, 333, 339-40, 345-6, 353, 359, 370, 475-6
hormonal   332, 365-6, 418
hormonal activity   30, 46, 59-60, 63-4, 116, 145, 291, 354, 456
hormonal changes   59-60, 337-8
hormonal imbalances   37-8, 182, 191, 219, 280, 324, 401, 433, 437
hormonal level   47, 88
hormonal secretions   415
hormonal upsets   272-3
hormone activity, reproductive   107, 332
hormone imbalance   80, 106, 134, 169, 172, 175-6, 210, 247, 271, 273, 281, 308, 480
hormone production   79, 88, 91, 103, 118-19, 188, 192, 273, 363, 380, 449, 465

Hormone, progesterone   269, 278

hormone treatments   377, 427
hormones   21-3, 39-40, 57, 61, 63-4, 72-3, 80-1, 88-91, 98-9, 116, 118-20, 145, 171, 232-3, 269-71, 442
  fertility-inhibiting   119
  male   118, 145, 240, 293, 356-7, 363
  steroid   292
Hot tubs   70, 358, 360, 444, 448
human growth hormone (HGH)   363
hypothalamus   21, 64, 90, 100, 107, 119, 465

I

ibuprofen   212-13, 315-16
ice cream   9, 133-4, 157, 170-2, 176, 246
ICSI (See also Injection, intracytoplasmic sperm) 355, 454
IFRS (Inflammatory Food Rating System)   167
IGA   156
infection   13, 27, 36, 38, 41, 47, 51, 68, 71, 155, 235, 268, 284, 341, 445, 453-4
infertility   15-17, 80-1, 116, 151-3, 164-5, 256, 273, 284-5, 320, 323-4, 327, 348, 367-8, 380-1, 392-3, 414-16
  male   360, 376, 378-9, 468
  ovulatory-based   174
  risk of   82, 98, 247, 308, 380, 401
  tubal factor   308
infertility treatments   15, 462, 467, 480
inflammation   8, 41, 81, 83, 103-4, 133, 156, 161-2, 167, 194, 277, 402-3, 408-10, 420, 431
inflammatory compounds   81-3, 103, 160, 173, 190, 275
injection, intracytoplasmic sperm (ICSI)   355, 454
inositol   425
insemination   11, 137, 470-3, 475-6
insulin   78, 145, 169, 173, 261, 417, 419-21, 426, 434, 436-7
insulin resistance   95, 145, 161, 164, 169, 180, 190, 210, 220, 222, 247, 261-4, 416-19, 424-6, 430-1, 433-4

intercourse 27, 56, 63, 66, 70-1, 75, 371, 449-50
intrauterine insemination (*see also* IUI) 472
intuition 42-3, 344
iron 39, 152, 155, 223, 231, 253, 255-8, 295, 388
 elemental 258
iron deficiency 39, 155, 223, 255
iron supplements 223, 255-8
irregular ovulation 28, 315
irregular periods 40, 416
isoflavone (*see also* Soy, Red Clover) 190-1, 202, 280
IUI 472
IVF 170, 200-1, 214, 375, 454-7, 459-60, 462, 464, 475-6
 traditional 454-5, 458-60, 462, 464, 474
 undergoing 464, 466, 468-9, 475

J

Journal, Fertility and Sterility - 115, 119, 228, 261, 361, 385, 408, 458, 463, 465, 467

K

Knit To Quit 306
knitting 122, 129, 306

L

L-arginine 205, 382, 428
L-Ascorbic Acid 230 (*see also* Vitamin C)
L-Carnetine 382
Lauersen, Niels H MD 3, 7, 480, 483
Lavender and aromatherapy 136, 306
leptin 89-90, 425
LH (luteinizing hormone) 21, 40, 57, 61, 90, 100, 102, 116, 118, 152, 175, 192, 219, 233, 270, 428
LH surges 57-8

lifestyle (and fertility) 16-17, 30, 34-5, 97, 122, 139, 155, 208, 319, 369, 393, 412, 438, 452-3
lifestyle changes (and fertility) 15, 17, 30, 47, 301, 349, 353, 394, 438-9, 446, 452, 474
lifestyle factors (and fertility) 15-17, 30, 43, 165, 180, 349, 353, 390
lifestyle habits (and fertility) 15-16, 28, 392
Lilly of the valley and aromatherapy 136
Lipton Diet Green Tea 310
loss, fetal 337-8
love 10, 44, 48-9, 51, 63-70, 73-4, 93, 104, 111, 139, 148, 162, 167, 204, 209, 447-9
 making 26-7, 44-5, 49, 54, 57-8, 60, 62-3, 65-7, 69, 75, 77, 137, 447-9, 473
low fat dairy products 171-2
lubricants 69, 447
lupin 148, 177
luteal phase insufficiency 269, 271
lutein 192-3, 217
luteinizing hormone 21, 57, 192, 215, 219, 270, 428 (*see also* LH)
lycopene 192-3, 217, 374, 378, 401

M

Maca root, and male fertility 388
magnesium 75-6, 205, 230-1, 248-51, 295, 388
making Babies 1, 3-4, 7, 63, 65, 336, 370, 449, 472, 474, 476, 478, 482
making love 26-7, 44-5, 49, 54, 57-8, 60, 62-3, 65-7, 69, 75, 77, 137, 447-9, 473

male fertility 28, 79, 122, 192, 203, 224, 242, 337-9, 349-51, 362-6, 371, 373-5, 380-2, 384-5, 387-9, 428
male fertility check up - 371
male fertility factors 455
male impotency and infertility 367

Maloney, Carolyn, Rep 340
marijuana 319, 362-3
massage therapy 137
medications 10, 35, 40, 213, 225, 238, 261, 274, 276, 313-16, 363-4, 426-7, 432, 436-7, 444, 456-7
  allergy 267, 318
  over-the-counter 268, 276, 309, 313-15, 364
medicine, cough 55, 444
meditation 107, 119-22, 127-8, 131, 306, 391, 411, 445
menopause 79, 255, 272-4, 285-6
menopause symptoms 272-3, 281, 285-6
menstrual cycle 13, 21, 45, 52-3, 59, 61, 63-4, 73, 80, 88-9, 106, 110, 131, 152, 299, 428-9
menstrual irregularities 337-8, 434-5
metabolism 98-102, 161, 237, 292, 319, 420
milk 76, 134, 170-2, 225, 237, 246
mindful meditation 127-8
mineral deficiency 245
Minerals 9, 39, 75, 150, 152, 196, 205, 210, 231, 244-6, 251-3, 256-61, 265, 295-6, 385, 423
  - Daily Fertility Calcium Requirements 248
  - Daily Fertility Iron Requirements 258
  - Daily Fertility Magnesium Requirements 251
  - Daily Fertility Selenium Requirements 260
  - Daily Fertility Zinc Requirements 254

miscarriage, risk of 39, 91, 109, 115, 151, 154, 190, 203, 252, 276, 278, 294, 309, 317, 319, 475-6
mother nature 7, 12, 14-15, 27, 29, 56, 178-9, 186, 188, 267-8, 291, 359, 440-7, 450, 457, 478
mucous 53-5, 318, 448, 470
  cervical 52, 472
MUFAs (Mono unsaturated fatty acids) 159-60
Multi Vitamins 9, 210, 258-9, 443

muscles 87, 103, 108, 110, 125, 218, 223, 249, 255, 276, 411

N

NAC 426-7
National Foundation for Celiac Awareness 150
natural compounds 180, 183, 186-7, 196, 198, 267, 272
natural conception 63, 137, 214, 228, 319, 436, 453, 455, 460, 477
natural cycle IVF 457-60, 462, 478
natural fertility boosters 180, 287
natural treatments 4, 142, 267-8, 478-80
Nature's Secrets 1, 3-4, 7, 336, 370, 472, 474, 476, 478, 482
NCCAOM 277
nervous system, sympathetic 434-5
New Hope Fertility 460
New Hope Fertility Clinic in New York City 458
niacin 177, 219 (*see also* Vitamin B6)
nicotine patch, and fertility 304
NSAIDs 213, 315-17
nutrient supplements 208, 243, 423
nutrients 150, 153-4, 178, 187-8, 194, 211-12, 217-21, 223-4, 226-8, 261-3, 265, 287-9, 294-9, 378-9, 382-4, 423-9
  carotinoid 215, 217
  essential 215-16, 373, 383
  important fertility 220
  powerful fertility 226
Nutrients for male fertility 382
nutritional fertility goals 443
nuts 76, 134, 159, 168, 174, 179-80, 189, 200-2, 242, 254, 258, 357

O

oats 144, 158, 177
obesity 84, 86, 380, 427, 437
Omega 3 9-10, 160-3, 200, 203, 287-90, 292, 376, 386, 403, 408, 420, 431
Omega 6 160-3, 386

omentum   82
onions   168, 185-6, 191, 198, 201, 376, 403-4
optimal fertility weight   92
ORAC points   185-6
ORAC Score   184-5
organs, reproductive   21, 38, 106, 108, 226, 233, 255-6, 339, 343, 465
orgasm   76, 205-6, 351
Ova Cue, fertility monitor   60
ovarian cysts   36-7, 41, 429
ovaries   20-5, 39, 41, 44, 57, 79-80, 100, 145-6, 226, 239-40, 398, 415-18, 436-7, 454-5, 461, 465-6
overweight (and fertility)   37, 66, 79-84, 86, 89-90, 97, 103, 105, 110, 172, 190, 241, 263, 359, 380-1, 424
ovulating   26, 28, 41, 56, 63, 73, 100, 152, 161, 176, 194, 273, 287, 293, 436, 444
Ovulation (ovulate)   21-3, 25-7, 44-64, 70, 76, 100, 118, 146, 173, 175-6, 182, 190, 219-20, 226-7, 255-6, 272-4, 279-80, 315-16, 437, 453-6
ovulation prediction   45-6, 60-2
ovulation prediction kit   58, 447
ovulation prediction methods   46-8, 52, 57, 59, 61, 446
oxidative stress   182, 187, 189, 196, 356, 405-6
oxytocin   126
oysters   205, 251, 254, 258, 260

P

Pain medications (and infertility)   315-16
pain relievers   314-16, 444
palmetto   388, 427-8
Panax Ginseng, and male fertility   388
Panty liners   340
Pap smear   39, 41
papayas   193, 403-4, 406
partner smells   72-3
partner's sperm   20-5, 45, 53-4, 57, 75, 215, 235, 415, 453-5, 470-2
pasta   134, 143-4, 155, 157, 409, 419, 421-2

PBDEs   322, 330-1
PCBs   322, 337
PCOS (Poly cystic ovarian syndrome)   11, 28, 41, 81, 146, 161, 190-1, 201-2, 234, 247, 262, 264, 281, 286-7, 414-38, 461
   - symptoms of   270, 418, 420, 427, 432
peanuts   174, 202, 251, 254, 357, 366, 402, 406
penis   68, 350-2, 372, 449
personal care products & fertility   10, 322, 340, 366
pesticides   180, 322-4, 333, 337-8, 365
Phenolic acids   189
physical activity   35, 97, 101, 306
phytoestrogens   357, 366
phytonutrients   9, 186-9, 192-3, 198-9, 201, 270, 273, 379
   fertility-boosting   193
phytosterols   201
placenta   154, 161, 275
plant estrogens   175, 190, 202, 280, 357
plastic containers   329
PMS (pre menstrual syndrome)   40, 134, 202, 210, 216, 218-20, 222, 234, 247, 270-1, 275, 278, 291, 299, 480
pollen, bee   282-5
Poly Cystic Ovarian Syndrome (See also PCOS)   11, 28, 41, 81, 146, 210, 212, 222, 247, 415, 461
potassium   39, 75-6, 205-6
pregnancy   12-13, 26-7, 65-7, 107-9, 161-2, 212-13, 216-17, 222-5, 227-9, 248, 256-8, 266-70, 303-5, 440, 454-6, 475-6
   healthy   27, 38, 41, 45, 105, 108-9, 156, 178, 219, 226, 268, 309, 476
pregnancy rates   67, 114-15, 127, 137, 201, 228, 269, 293, 296-7, 317, 408, 450, 458, 460, 462, 464
pregnancy success   15, 18, 66, 119, 440
proanthocyanidin   190
progesterone   21-3, 40, 57, 102, 175, 192, 202-3, 216, 219, 228, 252, 269-71, 278, 296, 400, 475
progesterone supplements, natural   475
prolactin   100, 152, 270, 416, 428
Promensil   280-1

propolis, bee   284-5, 408
proteins   81, 118, 143, 150, 152, 173-6, 178, 202, 205, 256, 265, 285, 375, 386, 410, 424
Proven fitness plan   97, 99, 101, 103, 105, 107, 109, 111
PUFAs, (poly unsaturated fats)   160
pumpkin seeds   203

Q

quercertin   190-1
quit smoking   305-6, 355

R

Raspberry Leaf   278-9
red blood cells   39, 211, 223, 255-7
Red Clover   279-81, 366
red meat   160, 167, 169, 172-4, 256-8, 377, 400, 402, 404
regular exercise   96, 106
relaxation (and relax) 66,   107-8, 115, 121-3, 124-5,127, 129, 131, 135-40, 206, 239, 248-9, 278, 392, 411-12,446-
Remifemin   274
reproduction   40, 90, 107, 117, 119, 194, 196, 291-2, 343
reproductive health   4, 16, 33, 36, 97, 273, 275, 277, 365-6, 380, 438, 445
reproductive hormones   40, 48, 91, 102, 110, 119, 125, 129, 139, 143, 169, 171, 219, 279, 308, 332
reproductive system   13, 28-9, 47, 55, 57, 106, 108, 116, 137, 143, 190, 203, 350-1, 390, 398-9, 471-2
  male   352, 358, 385, 388
reproductive tract   45, 66, 68, 71, 75, 449, 470, 472
rice, white   147-8, 419, 421
royal bee jelly   10, 282, 285-6
running and fertility   35, 87, 99, 101-2, 110, 132, 198

S

saliva   59-60, 68, 120
saturated fats   169-70, 172, 180, 202, 420
saw palmetto , and male fertility   388, 427
second hand smoke   35, 209, 260, 304-5, 338, 427, 476
selection, natural gender   74-6
selenium   203, 259-60, 295, 374, 376, 385, 389, 428
Sensory Perception Fertility Exercise   132
Sensory perception relaxation   131
serotonin   135, 219
sex   7-8, 21-2, 26, 56, 63, 65, 70, 74-6, 204-5, 293, 318, 351, 356, 375, 390, 467
  oral , anal   68
sex toys   68-9
Shikhman, Alex MD   152-4
silent fertility robbing infections   445
skin   37, 70, 82, 84, 127, 130, 201, 204, 218, 222, 225, 232, 236, 240, 331-2, 334
sleep   28, 35, 50, 94, 114, 207, 210, 343, 448
smell   71-3, 131, 135, 218, 290, 305, 341, 347
smoking   15, 35, 43, 50, 147, 229, 301-6, 353-5, 380, 476
snacks, super fertility   379
soaps   52, 68-9, 71, 333-4
soda   9, 148, 209, 251, 309, 328
Soft Talk Fertility Exercise   125
Somer, Elizabeth, RD   163
soy   148, 157, 163-4, 175-7, 191, 202, 280, 366, 404
soybeans   174, 254, 279-80, 375
sperm   24, 26, 28-9, 45, 66-70, 73-6, 350-5, 357-9, 361-6, 373-4, 376-9, 381-6, 388-91, 454-7, 468, 470-3
  abnormal   338, 362, 383
  defective   153, 349, 358, 375, 377
  mature   353
  transport   28, 368

sperm, healthy   27, 118, 192, 363, 376, 430, 467-8
sperm abnormalities   375-6, 468
sperm assassins   354, 356, 358, 360, 362, 365
sperm concentrations   374, 381, 449
sperm count   67, 113, 178, 224, 332, 356-7, 359, 361-3, 365, 374-5, 381-5, 390-1
  low   67, 70, 224, 374, 472
  very low   391, 430, 472
Sperm-Happy Meals   10, 375
sperm motility   70, 224, 332, 354, 376, 381, 383, 388, 467-8, 470, 472
sperm production   27, 73, 79, 153, 182, 240, 254, 342, 354-7, 359-61, 363, 372, 375, 381-3, 385-6, 444
sperm quality   29, 353
sperm sample   467-8
sperm tail   350, 362
spermatids   350
spironolactone   432
stomach   82, 198, 218, 225, 230-1
stress   8, 50, 62, 69, 95, 106-8, 111, 113-23, 127-34, 136-40, 206-7, 249-50, 301, 306, 390-3, 410-12
  acute   8, 117, 119
  prolonged   390
Stress busters   123, 125-7, 129, 131, 133, 135, 137-8
stress hormones   95, 108, 116-17, 120, 123, 125, 134, 136, 250
  production of   125-6, 133-4, 137, 410
stress reduction program   123-4
stress responses   30, 131, 135, 250
  body's   135
stressors   95, 113, 115-16, 249, 445
stretching   105-6, 397
sugar levels   144, 220, 421, 424, 433
sugars   95, 143-5, 147, 165, 169, 220, 261, 264, 285, 290, 417-21, 441
sun   180-1, 187, 232-4, 236-40, 276, 404, 429-30
Sun and male fertility   240
Sunscreen   237-8, 430
Super Fertility Food Boosters   9, 194
Super Fertility Nutrients   215, 219, 223, 226, 232
Super Protein Fertility Power   9, 173

Supplements   163, 199, 208, 215-18, 224-5, 227-8, 230-1, 236-8, 243, 263-5, 286-92, 294-7, 378-9, 406-8, 423-6, 429-31 (see also fertility supplements)
  bee pollen   282-3
  chromium   262, 264, 424
  fish oil   288-9, 431
  high potency vitamin/mineral   283
  high potency vitamin-mineral   299
  multi-vitamin   245
surgery   155, 292, 436-7
synthetic estrogens   324, 366-7, 377
system, immune   127, 201, 219, 235, 284, 396, 444

T

tampons   340-1
temperature   48-51, 70, 358, 360, 445
temperature changes   51-2
testicles   70, 350, 352-3, 356, 358-61, 372, 380, 384-5
  hot   358-9, 361
testosterone   73, 118, 145, 240, 356, 363, 375, 381-3, 385, 388, 417, 427, 432, 435, 437
tests, fertility and saliva   60
thyroid   8, 90, 98-100, 102
thyroid hormones   40, 100-1, 331
tomato soup   378
tomatoes   148, 193, 254, 328, 374
touch   53-4
toxins   108, 150, 181, 288, 303-4, 339, 376, 379
tranquillizers, and fertility   131, 319, 444
trans fats   164-7, 169, 172, 404-5, 420, 422
Triclosan   331-5
twins   9, 214, 457
type 2 diabetes   78, 103, 164, 210, 263, 281, 417-18, 424

U

underweight and infertility,   79, 86, 88-9, 103, 106, 172, 442

unexplained infertility   13-14, 16, 29, 64, 104, 113, 149-51, 153, 155-6, 182, 221-2, 271, 353, 384, 467-8, 471-2
urine   57, 61, 71, 222, 322, 327, 333
uterine lining   216, 278, 475
uterus   22-4, 28, 70, 76, 81, 106, 182, 194-5, 215-16, 269-70, 274-8, 291-2, 396, 398-9, 461, 472-3

V

vagina   22, 38, 52-3, 66, 68-71, 340-1, 449, 471-3
vanilla, and aromatherapy   136, 306, 311, 379
vegetables   9, 144, 147, 157, 178-80, 185-9, 193-4, 196-8, 217-18, 258, 264-5, 400-1, 406-7, 420-1, 423, 441-2 (see *individual* vegetables)
  cruciferous   196-7
  green   193, 224
vibrators   69
vitamins   9, 152, 183-4, 187,196, 205-8, 211, 215-19, 223-4, 226-43, 257-9, 282-3, 294-6, 347, 377-9, 382-4, 405-7, 423-5, 429-30
  complex   221-3
  prenatal   154, 209, 221-2, 257-8, 407, 444, 475
Vitamin A   192, 215-18, 379, 383, 406
Vitamin B6   203, 206, 219-22, 378, 383
  taking extra   220
Vitamin B12   223-5, 383
Vitamin B Complex   219, 221-3, 243,283,347,383, 444,448
Vitamin Bath   9, 227
Vitamin C   9, 70, 184, 187, 226-31, 241, 243, 253, 257, 377, 383-4, 401, 406, 444, 448
Vitamin D   40, 232-40, 247, 347, 378-9, 384, 424, 429-30
Vitamin D deficiency   236-7
Vitamin E   183-4, 203, 205, 210, 241-2, 289, 291, 295, 384-5, 406
  vitex   269, 428-9
Vitex   269, 428-9 (see *also* Chasteberry)

W

walnuts   134, 160-1, 163, 167-8, 177, 189, 200, 242, 403, 420
WebMD   481
weight   8, 30, 35, 78-9, 83-93, 97, 101-2, 104-6, 110, 132-3, 158, 359, 379-81, 425-6, 435, 442
  gain   93, 97, 99, 442
  normal   84, 86, 88, 103-4, 106
weight control   11, 79, 81, 83, 85, 87, 89, 91, 93-5, 141, 301
weight loss   90-1, 103, 111, 225, 433
wheat   144, 150, 155, 409-10
wheat germ   157, 203, 213, 260
whole grains   94, 134, 144, 147, 180, 258, 260, 264, 377-8, 403, 410
wine & fertility   10
wine, red   206, 264, 307, 357, 366
www.FertilityDietGuide.com   148, 403
www.GreenFertility.com   370, 473

Y

yoga   106-9, 119-22, 131, 138, 306, 391, 411, 445
Yoga & Fertility   8
yogurt   134, 164, 170-1, 234, 237, 248, 254, 379, 403, 422

Z

zeaxanthin   192
Zerofon   343
Zerocom   343
zinc   203, 205, 252-4, 295, 375, 378, 383, 385, 388-9, 406-7, 428
  elemental   253
zinc supplements   253, 406-7
Zyban   305

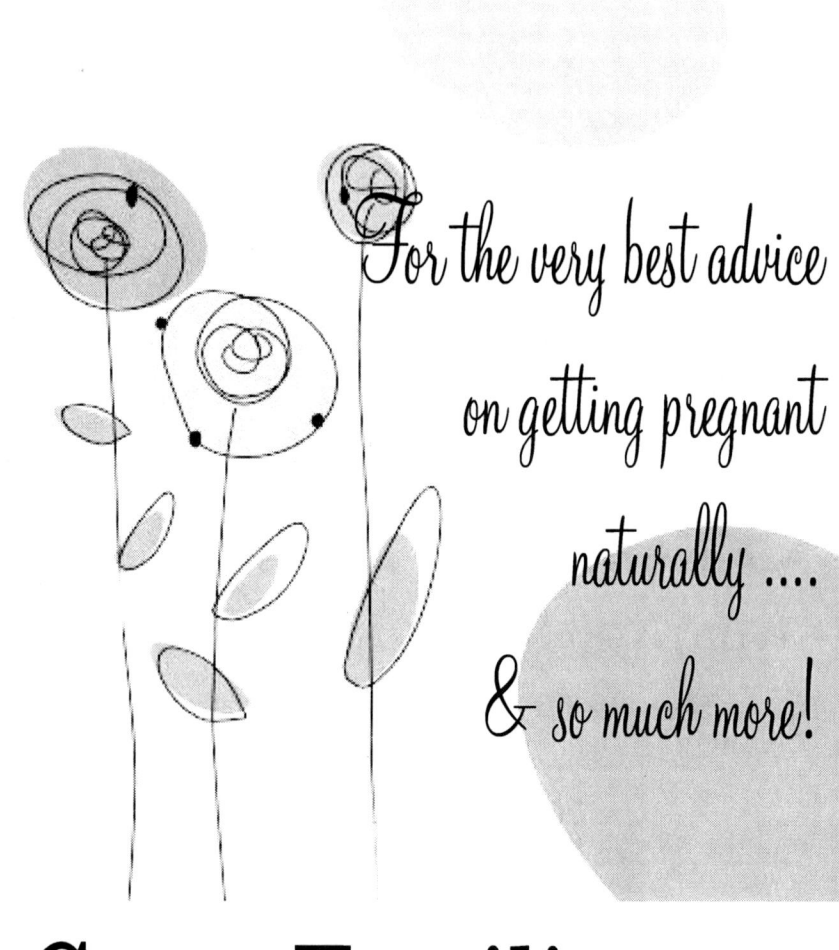

For the very best advice on getting pregnant naturally....
& so much more!

GreenFertility.com

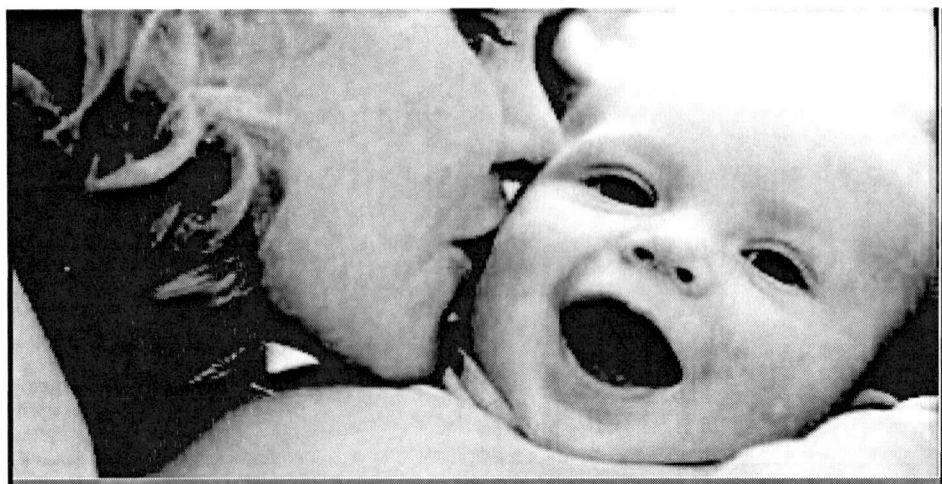

The Classic Best Seller - Completely Revised & Updated

Getting Pregnant

WHAT YOU NEED TO KNOW RIGHT NOW!

BREAKTHROUGH TECHNIQUES FOR TREATING INFERTILITY PLUS:

How To Get Pregnant Fast
Six New Ways To Avoid Miscarriage
The New IVF - How It Can Help You
Gender Selection: What You Should Know
New Treatments for Male Fertility
7 Super Fertility Threats & How To Avoid Them
Your Fertility From 9 - 5
And So Much More!

By Niels H. Lauersen, M.D., Ph.D.
& Colette Bouchez

Getting Pregnant:
What You Need To Know Now!

From the authors of "Green Fertility" and "Eat, Love, Get Pregnant" comes a classic, best selling book on getting pregnant for over two decades! Now fully updated, discover why tens of thousands of couples already call this book their "Fertility Bible"!

Voted # 1 by New Moms
Getting Pregnant
is the only book to combine
the latest technologies
with the best self-help advice
to give you every option
for getting pregnant fast!

A small fraction of what you'll find in Getting Pregnant:

- Six ways to avoid miscarriage
- Seven fertility threats - and how to avoid them.
- What to do today - to double your chances for conception tomorrow!
- How to get pregnant after age 40!
- 8 brand new fertility drugs - and how they can help you.
- The new 15 minute in-office procedure that can double your conception odds immediately!
- The latest versions of GIFT, IVF and ICSI
- AND SO MUCH MORE!

Visiting GetPregnantFast.net to discover how to purchase this amazing book in print or as an e-book! Also find it at fine bookstores worldwide - including online at Amazon.com, BarnesandNoble.com, Borders.com and many more!

GettingPregnantNow.org

Helping couples get pregnant for over 20 years!

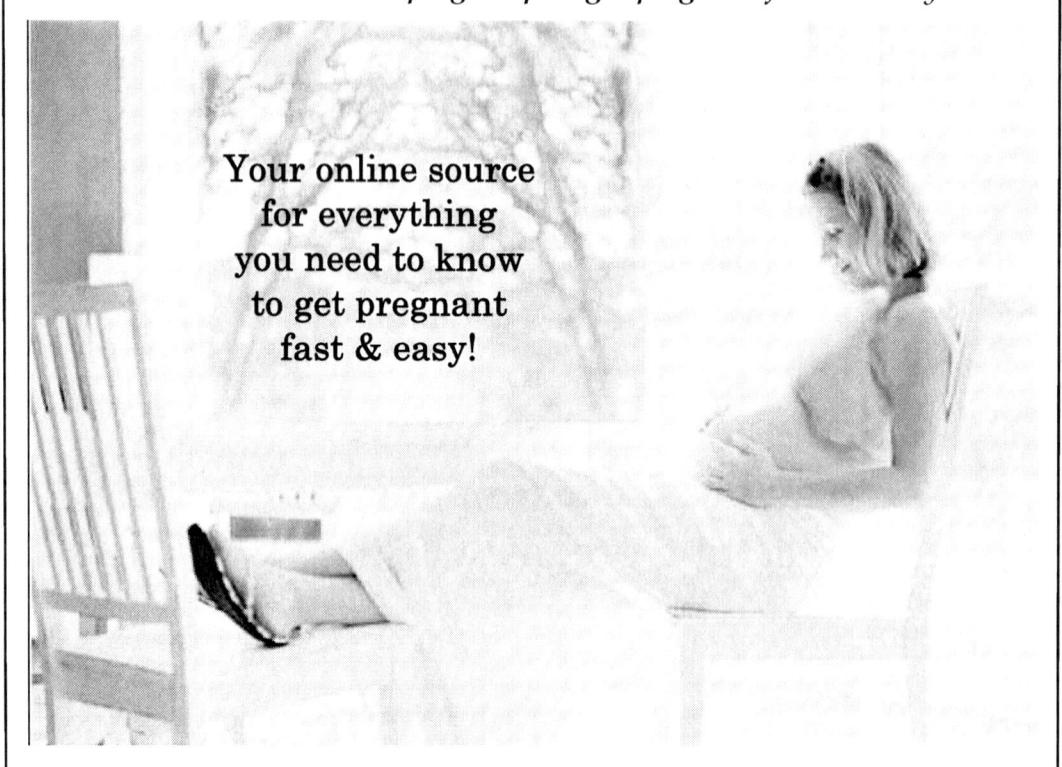

Your online source
for everything
you need to know
to get pregnant
fast & easy!

From the best self help fertility boosters to the most sophisticated medical fertility treatments you'll find all the information you need to make your pregnancy dreams come true!

Plus: Ask The Fertility Expert - Get a free personalized email answer to any question about getting pregnant direct to you from a fertility doctor!

Don't wait another second!
Visit GettingPregnantNow.org -
It's the website that will change your life!

Eat Love Get Pregnant
The Natural, Easy Proven Way To Make A Baby Fast!

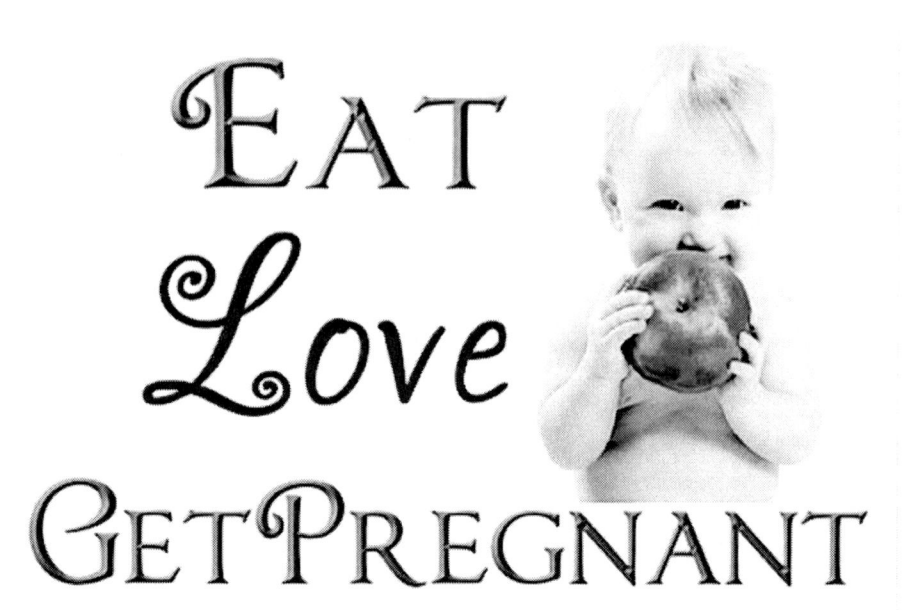

By Niels H. Lauersen M.D., Ph.D.
& Colette Bouchez

By the authors
of "Green Fertility" & "Getting Pregnant"
comes this revolutionary new
guide to the foods that will help you get pregnant
fast, easy & naturally!

Including: Over 200 Delicious Fertility Foods!

Available Late-Fall 2010
From IvyLeaguePress.com

PamperingMom.com

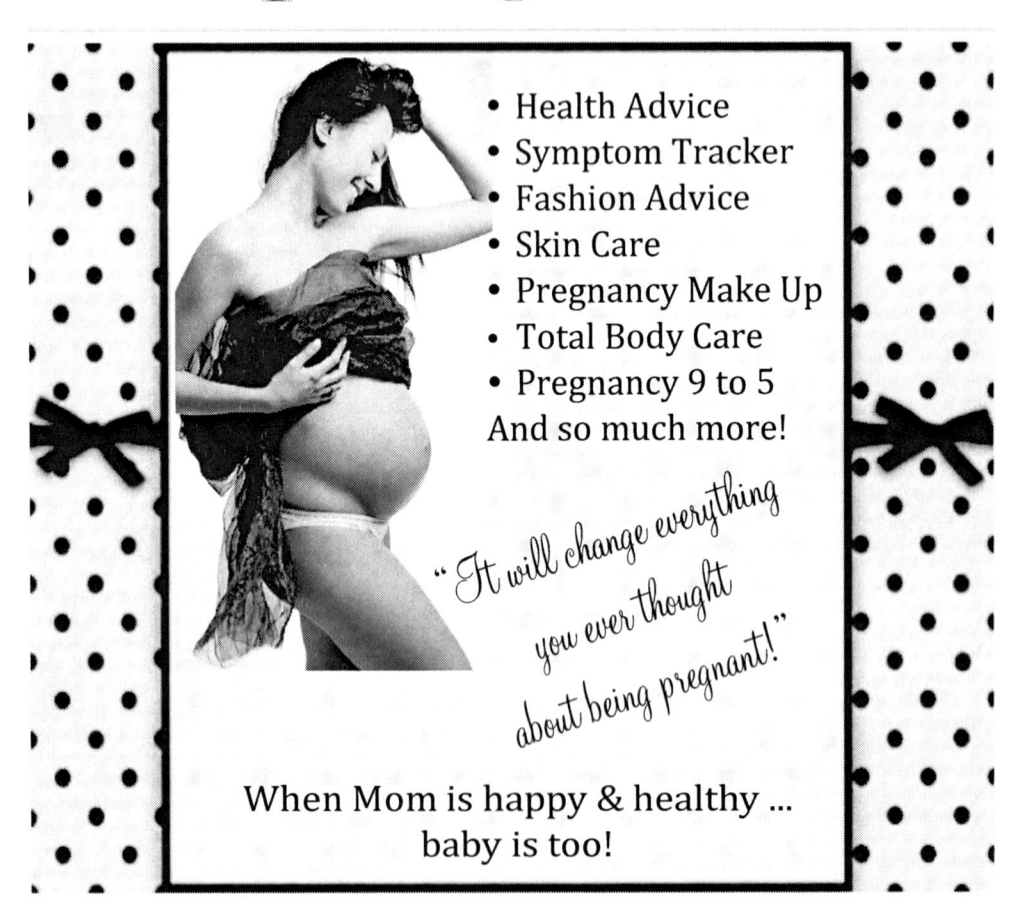

- Health Advice
- Symptom Tracker
- Fashion Advice
- Skin Care
- Pregnancy Make Up
- Total Body Care
- Pregnancy 9 to 5

And so much more!

"It will change everything you ever thought about being pregnant!"

When Mom is happy & healthy ... baby is too!

Now comes the only pregnancy web site to put Mom on center-stage
with 24-7 advice on how to look & feel fabulous
from First Trimester To Labor & Delivery - *& beyond!*

www.PamperingMom.com

Natural Gemstone Fertility Jewelry

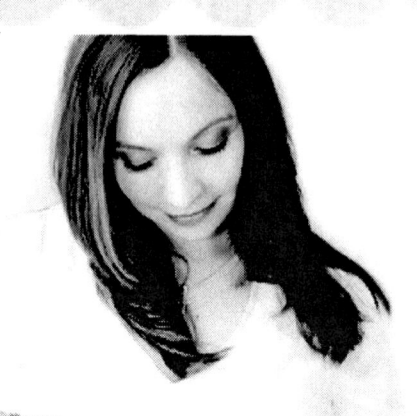

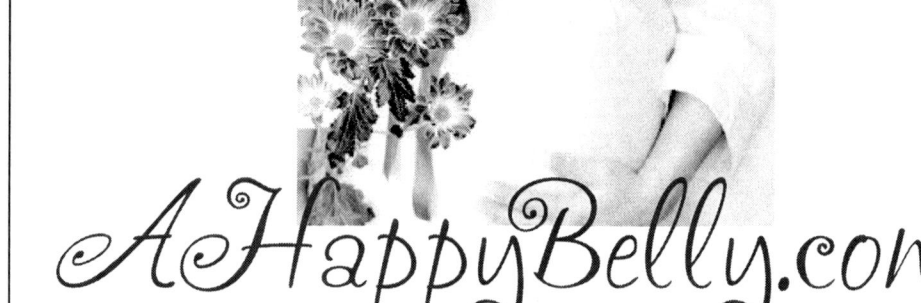

AHappyBelly.com

Look fabulous ...get pregnant faster ... have a healthy baby!

Tap into the centuries old wisdom of natural gemstone
jewelry designed to help encourage fertility and foster
a healthy, happy pregnancy!
Lead-free · natural gemstones · healthy, gorgeous designs
become a lasting memento of your pregnancy !

AHappyBelly.com

Other books by Niels H. Lauersen, M.D., Ph.D.

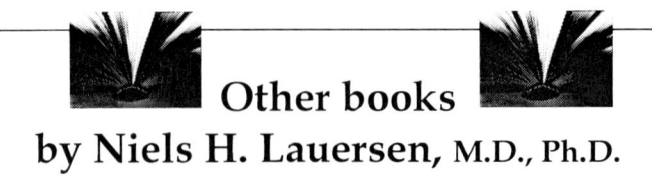

It's Your Body
Listen To Your Body
PMS & You
Childbirth With Love
The Endometriosis Answer Book
It's Your Pregnancy
Getting Pregnant
You're in Charge
The Breast Book
The New Fertility Diet Guide
Eat, Love, Get Pregnant
Green Fertility

Other books by Colette Bouchez

Getting Pregnant
The V Zone
Is It Healthy - Is It Harmful?
Your Perfectly Pampered Pregnancy
Your Perfectly Pampered Menopause
The Hot Flash Solution
The New Fertility Diet Guide
Eat, Love, Get Pregnant
Green Fertility

Visit IvyLeaguePress.com for more information on purchasing any of these books.

CPSIA information can be obtained at www.ICGtesting.com
Printed in the USA
BVOW061037051211

277620BV00005B/47/P